Rethinking MSM, Trans* and other Categories in HIV Prevention

As the HIV epidemic moves into its fourth decade, it is clear that the global response has failed to adequately address the needs of a wide range of vulnerable populations and groups. Chief among these are gay, bisexual and other men who have sex with men, and transgender persons, who globally face the disproportional burden of HIV infection.

This book rethinks HIV prevention and health promotion for sexual and gender minorities – in both the industrialised societies of the West, as well as in the developing nations of the Global South. The chapters it contains offer a critical analysis of past and present HIV research employing categories to designate gay and other men who have sex with men, transgender persons and/or other persons and communities with diverse gender and sexual identities.

Contributors question the politics of many of the existing classifications and categories in HIV research and argue for a more sophisticated analysis of gender and sexual diversity in order to tackle the social and political barriers that impede the design of successful HIV prevention and health promotion approaches.

The chapters in this book were originally published as a special issue of *Global Public Health*.

Amaya Perez-Brumer is a PhD candidate in the Department of Sociomedical Sciences at Columbia University, USA.

Richard Parker is Professor Emeritus of Sociomedical Sciences and Anthropology at Columbia University, USA, and Director of the Associação Brasileira Interdisciplinar de AIDS (ABIA), Brazil.

Peter Aggleton is Scientia Professor Emeritus of Education and Health at UNSW Sydney, and an Honorary Distinguished Professor in the Research School of Social Sciences at The Australian National University, Canberra, Australia.

Rethinking MSM, Trans* and other Categories in HIV Prevention

Edited by
Amaya Perez-Brumer, Richard Parker and Peter Aggleton

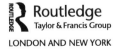

LONDON AND NEW YORK

First published 2018
by Routledge
2 Park Square, Milton Park, Abingdon, Oxon, OX14 4RN, UK

and by Routledge
711 Third Avenue, New York, NY 10017, USA

Routledge is an imprint of the Taylor & Francis Group, an informa business

© 2018 Taylor & Francis

All rights reserved. No part of this book may be reprinted or reproduced or utilised in any form or by any electronic, mechanical, or other means, now known or hereafter invented, including photocopying and recording, or in any information storage or retrieval system, without permission in writing from the publishers.

Trademark notice: Product or corporate names may be trademarks or registered trademarks, and are used only for identification and explanation without intent to infringe.

British Library Cataloguing in Publication Data
A catalogue record for this book is available from the British Library

ISBN 13: 978-1-138-55775-8

Typeset in Minion Pro
by diacriTech, Chennai

Publisher's Note
The publisher accepts responsibility for any inconsistencies that may have arisen during the conversion of this book from journal articles to book chapters, namely the possible inclusion of journal terminology.

Disclaimer
Every effort has been made to contact copyright holders for their permission to reprint material in this book. The publishers would be grateful to hear from any copyright holder who is not here acknowledged and will undertake to rectify any errors or omissions in future editions of this book.

Contents

Citation Information ix
Notes on Contributors xiii

Introduction: The trouble with 'Categories': Rethinking men who have sex with men, transgender and their equivalents in HIV prevention and health promotion 1
Richard Parker, Peter Aggleton and Amaya Perez-Brumer

1 In the name of brevity: The problem with binary HIV risk categories 6
Rachel L. Kaplan, Jae Sevelius and Kira Ribeiro

2 The conflation of gender and sex: Gaps and opportunities in HIV data among transgender women and MSM 17
Tonia Poteat, Danielle German and Colin Flynn

3 Towards 'reflexive epidemiology': Conflation of cisgender male and transgender women sex workers and implications for global understandings of HIV prevalence 31
Amaya Perez-Brumer, Catherine E. Oldenburg, Sari L. Reisner, Jesse L. Clark and Richard Parker

4 A global research synthesis of HIV and STI biobehavioural risks in female-to-male transgender adults 48
Sari L. Reisner and Gabriel R. Murchison

5 'Men who use the Internet to seek sex with men': Rethinking sexuality in the transnational context of HIV prevention 70
Rusty Souleymanov and Yu-Te Huang

6 From marginal to marginalised: The inclusion of men who have sex with men in global and national AIDS programmes and policy 84
Tara McKay

CONTENTS

7 From MSM to heteroflexibilities: Non-exclusive straight male identities and their implications for HIV prevention and health promotion 105
Héctor Carrillo and Amanda Hoffman

8 What is in a label? Multiple meanings of 'MSM' among same-gender-loving Black men in Mississippi 119
Nhan Truong, Amaya Perez-Brumer, Melissa Burton, June Gipson and DeMarc Hickson

9 Switching on after nine: Black gay-identified men's perceptions of sexual identities and partnerships in South African towns 135
Joanne E. Mantell, Jack Ume Tocco, Thomas Osmand, Theo Sandfort and Tim Lane

10 Intersections and evolution of 'Butch-trans' categories in Puerto Rico: Needs and barriers of an invisible population 148
Alíxida G. Ramos-Pibernus, Sheilla L. Rodríguez-Madera, Mark Padilla, Nelson Varas-Díaz and Ricardo Vargas Molina

11 'You should build yourself up as a whole product': Transgender female identity in Lima, Peru 163
Lealah Pollock, Alfonso Silva-Santisteban, Jae Sevelius and Ximena Salazar

12 HIV vulnerability and the erasure of sexual and gender diversity in Abidjan, Côte d'Ivoire 176
Matthew Thomann

13 Gender identity, healthcare access, and risk reduction among Malaysia's *mak nyah* community 192
Britton A. Gibson, Shan-Estelle Brown, Ronnye Rutledge, Jeffrey A. Wickersham, Adeeba Kamarulzaman and Frederick L. Altice

14 The limitations of 'Black MSM' as a category: Why gender, sexuality, and desire still matter for social and biomedical HIV prevention methods 208
Jonathan Garcia, Richard Parker, Caroline Parker, Patrick A. Wilson, Morgan Philbin and Jennifer S. Hirsch

15 Sexual identities and sexual health within the Celtic nations: An exploratory study of men who have sex with men recruited through social media 231
Kareena McAloney-Kocaman, Karen Lorimer, Paul Flowers, Mark Davis, Christina Knussen and Jamie Frankis

CONTENTS

16 'I am not a man': Trans-specific barriers and facilitators to PrEP acceptability among transgender women 242
Jae Sevelius, JoAnne Keatley, Nikki Calma and Emily Arnold

17 'Proyecto Orgullo', an HIV prevention, empowerment and community mobilisation intervention for gay men and transgender women in Callao/Lima, Peru 258
Andres Maiorana, Susan Kegeles, Ximena Salazar, Kelika Konda, Alfonso Silva-Santisteban and Carlos Cáceres

Index 275

Citation Information

The chapters in this book were originally published in *Global Public Health*, volume 11, issue 7–8 (August–September 2016). When citing this material, please use the original page numbering for each article, as follows:

Introduction
The trouble with 'Categories': Rethinking men who have sex with men, transgender and their equivalents in HIV prevention and health promotion
Richard Parker, Peter Aggleton and Amaya Perez-Brumer
Global Public Health, volume 11, issue 7–8 (August–September 2016) pp. 819–823

Chapter 1
In the name of brevity: The problem with binary HIV risk categories
Rachel L. Kaplan, Jae Sevelius and Kira Ribeiro
Global Public Health, volume 11, issue 7–8 (August–September 2016) pp. 824–834

Chapter 2
The conflation of gender and sex: Gaps and opportunities in HIV data among transgender women and MSM
Tonia Poteat, Danielle German and Colin Flynn
Global Public Health, volume 11, issue 7–8 (August–September 2016) pp. 835–848

Chapter 3
Towards 'reflexive epidemiology': Conflation of cisgender male and transgender women sex workers and implications for global understandings of HIV prevalence
Amaya Perez-Brumer, Catherine E. Oldenburg, Sari L. Reisner, Jesse L. Clark and Richard Parker
Global Public Health, volume 11, issue 7–8 (August–September 2016) pp. 849–865

Chapter 4
A global research synthesis of HIV and STI biobehavioural risks in female-to-male transgender adults
Sari L. Reisner and Gabriel R. Murchison
Global Public Health, volume 11, issue 7–8 (August–September 2016) pp. 866–887

CITATION INFORMATION

Chapter 5
'Men who use the Internet to seek sex with men': Rethinking sexuality in the transnational context of HIV prevention
Rusty Souleymanov and Yu-Te Huang
Global Public Health, volume 11, issue 7–8 (August–September 2016) pp. 888–901

Chapter 6
From marginal to marginalised: The inclusion of men who have sex with men in global and national AIDS programmes and policy
Tara McKay
Global Public Health, volume 11, issue 7–8 (August–September 2016) pp. 902–922

Chapter 7
From MSM to heteroflexibilities: Non-exclusive straight male identities and their implications for HIV prevention and health promotion
Héctor Carrillo and Amanda Hoffman
Global Public Health, volume 11, issue 7–8 (August–September 2016) pp. 923–936

Chapter 8
What is in a label? Multiple meanings of 'MSM' among same-gender-loving Black men in Mississippi
Nhan Truong, Amaya Perez-Brumer, Melissa Burton, June Gipson and DeMarc Hickson
Global Public Health, volume 11, issue 7–8 (August–September 2016) pp. 937–952

Chapter 9
Switching on after nine: Black gay-identified men's perceptions of sexual identities and partnerships in South African towns
Joanne E. Mantell, Jack Ume Tocco, Thomas Osmand, Theo Sandfort and Tim Lane
Global Public Health, volume 11, issue 7–8 (August–September 2016) pp. 953–965

Chapter 10
Intersections and evolution of 'Butch-trans' categories in Puerto Rico: Needs and barriers of an invisible population
Alíxida G. Ramos-Pibernus, Sheilla L. Rodríguez-Madera, Mark Padilla, Nelson Varas-Díaz and Ricardo Vargas Molina
Global Public Health, volume 11, issue 7–8 (August–September 2016) pp. 966–980

Chapter 11
'You should build yourself up as a whole product': Transgender female identity in Lima, Peru
Lealah Pollock, Alfonso Silva-Santisteban, Jae Sevelius and Ximena Salazar
Global Public Health, volume 11, issue 7–8 (August–September 2016) pp. 981–993

CITATION INFORMATION

Chapter 12
HIV vulnerability and the erasure of sexual and gender diversity in Abidjan, Côte d'Ivoire
Matthew Thomann
Global Public Health, volume 11, issue 7–8 (August–September 2016) pp. 994–1009

Chapter 13
Gender identity, healthcare access, and risk reduction among Malaysia's mak nyah community
Britton A. Gibson, Shan-Estelle Brown, Ronnye Rutledge, Jeffrey A. Wickersham, Adeeba Kamarulzaman and Frederick L. Altice
Global Public Health, volume 11, issue 7–8 (August–September 2016) pp. 1010–1025

Chapter 14
The limitations of 'Black MSM' as a category: Why gender, sexuality, and desire still matter for social and biomedical HIV prevention methods
Jonathan Garcia, Richard Parker, Caroline Parker, Patrick A. Wilson, Morgan Philbin and Jennifer S. Hirsch
Global Public Health, volume 11, issue 7–8 (August–September 2016) pp. 1026–1048

Chapter 15
Sexual identities and sexual health within the Celtic nations: An exploratory study of men who have sex with men recruited through social media
Kareena McAloney-Kocaman, Karen Lorimer, Paul Flowers, Mark Davis, Christina Knussen and Jamie Frankis
Global Public Health, volume 11, issue 7–8 (August–September 2016) pp. 1049–1059

Chapter 16
'I am not a man': Trans-specific barriers and facilitators to PrEP acceptability among transgender women
Jae Sevelius, JoAnne Keatley, Nikki Calma and Emily Arnold
Global Public Health, volume 11, issue 7–8 (August–September 2016) pp. 1060–1075

Chapter 17
'Proyecto Orgullo', an HIV prevention, empowerment and community mobilisation intervention for gay men and transgender women in Callao/Lima, Peru
Andres Maiorana, Susan Kegeles, Ximena Salazar, Kelika Konda, Alfonso Silva-Santisteban and Carlos Cáceres
Global Public Health, volume 11, issue 7–8 (August–September 2016) pp. 1076–1092

For any permission-related enquiries please visit:
http://www.tandfonline.com/page/help/permissions

Notes on Contributors

Peter Aggleton is Scientia Professor Emeritus of Education and Health at UNSW Sydney, and an Honorary Distinguished Professor in the Research School of Social Sciences at The Australian National University, Canberra, Australia. He is editor-in-chief of the journals *Culture, Health & Sexuality and Sex Education.*

Frederick L. Altice is Professor of Medicine and of Epidemiology at Yale University School of Medicine, USA.

Emily Arnold is Associate Professor of Medicine at the University of California, San Francisco, USA.

Shan-Estelle Brown is a postdoctoral research associate at the Department of Internal Medicine - AIDS Program, Yale University School of Medicine, USA.

Melissa Burton is an IMG-Crown Energy Services Contractor for U.S. Department of Energy, USA.

Carlos Cáceres is Professor of Public Health at the Universidad Peruana Cayetano Heredia (UPCH) and Founding Director of the UPCH Centro de Investigación Interdisciplinaria en Sexualidad, Sida y Sociedad (Sexuality and Human Development Research Group).

Nikki Calma is Program Manager of Trans: Thrive at API Wellness, USA.

Héctor Carrillo is Associate Professor of Sociology and Gender & Sexuality Studies, Northwestern University, USA.

Jesse L. Clark is Associate Professor-in-Residence in the Department of Medicine, Division of Infectious Disease and Department of Family Medicine, and a member of the Center for HIV Identification, Prevention and Treatment Services at the University of California, Los Angeles.

Mark Davis is Associate Professor at Monash University, Australia.

Paul Flowers is Professor of Sexual Health Psychology at Glasgow Caledonian University, UK.

Colin Flynn is Chief at the Center for HIV Surveillance, Epidemiology and Evaluation, Maryland Department of Health, USA.

NOTES ON CONTRIBUTORS

Jamie Frankis is Senior Lecturer in Research Methods at Glasgow Caledonian University, UK.

Jonathan Garcia is Assistant Professor at the School of Biological and Population Health Sciences, Oregon State University, USA.

Danielle German is Assistant Professor at the Department of Health, Behavior and Society, Johns Hopkins Bloomberg School of Public Health, USA.

Britton A. Gibson is a public health researcher and medical student at Yale University School of Medicine USA.

June Gipson is President of My Brother's Keeper, USA, a non-profit organisation designed to enhance the health and well-being of minorities through leadership in public and community health practices.

DeMarc Hickson is Visiting Associate Professor at the Department of Epidemiology and Biostatistics, Jackson State University, USA. He is also Chief Operating Officer at My Brother's Keeper, USA.

Jennifer S. Hirsch is Professor of Sociomedical Sciences at Columbia University, USA.

Amanda Hoffman is Project TEAL director at the Institute of Policy Research, Northwestern University, USA.

Yu-Te Huang is a doctoral student at the Factor-Inwentash Faculty of Social Work, University of Toronto, Canada.

Adeeba Kamarulzaman is Dean of the Faculty of Medicine and Professor of Medicine and Infectious Diseases at the University of Malaya, Malaysia.

Rachel L. Kaplan is Assistant Professor at the Department of Obstetrics, Gynaecology & Reproductive Sciences, Bixby Center for Global Reproductive Health, University of California, USA.

JoAnne Keatley directs the Center of Excellence for Transgender Health, University of California, San Francisco, USA.

Susan Kegeles is Professor of Medicine of University of California, San Francisco, USA.

Christina Knussen is an academic researcher and lecturer at the Glasgow Caledonian University, UK.

Kelika Konda is Adjunct Assistant Professor at the David Geffen School of Medicine at University of California, Los Angeles and External Research Professor at the Universidad Peruana Cayetano Heredia, Peru.

Tim Lane is Associate Professor at the Center for AIDS Prevention Studies and Global Health Sciences, University of California, San Francisco, USA.

Karen Lorimer is a senior research fellow in Public Health at the School of Health and Life Sciences, Glasgow Caledonian University, UK.

NOTES ON CONTRIBUTORS

Andres Maiorana is a qualitative research analyst at the Center for AIDS Prevention Studies, University of California, San Francisco, USA.

Joanne E. Mantell is a Research Scientist at the HIV Center for Clinical and Behavioral Studies and Professor of Clinical Psychology at Columbia University, USA.

Kareena McAloney-Kocaman is a lecturer in Applied Health Psychology at the School of Health and Life Sciences, Glasgow Caledonian University, UK.

Tara McKay is Assistant Professor of Medicine, Health, and Society at Vanderbilt University, USA.

Gabriel R. Murchison is Senior Research Manager at Human Rights Campaign Foundation, USA.

Catherine E. Oldenburg is Assistant Professor at the Proctor Foundation Faculty, University of California, San Francisco, USA.

Thomas Osmand is a research specialist at Center for AIDS Prevention Studies, University of California, San Francisco, USA.

Mark Padilla is Associate Professor at the Department of Global and Sociocultural Studies, Florida International University, USA.

Caroline Parker is a PhD candidate in the Department of Sociomedical Sciences at Columbia University, USA.

Richard Parker is Professor Emeritus of Sociomedical Sciences and Anthropology at Columbia University, USA, and Director of the Associação Brasileira Interdisciplinar de AIDS (ABIA), Brazil.

Amaya Perez-Brumer is a PhD candidate in the Department of Sociomedical Sciences at Columbia University, USA.

Morgan Philbin is Assistant Professor at the Mailman School of Public Health, Columbia University, USA.

Lealah Pollock is Assistant Professor at the School of Medicine, University of California, San Francisco, USA.

Tonia Poteat is Assistant Professor at Department of Epidemiology, Johns Hopkins Bloomberg School of Public Health, USA.

Alíxida G. Ramos-Pibernus is Project Director of TRANSforma-2 at University of Puerto Rico, Medical Sciences Campus, USA.

Sari L. Reisner is Assistant Professor of Pediatrics at Harvard Medical School and Boston Children's Hospital and Assistant Professor in the Department of Epidemiology at Harvard T.H. Chan School of Public Health, USA.

Kira Ribeiro is a PhD student at the Centre de Recherches Sociologiques et Politiques de Paris, University of Paris 8, France.

NOTES ON CONTRIBUTORS

Sheilla L. Rodríguez-Madera is Associate Professor of Psychology at the University of Puerto Rico, USA.

Ronnye Rutledge is a medical student at Yale University School of Medicine USA.

Ximena Salazar is an anthropologist and senior research at the Universidad Peruana Cayetano Heredia Centro de Investigación Interdisciplinaria en Sexualidad, Sida y Sociedad (Sexuality and Human Development Research Group) in Lima, Peru.

Theo Sandfort is Professor of Clinical Sociomedical Sciences at Columbia University, USA.

Jae Sevelius is Associate Professor at the Center for AIDS Prevention Studies (CAPS) in the Department of Medicine at the University of California, San Francisco, USA.

Alfonso Silva-Santisteban is a physician researcher at the Universidad Peruana Cayetano Heredia Centro de Investigación Interdisciplinaria en Sexualidad, Sida y Sociedad (Sexuality and Human Development Research Group) in Lima, Peru.

Rusty Souleymanov is a PhD candidate and a course instructor at the Factor-Inwentash Faculty of Social Work, University of Toronto, Canada.

Matthew Thomann is Visiting Assistant Professor at Kalamazoo College, USA.

Jack Ume Tocco is a postdoctoral research fellow at the HIV Center for Clinical and Behavioral Studies, USA.

Nhan Truong is a postdoctoral research fellow at the Center for Research on Sexuality and Sexual Health, San Diego State University, USA.

Nelson Varas-Díaz is Professor at the Department of Global and Sociocultural Studies, Florida International University, USA.

Ricardo Vargas Molina is a project coordinator at the School of Public Health, University of Puerto Rico, USA.

Jeffrey A. Wickersham is Assistant Professor of Medicine at Yale University School of Medicine, USA.

Patrick A. Wilson is Associate Professor of Sociomedical Sciences and the Director of the SPHERE (Society, Psychology, and Health Research) Lab at Columbia University.

INTRODUCTION

The trouble with 'Categories': Rethinking men who have sex with men, transgender and their equivalents in HIV prevention and health promotion

Richard Parker, Peter Aggleton and Amaya G. Perez-Brumer

ABSTRACT
This double Special Issue of *Global Public Health* presents a collection of articles that seek more adequately to represent sexual and gender diversities and to begin to rethink the relationship to HIV prevention and health promotion – in both the resource rich nations of the global North, as well as in the more resource constrained nations of the global South. Reckoning with the reality that today the global response to HIV has failed to respond to the needs of gay, bisexual and other men who have sex with men, and transgender persons, we turn our attention to processes and practices of categorisation and classification, and the entanglement of the multiple social worlds that constitute our understanding of each of these categories and people within the categories. Jointly, these articles provide critical perspectives on how defining and redefining categories may impact the conceptual frameworks and empirical evidence that inform global understandings of HIV infection, those communities most vulnerable, and our collective response to the evolving HIV epidemic.

As the HIV epidemic moves deeper into its fourth decade, it has become clear that the global response has failed adequately to address the needs of a wide range of vulnerable populations and groups. Chief among these are gay, bisexual and other men who have sex with men, and transgender persons, who face a disproportionate burden of HIV infection globally. Also included are women, men and transgender persons who, regularly or occasionally, transact or sell sex. Global estimates have reported the staggering burden of HIV infection disproportionately concentrated among members of each of these groups, in many cases rates of infection that, contrary to rhetoric of the 'End of AIDS' (Piot et al., 2015; UNAIDS, 2015), are in fact rising rapidly (Baral et al., 2013; Beyrer et al., 2012; Oldenburg et al., 2014; Shannon et al., 2015).

While awareness of these trends and associated needs has been demonstrated in the recent designation of these groups as 'key populations' at risk of being 'left behind' in the global response to the epidemic (UNAIDS, 2014), relatively little research has sought to understand the intersections between gender, sexuality, age, ethnicity, class and social context for members of these groups, and their possible links to vulnerability and risk for HIV acquisition and transmission. Instead, the focus has predominantly been on epidemiological assessments of risk practices and behaviours along with the prevalence and incidence of HIV. This latter kind of research, while valuable, runs the risk of being superficial: describing rather than explaining, and offering only the shallowest of intervention and programmatic possibilities.

In seeking to assess the current state of scholarship on these issues, it is striking how little recent research attention has focused on the 'categories' that have been used to investigate supposedly key populations – especially in relation to communities and groups with sexualities and genders that do not easily fit within dominant biomedical or epidemiological systems of classification. The use of generic categories, such as, 'MSM' (i.e. men who have sex with men), 'TGW' (or TW as an acronym for transgender women), or, more recently, 'Trans*' (i.e. to denote transgender as an umbrella term), offers a means of circumnavigating the complicated social, cultural and behavioural realities such categories mask – obscuring the porous margins of these classifications, the important diversities that exist within categories, and the intersections between them.

Speaking to these limitations, over the history of the response to the epidemic, a small but important literature has emerged examining the politics of language, processes and practices of categorisation and classification, and the entanglement of the multiple social worlds that constitute our understanding of each of these categories, people within the categories, and responses to the HIV epidemic (Aggleton & Parker, 2015; Boellstroff, 2011; Epstein, 1999; Parker, 1999; Sontag, 2001; Treichler, 1987; Young & Meyer, 2005). However, to date these insights have had minimal influence on the homogenising deployment of umbrella categories, and today within the domain of global public health there remains a marked lack of understanding concerning the heterogeneity that characterises each of these populations (and which is largely erased by the use of broad-brush categories such as 'MSM' or 'Trans*').

Not surprisingly therefore there still exists much confusion as to the distinctions, if any, between terms such as transgender and transsexual, and/or context-specific notions such as *bakla*, *travesti* (see Pollock et al. and Maiorana et al., in this issue), *hijra*, *kathoey*, *kothi*, *mak nyah* (see Gibson et al., in this issue). Associated with this, is lack of clarity about how best to implement culturally relevant HIV prevention and health promotion strategies that engage with the identities and subjectivities that exist within each key population category.

In the past decade, this limited recognition of the lived realities of affected individuals and communities has narrowed the scope of possibility when developing meaningful policies and programs. This is most clearly evidenced by the disconnect between astounding biomedical advance in HIV treatment and prevention (e.g. pre-exposure prophylaxis (PrEP), post-exposure prophylaxis, microbicides, etc.) and the growing burden of HIV infection in key population groups. Aiming to address this gap, this double Special Issue of *Global Public Health* presents a collection of articles that seek more adequately to represent sexual and gender diversities and to begin to rethink their relationship to HIV prevention and health promotion – in both the resource rich nations of the global North, as well as in the more resource constrained nations of the global South.

A common denominator across all the different contributions is the emphasis given to the importance of understanding sexual and gender diversity – and awareness that the application of this knowledge is crucial for successful public health efforts, as well as for tackling the social and political barriers that impede the design of more effective policies and programs.

All of the papers included in this Special Issue exemplify practical applications of critical perspectives on how redefining categories may impact the empirical and conceptual evidence that informs global understandings of HIV infection prevalence and our collective response to the evolving epidemic. With direct application to contemporary public health, many of the papers included here seek to develop an understanding of the 'trouble' with categories on a global level via macro-synthesis (see McKay; Reisner & Murchison; Souleymanov & Huang; Perez-Brumer et al., in this issue). Other papers offer case studies based on research carried out in specific communities or countries: in the global North, especially in the USA (see Carrillo & Hoffman; Garcia et al.; Kaplan et al.; Poteat et. al; Sevelius et al.; Truong et al.; Ramos-Pibernus et al.) and in a range of Celtic nations, including, Northern Ireland, the Republic of Ireland, Scotland and Wales (see McAloney-Kocaman et al.), as well as in the global South, in countries as different as Côte d'Ivoire (Thomann), Malaysia (Gibson et al.), Peru (Pollock et al.; Maiorana et al.) and South Africa (Mantell et al.).

Across such a wide range of different countries, it becomes clear that the challenges and limitations of applying dominant epidemiological and biomedical categories is a tension faced by public health researchers and practitioners globally.

Throughout this set of articles, a number of key patterns and issues emerge highlighting important opportunities for future research. Critical analytical and historical research into the categories used to designate gay and other men who have sex with men and/or transgender persons illustrate the ongoing tensions within binary notions of gender and sex and their application to contemporary HIV prevention and promotion efforts in the USA (Kaplan et al.; Poteat et al.) and globally (McKay; Perez-Brumer et al.). Building out these tensions, and commenting on the growing visibility of persons representing a spectrum of identities in which female identity or 'femininity' is prominent, authors underscore the need to think beyond 'transgender' to inform new more culturally relevant public health HIV strategies (Pollock et al.; Gibson et al.; Sevelius et al.; and Maiorana et al.). Further troubling the existing use of these categories, other authors highlight obscured and emerging groups, communities and populations to deepen our understandings of fluidity and complexity in expressions of sexuality and gender. They do this through studies of transgender men and *buchas* (Reisner & Murchison; Ramos-Pibernus et al.); through enquiry into the influence of time (over the 24-hour cycle of each day) on sexual expression and behaviours in the case of *after-nines* (Mantell et al.); and through research into the growing role of the Internet in destabilising the category 'MSM' (Souleymanov & Huang). Primarily within a US-context, Truong et al., Garcia et al., and Carrillo and Hoffman argue for the importance of race and ethnicity as providing a key intersection for re-conceptualising notions of risk and vulnerability to HIV among men traditionally denoted by the master category 'MSM'.

Taken together, the diverse articles in this Special Issue of *Global Public Health* underscore the need to continually develop more critical analyses of the ways in which the categories and classifications used in HIV research (and in global health research more broadly) carve up the realities of gender and sexuality in specific ways that often have little to do with the lived experience of those they seek to describe and analyse. While Sevelius et al. and Garcia et al. push readers to specifically engage with the limitations of 'MSM' and 'transgender' in direct relation to PrEP, in many ways, all authors argue that future success in the implementation of HIV prevention strategies depend on an critical engagement with the dominant classifications related to gender, sexuality, behaviours and identities that are used in HIV research and practice today.

In the midst of the fourth decade of the HIV epidemic, as rates of HIV infection continue disproportionately to impact on gay, bisexual and other men who have sex with men and transgender persons, the need to more effectively engage and serve their needs should be obvious. Yet doing this requires a move beyond patronising platitudes about the risk of these populations are being 'left behind'. Crucially, it requires the recognition of community-based expertise (Maiorana et al.) and the development of reflexive research (Perez-Brumer et al.; Poteat et al.) to more adequately characterise the richness and diversity of sexual and gender minorities (Carrillo & Hoffman; Garcia et al.; Mantell et al.; Thomann; Truong et al.), and to more effectively inform policies and programmes (McKay) to meet their needs. Perhaps most of all, it requires us to move beyond the overly neat analytic distinctions between sexual orientation and gender identity that prevail in much of this field of work. While all of the articles in this Special Issue raise important questions about this, Carrillo and Hoffman; Kaplan; Mantell et al.; and Thomann provide especially good examples in this regard.

Our hope is that the papers published in this Special Issue represent at least a small step in the direction of challenging practitioners in the arena of global HIV research and practice not only to recognise the limitations of existing classifications and categories to HIV but also to move forward by applying new and deeper understandings of sexual and gender diversity, methods, and intervention to existing analysis and research.

Disclosure statement

No potential conflict of interest was reported by the authors.

References

Aggleton, P., & Parker, R. (2015). Moving beyond biomedicalization in the HIV response: Implications for community involvement and community leadership among men who have sex with men and transgender people. *American Journal of Public Health*, *105*(8), 1552–1558. doi:10.2105/AJPH.2015.302614.

Baral, S. D., Poteat, T., Strömdahl, S., Wirtz, A. L., Guadamuz, T. E., & Beyrer, C. (2013). Worldwide burden of HIV in transgender women: A systematic review and meta-analysis. *The Lancet Infectious Diseases*, *13*(3), 214–222. doi:10.1016/S1473-3099(12)70315-8.

Beyrer, C., Baral, S. D., van Griensven, F., Goodreau, S. M., Chariyalertsak, S., Wirtz, A. L., & Brookmeyer, R. (2012). Global epidemiology of HIV infection in men who have sex with men. *The Lancet*, *380*(9839), 367–377. doi:10.1016/S0140-6736(12)60821-6.

Boellstroff, T. (2011). But do not identify as gay: A proleptic genealogy of the MSM category. *Cultural Anthropology*, *26*(2), 287–312. doi:j.1548-1360.2011.01100.x.

Epstein, S. (1999). *Impure science: AIDS, activism and the politics of knowledge*. Berkeley: University of California Press.

Gibson, B. A., Brown, S., Rutledge, R., Wickersham, J. A., Kamarulzaman, A., & Altice, F. L. (this issue). Gender identity, healthcare access, and risk reduction among Malaysia's *mak nyah* community. *Global Public Health*. doi:10.1080/17441692.2015.1134614

Maiorana, A., Kegeles, S., Salazar, X., Konda, K., Silva-Santisteban, A., & Cáceres, C. (this issue). 'Proyecto Orgullo', an HIV prevention, empowerment and community mobilisation intervention for gay men and transgender women in Callao/Lima, Peru. *Global Public Health*. doi:10.1080/17441692.2016.1161814

McKay, T. (this issue). From marginal to marginalised: The inclusion of men who have sex with men in global and national AIDS programmes and policy. *Global Public Health*. doi:10.1080/17441692.2016.1143523

Oldenburg, C. E., Perez-Brumer, A. G., Reisner, S. L., Mattie, J., Bärnighausen, T., Mayer, K. H., & Mimiaga, M. J. (2014). Global burden of HIV among men who engage in transactional sex: A systematic review and meta-analysis. *PloS One*, 9(7), e103549. doi:10.1371/journal.pone.0103549.

Parker, R. G. (1999). *Beneath the equator: Cultures of desire, male homosexuality, and emerging gay communities in Brazil*. New York, NY: Routledge.

Perez-Brumer, A. G., Oldenburg, C. E., Reisner, S. L., Clark, J. L., & Parker, R. G. (this issue). Towards 'reflexive epidemiology': Conflation of cisgender male and transgender women sex workers and implications for global understandings of HIV prevalence. *Global Public Health*. doi:10.1080/17441692.2016.1181193

Piot, P., Abdool Karim, S. S., Hecht, R., Legido-Quigley, H., Buse, K., Stover, J., … Goosby, E. (2015). Defeating AIDS – advancing global health. *The Lancet*, 386(9989), 171–218. doi:10.1016/S0140-6736(15)60658-4.

Pollock, L., Silva-Santisteban, A., Sevelius, j., & Salazar, X. (this issue). 'You should build yourself up as a whole product': Transgender female identity in Lima, Peru. *Global Public Health*. doi:10.1080/17441692.2016.1167932

Reisner, S. L., & Murchison, G. R. (this issue). A global research synthesis of HIV and STI biobehavioural risks in female-to-male transgender adults. *Global Public Health*. doi:10.1080/17441692.2015.1134613

Shannon, K., Strathdee, S. A., Goldenberg, S. M., Duff, P., Mwangi, P., Rusakova, M., … Boily, M. C. (2015). Global epidemiology of HIV among female sex workers: Influence of structural determinants. *The Lancet*, 385(9962), 55–71. doi:10.1016/S0140-6736(14)60931-4.

Sontag, S. (2001). *Illness as metaphor and AIDS and its metaphors*. New York, NY: Palgrave Macmillan.

Souleymanov, R., & Huang, Y.-T. (this issue). 'Men who use the Internet to seek sex with men': Rethinking sexuality in the transnational context of HIV prevention. *Global Public Health*. doi:10.1080/17441692.2016.1180701

Treichler, P. A. (1987). AIDS, homophobia and biomedical discourse: An epidemic of signification. *Cultural Studies*, 1(3), 263–305. doi:10.1080/09502388700490221.

UNAIDS. (2014). *Infographic: 12 key populations being left behind*. Retrieved April 25, 2016, from http://www.unaids.org/sites/default/files/12_Populations_en_0.pdf.

UNAIDS. (2015). *On the fast-track to end AIDS: World AIDS day 2015*. Retrieved April 25, 2016, from http://www.unaids.org/wad2015/.

Young, R. M., & Meyer, I. H. (2005). The trouble with 'MSM' and 'WSW': Erasure of the sexual-minority person in public health discourse. *American Journal of Public Health*, 95(7), 1144–1149. doi:10.2105/AJPH.2004.046714

In the name of brevity: The problem with binary HIV risk categories

Rachel L. Kaplan, Jae Sevelius and Kira Ribeiro

ABSTRACT
According to the 'Consolidated Guidelines on HIV Prevention, Diagnosis, Treatment and Care for Key Populations' there are five groups of people at elevated risk of HIV, including 'transgender women or transgender men who have receptive anal sex with men'. Although cost effectiveness strategies and best practice lessons recommend targeting specific populations for HIV prevention, existing risk categories lack specificity, and may in fact cause further confusion. Existing categories of risk often perpetuate notions of gender and sexuality that can erroneously exclude, alienate, and stigmatise those who are at the highest risk and thus should be prioritised. We review the troubled history of the MSM category and the problematic conflation of trans feminine individuals and MSM in much of the existing HIV literature, and how this practice has stymied progress in slowing the HIV epidemic in the most at-risk groups, including those who do not fit neatly into binary notions of gender and sex. We draw from examples in the field, specifically among trans feminine people in Beirut and San Francisco, to illustrate the lived experiences of individuals whose identities may not fit into Euro-Atlantic constructs of HIV prevention categories.

Defining categories, erasing bodies: the troubled history of 'MSM'

The seeming self-evidence of the phrase 'men who have sex with men' and its acronym 'MSM', could easily lead one to think that it constitutes a purely descriptive category, whose meaning is simple, well defined, and stable. However, exploring the history of this category rapidly reveals how its uses and meanings are frequently questioned and continuously shifting. In the paper 'But do not identify as gay: A proleptic genealogy of the MSM category', Boellstorff (2011) illustrates how the MSM category underwent successive transformations to anticipate its own failure and stabilise a definition that continues to face crises. By examining how the meaning of 'MSM' has shifted throughout the years to the point where it now sometimes refers to an identity or a community, Boellstorff points out how 'MSM' is more than an acronym describing a simple and easily identifiable behaviour.

According to Young and Meyer (2005), the terms MSM and WSW, though sometimes useful and accurate, can also render invisible important information on identity, community, and sexual culture. By separating people from their contexts in order to define them solely by their practices, the MSM acronym can actually prevent health professionals from reaching communities at risk for HIV. The lived experiences of people self-identifying as gay are not the only ones that fail to be captured by the use of the MSM category. In the same vein, others (Namaste et al., 2007) have pointed out that though 'MSM' aims to include all kinds of men – independent of their sexual orientation or identity – it does so by effectively erasing the specificities of bisexual lives. By only focusing on sex bisexual men have with men, the MSM category does not account for the complexity of HIV transmission and prevention for bisexual men.

The trouble with 'MSM' does not only lie in the way this category excludes certain men, certain communities, and certain identities. It also lies in the way it includes, by force, certain populations by defining them as 'men who have sex with men'. According to Khan and Khan (2006), it may be inappropriate to talk about 'men who have sex with men' in some non-Euro-Atlantic contexts. In fact, many organisations prefer the phrase 'males who have sex with males' to account for a myriad of male identities – 'man' only being one of them. By taking a look outside of the Euro-Atlantic context from which the MSM category emerged, it is possible to see how the word 'men' is far from being a neutral term. Khan and Khan (2006) note that, though the phrase 'males who have sex with males' may seem less problematic, it still cannot account for people who do not fit within the male/female binary and their sexual partners.

These critiques reveal that the apparent explicitness of the MSM category relies on three main erroneous assumptions: (1) the assumption that 'men' is not an identity; (2) that we know the bodies we are talking about – that is, that the bodies of 'men', the 'male body' is something homogeneous, stable, and easily identifiable; and (3) that we know the sexual practices in which these bodies are engaged – that is, that the phrase 'men who have sex with men' is enough to describe a sexual behaviour.

Young and Meyer (2005) addressed and criticised the idea according to which 'men who have sex with men' could, in and of itself, appropriately describe sexual behaviour. As Patton (2002) notes, 'MSM' often supposes anal intercourse between men, even though those men may not engage in anal intercourse, especially in non-Euro-Atlantic contexts (Moody, 1988). By producing a largely implicit association between male–male sexuality and anal intercourse, the MSM category acts as a way to produce and naturalise homosexuality. Khan and Khan (2006) pointed out that the term 'men' – as well as 'male' – is far from being free of any notion of identity. In this paper, we draw on these critiques to analyse further the question of the body assumed by the MSM category. We argue that, by assuming a body without naming it, the use of the MSM category has stymied progress in slowing the HIV epidemic in some of the most at-risk groups, including those who do not fit neatly into binary notions of gender and sex.

Numerous works from anthropologists and feminist scholars have shown the variability of gender roles and norms throughout ages and cultures. Following the research of American sexologists John Money and Robert Stoller on intersex and transsexual individuals, Oakley (1972) introduced the distinction between sex and gender into Feminist Studies. Separating biological characteristics from identities, roles, or notions of femininity and masculinity allowed feminists to reveal the absence of causality between biology and social norms regarding sex. However, as early as the 1980s some feminists critiqued the way the distinction between sex and gender tended to reinforce the idea that gender was a social construct that submits to variation while sex was 'natural' and 'stable' (Dorlin, 2008). As the historicity of sex was being examined (Laqueur, 1990), scientific discourses on sex underwent the scrutiny of historians, philosophers, and social scientists. Feminist studies of science played an important role in demonstrating how the categories of sex constituted an arena of debate and struggle within biomedical sciences (Fausto-Sterling, 2000; Oudshoorn, 2001). Since the seventeenth century, Euro-Atlantic conceptualisations of sex have adopted a binary model. However, throughout history, successive definitions of sex – humeral, gonadic, hormonal, genetic – failed to prove the existence of two, and only two, perfectly distinct sexes. Epistemological changes in the definition of sex aimed to stabilise this binary model even though it cannot account for multiple forms of intersex, as well as for transgender bodies. Far from being an effective and universal concept, the binary of sex constitutes, for biomedical sciences themselves, an 'epistemological obstacle' (Dorlin, 2008).

More recently, critiques on the social construction of gender and sexuality have been effectively integrated into works on or with the MSM category, like the work of Young and Meyer (2005). However, critiques on the social construction of sex categorisation has yet to be really taken into account, even though it may help us understand some of the limits and problems related to the use of the MSM category. For example, if the sex binary itself regularly faces definitional crises, it is only logical that the MSM category would face similar issues regarding its own definition. In fact, we would like to argue that MSM's instability and inaccuracy is largely inherited from the sex categories upon which it is built. If the ability to know what 'male' is constitutes a challenge for modern science, it is no wonder that the ability to know whom 'men who have sex with men' are appears equally challenging.

This difficulty to define accurately what a 'man' is appears clearly in the way trans feminine individuals[1] have been included – or not – within the MSM category. Though excluded from the category at first, trans feminine people have been included because of what Boellstorff calls a 'biologized understanding of maleness' (2011, p. 296). Activists and scholars argued that 'MSM' didn't accurately describe trans feminine individuals for, though they were 'genetically male' (Kammerer, Mason, Connors, & Durkee, 2001), they did not live as men but as women (Hawkes, 2008). Including them within the MSM category not only negates their identity but also obscures specific issues, especially regarding the role of gender-based violence in HIV risk.

But the problem with defining trans feminine people as 'men' or 'males' does not only concern the social dimensions of HIV transmission and prevention. It is also about the very physicality and biology of HIV transmission and prevention. To include trans feminine individuals in the MSM category, one does not simply have to adopt a 'biologized understanding of maleness', as Boellstorff puts it. Whether we adopt a hormonal, genetic, or gonadic definition of sex – or a combination of these three criterion as it is often the case when it comes to assigning a sex to individuals who do not fit clearly in the sex binary – trans feminine people may, or may not, be considered male. In its 2006 Global Report, UNAIDS (2006, p. 110) defines 'men who have sex with men' as people engaging in male–male sex, including trans feminine individuals or, as they put it, 'transgendered males'. However, what is the definition of 'male' adopted here? Could a trans feminine person still be considered 'biologically male' while being on hormone replacement therapy? Could a trans feminine person still be considered 'biologically male' after an orchiectomy (the surgical ablation of testicles) or a vaginoplasty (the surgical construction of a vulva)? When does one begin or cease to be 'biologically male'? How does the erasure of surgically modified trans bodies prevent us from having access to accurate evaluation of HIV transmission post genital surgery?

These questions have particularly important implications when it comes to evaluating HIV transmission risk, developing HIV prevention programs, and implementing appropriate prevention tools. By subsuming vastly different bodies under the MSM category, we risk erasing important sexual practices and routes of HIV transmission. For example, by conflating MSM and trans feminine people, it becomes difficult to consider penile–vaginal penetration, thus erasing experiences of some post-operative trans feminine individuals. Similarly, how can we account for penile–vaginal penetration between trans-masculine people and non-transgender men within gay settings while acknowledging the fact that the MSM category implies, not only anal intercourse as Patton and other scholars have stated, but also a specific form of bodies labelled as male?

As specificities of the HIV epidemics within trans communities have become more and more apparent, a shift has appeared in the conflation of MSM and trans feminine people. Examining the more recent UNAIDS Global Reports offers interesting insight on this evolution. While the 2006 Global Report included trans feminine individuals in the MSM category, as they were considered 'biologically male', the 2010 Global Report used the phrase 'men who have sex with men and transgender people' (UNAIDS, 2010). Another shift appears in the 2013 Global Report as transgender women and MSM constitute two distinct categories (UNAIDS, 2013). As a result, this report extensively addresses challenges faced by transgender women and emphasises that gender inequalities and gender-based violence play an important role in the increased vulnerability of this population regarding HIV transmission. The 'Consolidated Guidelines on HIV Prevention, Diagnosis, Treatment and Care for Key Populations' further differentiate risk categories that honour differences in the specification of 'transgender women or transgender men who have receptive anal sex with men' (World Health Organization, 2014).

Even though these changes mark an extremely important shift in light of the disproportionate risk of HIV/AIDS among trans feminine people across the globe (Baral et al., 2013), it is essential to remember previous critiques on the use of categories in epidemiological research. Just as 'gay', 'man', and 'male' have raised definitional challenges and epistemological questions, 'trans woman' is a specific identity category, situated contextually and culturally in a particular place and time. The term 'trans woman' may refer to very different experiences, identities, or forms of embodiment and excludes trans feminine individuals who do not identify as women and/or do not embrace a binary definition of gender. While some people completely identify with the term, others may reject it altogether or use it strategically in order to make sense of their situation. In some non-Euro-Atlantic contexts, as well as some cultures within Euro-Atlantic environments, the category 'trans woman' may not make sense at all. Furthermore, attention should be given to the effects of using a category like 'trans woman' for the populations we want to reach. Do we – HIV researchers and scholars – effectively reach all parts of the trans community when using such a specific identity term? When we recruit 'trans women' as the target population, do we effectively reach trans populations most at risk for HIV, notably migrant trans feminine people engaged in sex work (Giami, Beaubatie, & Le Bail, 2011) who may not identify as 'trans' or as 'trans women'? What realities, narratives, bodies, sexualities, and practices are implied and prioritised by this category? Which ones are excluded or erased? How can we properly address the HIV epidemics among trans women and other trans people assigned male at birth without erasing the experiences of trans men and other trans people assigned female at birth? Answers to these interrogations are unclear and deserve further investigation. Though the use of categories is often challenging and can suffer severe limitations, keeping those interrogations in mind may keep us from erasing the broad diversity of bodies, identities, practices, and sexualities within trans communities and thus enable us to reach people in need of appropriate information, materials, and services.

Throughout the world, the risk of HIV infection among trans feminine individuals is 49 times higher than that of members of the general population (Baral et al., 2013). This staggering figure requires action. However, how is it possible to prioritise and address the health needs of a population with appropriate specificity while at the same time seeking to maximise inclusion and avoid perpetuation of the sex and gender binary? Further, how can health professionals describe and measure risk without reducing individuals to their physical bodies through language and summary? Although we do not yet have answers to these difficult questions, we draw on examples from the field to illustrate these complexities through the lived experiences of individuals whose identities may not fit into the male/female binary or Euro-Atlantic constructs of HIV prevention categories.

Examples from the field

Trans feminine individuals in the Middle East and North Africa: Beirut, Lebanon

To illustrate the complex history of HIV prevention categories that we have outlined and discussed above, we provide examples from the field that highlight some of the challenges associated with existing constructs of definition, recruitment, and description. Challenges in our decisions about expressing HIV risk categories extend beyond a Euro-Atlantic context and the English language. Until recently, HIV research among populations in the Middle East and North Africa (MENA) has often conflated trans feminine individuals and MSM (Mumtaz et al., 2010). In 2011, formative data were collected among a sample of 10 trans feminine people in Beirut, Lebanon to understand their lived experiences and risk behaviour (Kaplan et al., 2015). Recruitment took place through referrals from an LGBT organisation and from study participants. Interviews were then conducted by a social worker who was providing social support services to trans individuals. Unlike other contexts, such as India in which local terms approximate – to some degree – the North American usage of 'transgender' (Phillips et al., 2013), there is no equivalent term in Arabic that is used in Lebanon. Individuals use the term 'trans' due to a lack of local indigenous terminology; this gap has been identified as a need to be addressed within the trans community in Lebanon (El Khoury, 2014). In the above-described formative study, participants were recruited based on their understanding of the research team's use of the term 'transgender woman'. The participants used a range of words to express their identities including female, girl, woman, ladyboy, gay, transgender, and shemale transgender (Kaplan et al.,

2015). The research team believed that the participants understood the usage of 'transgender woman', but recruitment strategies, without the availability of a local term, had to rely on individuals' usage of terminology outside their first language. Further, although all participants indicated the preference for female pronouns to the interviewer (in Arabic the pronoun 'you' is gendered, therefore when speaking to or being spoken to directly, decisions about whether to use 'inteh' for 'you' [feminine] or 'intah' for 'you' [masculine], must be made), we cannot be certain that each individual necessarily agreed with or would identify herself with an identity of an individual who is assigned male at birth and has a female gender identity. In other words, participants were not asked if they agreed with the usage of the term 'transgender woman'; instead an open-ended question was used to allow participants to describe their gender identity without preconceived categories or identity labels. Thus as researchers, we impose our own definitions of the term 'trans' to recruit, define, and describe our target populations so that our audiences understand what we mean. However, is understanding actually taking place? What impact does this imposition have on individuals and communities with whom we work? How do these choices shape the way we attempt to approach important research questions?

The way in which the participants in the above-described study (Kaplan et al., 2015) defined their gender identity and comfort with it further elucidates the complexity of using terminology across different contexts and the problems with existing HIV risk categories. Participants were asked, 'How would you describe your gender identity? How comfortable are you with your gender identity?' and responded with a range of descriptions that speak to the diversity of gender experiences and expressions within and across times and places, as well as some of the motivational factors that are situated contextually. For example, some participants in the sample expressed frustration with existing labels and identity categories. One explained,

> I am a girl – a female. I don't like to identify as transsexual or transgender. I am not comfortable [with my gender identity] because I have a male sexual organ. I would prefer if I didn't have it. I would feel more comfortable with myself when I will do the sex change operation.

Another participant expressed being 'very comfortable' with her gender identity and identified as 'transgender', but said, 'I don't like the definitions of transgender or gay or any of all this to define myself'. Yet another participant seemed to view her identity as an unavoidable part of her:

> Being transgender is something I feel deep inside me and I can't deny it. It is a reality I live in every day. I face a lot of problems because of it, but I try my best to overcome those problems.

As mentioned, although participants all indicated the preference for the use of female pronouns, not all individuals wished to be perceived as women in all aspects of life.

The role of the family in overall health and well-being of trans feminine people was found to be integral in Lebanon (Kaplan et al., 2015). The importance of family support informed some participants' decisions about gender expression, which impacted gender identity. Fluidly identifying as 'ladyboy' or 'sometimes gay', one participant explained:

> I would like to look very feminine and have a whole body hair removal, but I don't want to have breasts or have any operation to change sex. If I want to go to [see] my parents, I can't be

dressed as a full woman. If my parents and family were not there, I would have nothing to lose.

This participant cites her need to see her parents as motivation for not dressing 'as a full woman'. Implied in the participant's response is that while she might want to dress 'as a full woman' when she sees her parents, she chooses to compromise that desire for another: familial support. Her comments about not wanting to 'have breasts' or 'any operation to change sex' suggest the need for further inquiry to understand better the motivations and desires of this population regarding accessing medical transition providers and procedures. These motivations and desires – and what is both at stake and necessary for independence – must be interpreted within an individual's and community's context.

Within the non-Euro-Atlantic context of Lebanon as well as other collectivist cultures, dependence on and priority for positive familial relationships may impact an individual's desire and motivation to 'transition' either medically or socially or both. Again, even the term 'transition' and what is understood, imposed, and implied by the term may not translate well across different contexts. These factors likely inform an individual's HIV risk in addition to vulnerability to other adverse health outcomes. For example, without the support and acceptance from the family of origin, a trans feminine individual might be unstably housed due to a lack of infrastructure in the form of formal support within a context that relies on the informal support of family. Threats of violence impact safety, which can in turn impact mental and physical health (Kaplan et al., 2015). Cultures across the MENA region have been described as adhering to often rigidly defined binary gender roles; Beirut is an example of 'hyperfemininity' and 'hypermasculinity' (El Feki, 2013; Saleh & Qubaia, 2015). Within these contexts, the experiences of the participants raise questions about the intersections of culture and gender expectations. Do trans feminine people in Lebanon and other parts of the MENA region embrace the female/male gender binary? How do they see themselves fitting or not fitting in existing paradigms of sex and gender? Do Middle Eastern trans feminine individuals view the gender binary as an imposition, which results in their resistance?

Trans feminine individuals in the United States: San Francisco, CA

San Francisco has long had a strong reputation for its liberal approach to self-expression and its political support of communities that have been historically marginalised, especially sexual and gender minorities. Recently, the context of living in San Francisco has changed due to the rising cost of living, an influx of high-profile tech companies, and decreasing diversity in its residents (Nevius, 2015).

However, San Francisco is currently leading the charge to increase access to transition-related health care for trans people, through innovative programs at the Department of Public Health (www.sfdph.org/dph/comupg/oprograms/THS/default2.asp) and at UCSF's Center of Excellence for Transgender Health (www.transhealth.ucsf.edu). While many trans people choose not to undergo surgery, some people who would historically not have had access to expensive transition-related surgeries that require specialists are now gaining access and realising their life-long dreams through programs such as these. With increased access to transition-related health care, trans feminine people can pursue hormones (and sometimes puberty blockers) from a young age, enabling some to avoid gender dysphoric experiences of puberty and young adulthood, and achieve a gender expression aligned with their identity without necessarily needing to have access to tremendous financial resources. In light of this shifting landscape of access to care for trans feminine individuals, options for various forms of gender expression and embodiment become possible. Not all trans people desire surgeries, and among those who do, many do not desire complete reconstruction of the appearance and function of the genitalia. Having choices about how one embodies and expresses gender identity allows for a myriad of possibilities that lie, both biologically and socially, outside of the gender binary. When we approach sexual health research using a binary lens that erases trans feminine individual's bodies and the sociocultural context of their experiences, it is no wonder that the data, the programs, and the outcomes so obviously miss the mark. In a qualitative study of the role of gender affirmation in sexual risk behaviour, 22 trans feminine people of colour described the unique cultural context of their experiences at the intersection of race and gender (Sevelius, 2013). Many participants discussed the safety that 'passing' as a non-trans woman affords, and while most did not feel that fully passing was accessible to them, it also was not a guarantee of protection:

> Even if you have the operation, you're still going to always be classified as male, no matter what ... That's the problem I have [even though I pass]. Once you get a sex change, you're still living a lie. And hopefully you don't get killed. A guy who finds out might forgive you, or he might just leave you. Or he might just set you up and have you killed. (African American, 35)

So while some trans feminine people aspire to achieve a binary-based gender expression and embodiment, whether for safety or as an authentic expression of their identity, the societal lens imposed upon them continues to negate their experience and contributes to their sense of vulnerability. Those who felt they did not pass described the pain of facing stigma and rejection on an almost daily basis, and when they did receive some social affirmation of their gender it was often grounded in sexual objectification from men. The objectification experiences were described as affirming in the sense that they felt validated through these experiences, but validation came with the price of feeling that they were not being valued as unique human beings with something beyond sex to offer the world. How can trans feminine individuals be true to themselves through expression and embodiment that is aligned with their authentic gender identity, when that very identity is largely not acknowledged as valuable or even possible? When their very existence is mostly erased or derided outside of sexual contexts, how is mental and sexual health possible for trans feminine people, especially trans feminine individuals of colour?

> You walk down the street after you done turned the trick and you feel like you're the grand diva 'cause somebody stopped 'cause you're pretty. But see what I realize is that it's not the beauty on the inside that they see. All they see you for is a piece of ass ... All they think that transgenders are good for is sex and drugs. (African American, 23)

The sociocultural framework of trans feminine individuals' lives cannot be completely understood using a binary lens of inquiry. The nuances of embodiment and expression, as well as intersections of gender with race, class, and other situating life contexts such as access to transition-related health care are readily erased when trans feminine people are defined by their birth sex, their genitalia, or their sexual practices. The conflation of trans feminine individuals with MSM has stymied progress in halting the epidemic and has categorically contributed to the disparities experienced by trans feminine people by erasing, marginalising, and misunderstanding the sociocultural context of their risk.

Conclusion

In this paper we have reviewed the troubled history of the MSM category and the problematic conflation of trans feminine individuals and MSM in much of the existing HIV literature. We have drawn examples from two settings in the field, Beirut and San Francisco, to illustrate how this practice has stymied progress in slowing the HIV epidemic in some of the most at-risk groups, including those who do not fit neatly into binary and Euro-Atlantic notions of gender and sex. Taking into account the sociocultural contexts of the individuals who are among the most at risk for HIV infection and other negative health sequelae will improve our abilities to recruit, measure, and report more effectively, accurately, and respectfully.

Here we have raised questions more than we have provided answers. We have established some of the problematic challenges with current approaches within cultural contexts in which we have expertise, but the best way forward remains murky. How might we proceed and strive to achieve both specificity and contextual relevance? Should we opt for referring to genitalia when describing risk categories and thereby prioritise bodies over cultures and contexts? Important shifts are taking place. What we used to consider highly specific risk categories are being challenged and/or becoming obsolete. The term '*unprotected* receptive anal intercourse' has recently been swapped out by some in favour of '*condomless* receptive anal intercourse' in light of strides in viral suppression and the protection that it affords. However, embedded in these terms are assumptions that still persist. The term 'receptive anal intercourse' tells us nothing about the penis – or other object – that is being inserted. Thus, even if we were to refer to types of sex that introduce higher risk profiles with purportedly more specificity, such as 'penile-anal sex', this terminology still erases individuals' experiences and sociocultural contexts including gender-based violence among trans women and what are likely to be different risk profiles among trans men who have had genital surgery.

Although we have struggled to construct the way forward and instead have deconstructed existing hegemony, we include the following concrete recommendations for health professionals, researchers, and scholars.

1. Do not conflate trans women with MSM. For studies that include trans, non-trans, and gender nonconforming participants, analyse data gathered from these groups separately and in meaningful ways.
2. When reporting sample demographics, include gender categories beyond the gender and sex binary.
3. When collecting data, use the two-step question for assessing gender categories (Tate, Ledbetter, & Youssef, 2013) to ensure that trans people are counted.

As researchers, we must make decisions about participation criteria that both includes and excludes people. However, when doing so, it is important to consider whether our terminology actually captures and reflects our intended meaning and that it encompasses our intended target population. With such staggering HIV risk and rates among trans feminine individuals, these decisions cannot be made lightly. We must ask ourselves whether we are perpetuating binaries through these decisions. Are we making assumptions about what it means to 'transition', to 'pass', and to use certain pronouns? Are we imposing Euro-Atlantic constructs of what it means to be trans on contexts that may or may not function in similar ways? Promising advances have been made in terms of both terminology and health care access; it is important to continue to query existing constructs and categories of HIV risk.

Note

1. Here we use the term 'trans feminine individual' to refer to people whose gender identity, expression, or behaviour is different from those typically associated with their binary sex of male assigned at birth. By using 'trans feminine individual' rather than 'trans woman' or 'transgender woman', we aim to broaden the meaning of trans experiences and not restrict our usage to any specific form of gender embodiment or identification.

Disclosure statement

No potential conflict of interest was reported by the authors.

Funding

This work was supported in part by the National Institutes of Mental Health [grant no. K08MH085566] (PI: Sevelius) and the National Institutes of Mental Health [grant no. 5R21MH093204-02] (PI: Wagner).

References

Baral, S. D., Poteat, T., Strömdahl, S., Wirtz, A. L., Guadamuz, T. E., & Beyrer, C. (2013). Worldwide burden of HIV in transgender women: A systematic review and meta analysis. *Lancet Infectious Diseases*, *13*, 214–222. doi:10.1016/S1473-3099(12)70315-8

Boellstorff, T. (2011). But do not identify as gay: A proleptic genealogy of the MSM category. *Cultural Anthropology*, *26*, 287–312. doi:10.1111/j.1548-1360.2011.01100.x

Dorlin, E. (2008). *Sexe, genre et sexualités*. Paris: Presses Universitaires de France.

El Feki, S. (2013). *Sex and the citadel: Intimate life in a changing Arab world*. New York, NY: Pantheon Books.

El Khoury, C. (2014). *The evidence of reality: A health needs assessment of trans* identified individuals* (Unpublished master's thesis). American University of Beirut & Marsa Sexual Health Center, Lebanon.

Fausto-Sterling, A. (2000). *Sexing the body: Gender politics and the construction of sexuality*. New York, NY: Basic Books.

Giami, A., Beaubatie, E., & Le Bail J. (2011). Caractéristiques sociodémographiques, identifications de genre, parcours de transition médicopsychologiques et VIH/sida dans la population trans. Premiers résultats d'une enquête menée en France en 2010. *Bulletin Epidemiologique Hebdomadaire*, *42*, 433–444.

Hawkes, S. (2008). *Prevention and treatment of HIV and other sexually transmitted infections among men who have sex with men and transgender populations*. Geneva: World Health Organization.

Kammerer, N., Mason, T., Connors, M., & Durkee R. (2001). Transgenders, HIV/AIDS, and substance abuse: From risk group to group prevention. In W. Bockting & S. Kirk (Eds.), *Transgender and HIV: Risks, prevention, and care* (pp. 13–38). New York, NY: Haworth Press.

Kaplan, R. L., Wagner, G. J., Nehme, S., Aunon, F., Khouri, D., & Mokhbat, J. (2015). Forms of safety and their impact on health: An exploration of HIV/AIDS-related risk and resilience among trans women in Lebanon. *Health Care for Women International*, 36, 917–935. doi:10.1080/07399332.2014.896012

Khan, S., & Khan, O. A. (2006). The trouble with MSM. *American Journal of Public Health*, 96, 765–766. doi:10.2105/AJPH.2005.084665

Laqueur, T. W. (1990). *Making sex: Body and gender from the Greeks to Freud*. Cambridge: Harvard University Press.

Moody, D. T. (1988). Migrancy and male sexuality in South African gold mines. *Journal of South African Studies*, 14, 178–193.

Mumtaz, G., Hilmi, N., McFarland, W., Kaplan, R. L., Akala, F. A., Semini, I., … Abu-Radad, L. J. (2010). Are HIV epidemics among men who have sex with men emerging in the Middle East and North Africa? A systematic review and data analysis. *PLoS Medicine*, 8, e1000444.

Namaste, V., Vukoy, T. H., Saghie, N., Jean-Gilles, J., Lafrenière, M., Leclerc, N., … Williamson, R. (2007). HIV and STD prevention needs of bisexual women: Results from Projet Polyvalence. *Canadian Journal of Communication*, 32, 357–381.

Nevius, C. W. (2015, April 24). Study finds S.F.'s ethnic diversity dwindling. *San Francisco Chronicle*. Retrieved from http://www.sfchronicle.com/bayarea/nevius/article/Study-finds-S-F-s-ethnic-diversity-dwindling-6222673.php

Oakley, A. (1972). *Sex, gender, and society*. London: Harper Colophone Books.

Oudshoorn, N. E. J. (2001). On bodies, technologies, and feminisms. In L. Schiebinger (Ed.), *Feminism in 20th century science, technology, and medicine* (pp. 199–213). Chicago, IL: University of Chicago Press.

Patton, C. (2002). *Globalizing AIDS*. Minneapolis: University of Minnesota Press.

Phillips, A.E., Molitor, J., Boily, M.C., Lowndes, C.M., Gurav, K., Blanchard, J., & Alary, M. (2013). Informal confidential voting interviewing in a sexual risk assessment of men who have sex with men (MSM) and transgenders (hijra) in Bangalore, India. *Sexually Transmitted Infections*, 89, 245–250. doi:10.1136/sextrans-2011-050373

Saleh, A.J., & Qubaia, A.A. (2015). *Transwomen's navigation of arrest and detention in Beirut: A case study*. Beirut: Civil Society Knowledge Center, Lebanon Support.

SeveliusJ. (2013). Gender affirmation: A framework for conceptualizing risk behavior among transgender women of color. *Sex Roles*, 68, 675–689. doi:10.1007/s11199-012-0216-5

Tate, C.C., Ledbetter, J.N., & Youssef, C.P. (2013). A two-question method for assessing gender categories in the social and medical sciences. *Journal of Sex Research*, 50, 767–776. doi:10.1080/00224499.2012.690110

UNAIDS. (2006). *Report on the Global AIDS Epidemic*. Geneva: Author. Retrieved from http://data.unaids.org/pub/report/2006/2006_gr_en.pdf

UNAIDS. (2010). *Report on the Global AIDS Epidemic*. Geneva: Author. Retrieved from http://www.unaids.org/globalreport/documents/20101123_GlobalReport_full_en.pdf

UNAIDS. (2013). *Report on the Global AIDS Epidemic*. Geneva: Author. Retrieved from http://www.unaids.org/sites/default/files/en/media/unaids/contentassets/documents/epidemiology/2013/gr2013/UNAIDS_Global_Report_2013_en.pdf

World Health Organization. (2014). *Consolidated guidelines on HIV prevention, diagnosis, treatment and care for key populations*. Geneva: Author.

Young, R. M., & Meyer, I. H. (2005). The trouble with 'MSM' and 'WSW': Erasure of sexual-minority person in public health discourse. *American Journal of Public Health*, 95, 1144–1149. doi:10.2105/AJPH.2004.046714

The conflation of gender and sex: Gaps and opportunities in HIV data among transgender women and MSM

Tonia Poteat, Danielle German and Colin Flynn

ABSTRACT

Historically, HIV studies have conflated men who have sex with men (MSM) with transgender (trans) women, explicitly excluded trans individuals, or included sample sizes of trans people that are too small to reach meaningful conclusions. Despite the heavy burden of HIV among trans women, conflation of this population with MSM has limited the information available on the social and behavioural factors that increase HIV vulnerability among trans women and how these factors may differ from MSM. Using data sets from quantitative studies among MSM ($n = 645$) and trans women ($n = 89$), as well as qualitative in-depth interviews with 30 trans women in Baltimore, we explore what these data tell us about similarities and differences in HIV vulnerability between the two groups and where they leave gaps in our understanding. We conclude with implications for data collection and intervention development.

Introduction

Globally, transgender (trans) women are one of the most vulnerable populations to HIV. A recent meta-analysis of HIV prevalence among trans women (Baral et al., 2013) found a pooled global prevalence of 19% with approximately 49 times the odds of infection compared to the general population. In the United States, the HIV prevalence was 22% (95% CI: 18.4–25.1) with 34 (95% CI: 31.2–37.5) times the odds of infection versus the general population. This overwhelming disparity highlights the urgent need for research to inform effective and appropriate HIV prevention, care, and treatment interventions for this population.

Historically, HIV studies have conflated men who have sex with men (MSM) and trans women, explicitly excluded trans individuals, or included sample sizes of trans people that were too small to reach meaningful conclusions. Studies published as recently as 2015, in well-respected peer-reviewed journals, combine MSM and trans women into one category for analysis and presentation of data (Muessig, Baltierra, Pike, LeGrand, & Hightow-Weidman, 2014; Peacock, Andrinopoulos, & Hembling, 2015; Zea et al., 2015).

Leaders in the trans community have called for an end to this conflation and for the recognition of trans women as a unique population, different from MSM. The World Health Organisation's 2014 consolidated guidelines for key populations state 'the high vulnerability and specific health needs of transgender people necessitate a distinct and independent status in the global HIV response' (World Health Organisation, 2014). At the same time, organisations like the US Food and Drug Administration consider trans women to be MSM for the purposes of identifying who should be excluded from donating blood based on elevated risk of HIV (Holden, 2015; The US Food and Drug Administration, 2014). This categorisation of trans women as MSM rests on the assumption that MSM and trans women share anatomy (i.e. penises) and sexual practices (i.e. anal intercourse), and it centres behaviour over identity in the calculation of HIV risk. However, as research among Black MSM has demonstrated, social consequences of oppressed identities may be more significant drivers of HIV disparities than traditional risk behaviours (Millett, Flores, Peterson, & Bakeman, 2007; Peterson et al., 2014). Other scholars have eloquently described how the use of behavioural labels in public health discourse about sexual minorities may undermine self-determined identities, obscure social meanings, and tell us very little about actual sexual practices (Young & Meyer, 2005). The same critiques apply to gender minorities.

These conflicting stances from well-respected health organisations raise not only issues of identity politics but also public health questions: What can currently available data tell us about the similarities and differences in HIV risk and vulnerabilities for trans women compared to non-transgender (cisgender) MSM? What data are missing? What does this mean for how data should be collected and for the appropriateness and effectiveness of current HIV interventions? In order to address these questions, we conducted a secondary analysis of data from three sources in the United States: the 2004–2005 Baltimore National HIV Behavioral Surveillance Survey; the 2004–2005 Baltimore Transgender Supplement Questionnaire (TSQ), and qualitative interviews with transgender adults, conducted as part of a larger study of gender, stigma, and HIV risk in Baltimore in 2010.

Methods

We used Intersectionality and Syndemic Theory to interpret the findings from this analysis. Intersectionality is a theoretical approach that foregrounds the intersection of multiple social identities that result in multiple and interdependent structural inequalities (Bowleg, 2012). Syndemic theory describes how multiple, co-occurring epidemics, concentrated within a specific population, interact and reinforce one another, giving rise to additional health problems (Singer, 2009).

Data sets

National HIV Behavioral Surveillance
The National HIV Behavioral Surveillance (NHBS) System, a collaboration between the Centers for Disease Control and Prevention (CDC) and 25 state and local health departments, surveys three populations in the United States: MSM, injection drug users, and 'high-risk' heterosexuals. Information is collected from these three populations during rotating 12-month cycles (Gallagher, Sullivan, Lansky, & Onorato, 2007). Recruitment

methods vary for each population, but standardised protocols and core questions are the same for each cycle. Participating health departments may include locally specific questions to address local needs. Questionnaires collect information about demographics, sexual behaviour, injection and non-injection drug use, and HIV testing.

During the June 2004 to April 2005 MSM data collection cycle (German et al., 2011), a small number of participants identified themselves as transgender. In order to be eligible, participants had to report being assigned male at birth (natal male), be 18 years of age or older, reside in the city's metropolitan area, and have sex with a man in the previous 12 months. Participants were recruited using venue-based, time-location sampling (TLS). All participants provided verbal informed consent, and data were collected via face-to-face interviews using handheld devices. Structured quantitative interviews lasted approximately one hour. After the interview, HIV-1 testing was done on serum samples that were sent to the state laboratory for analysis. Participants received $25 for completion of the survey and an additional $25 for HIV testing. Among the 694 eligible natal male participants who completed the 2004–2005 NHBS MSM questionnaire, 49 (7.6%) identified as transgender.

Transgender Supplement Questionnaire

TSQ participants were recruited using TLS and purposive sampling. Eligibility criteria were the same as for the NHBS with the additional requirement of a transgender identity. Data collection, HIV testing, and incentive payment were identical to NHBS with the exception of the use of paper questionnaires with several free lists and open-ended questions rather than completely structured questionnaires via handheld computers. The TSQ collected data on sexual behaviour, gender identity, expression, and use of transition-related interventions. Questions about sexual partners included multiple options to describe the gender expression as well as the gender identity of those partners (e.g. 'feminine men' and 'masculine men' were separate response options). It did not include questions about condom use, drug use, or injections of soft-tissue fillers such as silicone. Forty respondents completed the TSQ. Of those, five participants completed both the TSQ and the NHBS survey. Because the number of participants who completed both surveys was small with little overlap in the questions asked, the two samples were analysed separately.

Qualitative IDIs

Sex-stratified purposive sampling was used to identify transgender participants for in-depth interviews (IDIs) about stigma and HIV risk. Efforts were made to achieve variability along lines of race, engagement in medical care, and use of hormone therapy. Inclusion criteria for transgender participants included being 18 years of age or older, residing in the metropolitan area, and identifying as transgender or as a gender different from their birth sex. For this manuscript, the analysis was limited to participants who were assigned male at birth and identified as women and/or transgender.

One IDI was conducted with each of the 30 trans women participants between January 2011 and July 2011. All participants provided verbal informed consent; all interviews were audio recorded and transcribed verbatim. Each interview lasted between 45 and 180 minutes with an average duration of 90 minutes. The interviews elicited detailed narratives of individual experiences and perceptions. Specifically, participants were asked about their family and social life, gender identity, sexual orientation and practices, health care experiences, as well as experiences of stigma and discrimination. Participants received $25 for participation.

Analyses

NHBS

Data were downloaded daily from handheld devices onto a password protected study computer. The statistical software Stata© (version 11, StataCorp, College Station, TX) was used to calculate descriptive statistics. Chi square was used to test for differences in HIV risk behaviour and HIV test results, comparing trans women to MSM. Logistic regression modelling, controlling for demographic factors, was used to estimate odds ratios.

TSQ

Data from paper questionnaires were hand-entered into an Access database on a password protected study computer. Stata* was used calculate summary statistics. No MSM were included in this sample, therefore no comparative tests of association were conducted.

IDIs

Data for analysis included transcripts of audio recordings from IDIs. The first author coded the transcripts in the software program Atlas.ti* (version 6.2, Scientific Software Development GmbH, Eden Prairie, MN) using an a priori codebook based on the topics addressed in the NHBS and TSQ: sexuality, drug use, and HIV. Using constant comparison techniques (Crabtree & Miller, 1999) for thematic analysis, coded text was examined within and across participant transcripts for recurrent and salient themes. Memos were used throughout analysis to organise and document the analytic process.

Results

NHBS

Characteristics

Social and demographic characteristics of the sample are listed in Table 1. Compared to MSM, trans women were younger with an average age of 28 versus 34 years. Trans women were more likely to be Black and have a high school education or less. The two groups showed no statistically significant difference in housing stability. A higher proportion of trans women (25%) had been arrested in the previous 12 months compared to MSM (19%); however, this difference was not statistically significant ($p = .3$). While there was no difference in proportion of trans and MSM respondents who were insured, trans women (21%) were more likely than MSM (8%) to report Medicare as their insurer ($p = .002$).

Sexuality

Trans women were more likely than MSM to describe their sexual orientation as heterosexual or other ($p = .001$). Trans-identified respondents were not asked about condom use at last anal intercourse, and therefore no comparisons with MSM could be made. A similar proportion of MSM (84%) and trans women (79%) reported receiving free condoms in the

Table 1. Select characteristics of participants in NHBS and TSQ.

	NHBS: MSM N = 645	NHBS: Trans women N = 49	TSQ[a] N = 40
Mean age (range)*	34.3 (18–69)	28.3 (18–57)	28.8 (18–58)
Race, % *			
Black	62.5	79.6	75.0
White	31.1	18.4	22.5
Other	6.4	2.0	2.5
Education, % *			
Post-graduate	6.3	0.0	2.5
Any college	44.7	14.3	22.5
High school or less	49.0	85.7	75.0
Sexual orientation, % *			
Heterosexual or 'straight'	3.3	25.0	50.0
Homosexual, Gay, or Lesbian	63.1	35.4	32.5
Bisexual	31.8	10.4	17.5
Other	1.8	29.2	52.5
Condoms, %			
Received free condoms in last 12 months	83.8	78.7	
Used free condoms in last 12 months	79.4	91.9	
More likely to use if free	60.9	56.8	
Drug use, % *			
Ever injected drugs	17.2	20.8	
Non-injection drugs in last 12 months	49.0	39.6	
Amphetamine	17.4	20.0	
Crack cocaine	26.2	20.0	
Heroin	15.7	5.0	
Marijuana*	76.0	95.0	
Ecstasy*	18.6	40.0	
HIV, %			N = 21
Ever tested	86.8	87.8	–
Self-report HIV-positive	15.9	20.8	–
Laboratory confirmed HIV-positive	37.7	42.5	33.3
Unaware of HIV+ status	58.4	64.7	–

[a]TSQ participants were allowed to select more than one sexual orientation, therefore sum may be >100%.
*$p \leq .05$ for differences between MSM and transwomen in NHBS.

previous 12 months ($p = .4$). Among participants who had received free condoms in the previous 12 months, a greater proportion of trans women reported using them than MSM (92% vs. 79%, $p = .07$). Similar proportions of trans women (57%) and MSM (61%) reported that receipt of free condoms made it more likely that they would use them ($p = .6$). There was no significant difference in the proportion of trans women (12%) and MSM (16%) who reported ever being diagnosed with a sexually transmitted disease ($p = .5$).

Drug use

Twenty-one per cent of the trans women and 17% of MSM reported ever injecting drugs ($p = .5$). The average age of first injection was 21 years for trans women and 23 years for MSM ($p = 0.5$). All respondents denied injecting drugs in the preceding 12 months. Forty per cent of trans women and 49% of MSM had used non-injection drugs in the preceding 12 months. There was no difference between the two groups in frequency of non-injection use of amphetamines, crack, cocaine, downers, painkillers, hallucinogens, club drugs, heroin, or poppers. Among non-injecting drug users, 95% of trans women had used marijuana in the prior 12 months compared to 76% of MSM ($p = .05$). Forty per cent of trans women had used ecstasy in the past 12 months compared to 19% of MSM ($p = .02$). Power calculations for drug use analyses found 95% power to detect a difference between groups in marijuana use, 89% in ecstasy use, and less than 25% for all other drug use, suggesting that if significant differences existed in the use of these other drugs, our sample size was too small to detect it.

HIV

The majority of respondents (88%) had been previously tested for HIV with no difference in testing between trans women and MSM ($p = .9$). Twenty-one per cent of trans women and 16% of MSM reported having tested positive for HIV in the past ($p = .4$). Laboratory testing found 43% trans women and 38% MSM were HIV-positive ($p = .5$). Sixty-five per cent of trans women and 58% of MSM had unrecognised HIV infection. None of these differences were statistically significant with power less than 10%. In a multivariable logistic regression model that included race, age, gender identity and sexual orientation, transgender identity was not significantly associated with HIV status. Race was the strongest predictor of HIV; Black participants had 10 times the odds of HIV compared to white participants [CI: 6.3, 17.0, $p = .0001$].

TSQ

Gender affirmation

Demographic information for this sample can be found in Table 1. They are similar to the trans participants in the NHBS in age, race, and educational attainment. When asked what sex they would like to be seen by others, most participants wanted to be seen as female (33/39). When offered the opportunity to freely list as many labels for themselves as they wanted, the top three most commonly listed labels included female (80%), woman (75%), and feminine (75%); 73% also listed transgender. When asked to free list actions they had taken to support their gender transition, the most frequently listed actions included 'cross dressing' (80%), casual name change (80%), hormones or surgery (65%), and change of gender marker on legal identification (50%). Only one respondent reported having genital reconstruction surgery. Two-thirds of the respondents desired future gender transition. Of those who desired future transition, 73% wanted hormones or surgery. Desire for legal name change (55%), psychological counselling (52%), and cross dressing (45%) were also commonly reported. The most commonly listed reason (62%) for not having desired gender transition was lack of money to afford it; the next most common was inability to find providers in their area to help with transition (19%). Seventy-three per cent reported current or past use of feminising hormones; of those, 55% received these hormones by prescription from a licensed medical professional.

Sexuality and HIV

The great majority (88%) of respondents had sexual partners who were born male and who identified as masculine men, while 12% had feminine female partners. When choosing sexual partners for short-term or long-term relationships about half ($n = 17$) usually chose those with the same racial/ethnic identity as themselves and half chose those of any race/ethnicity ($n = 20$). Only two participants preferred partners of a different race or ethnicity. HIV test results were available for 21 of the 40 respondents, and one-third of them tested HIV-positive (33.3%).

IDIs

The average age of the trans women in the study was 39 years (range 21–66). Two-thirds identified as Black or African-American, the remainder identified as white. Most of the Black participants had exclusively male sexual partners, and most of the white participants had exclusively female sexual partners. Half had no more than a high school education. Twenty-six of the thirty trans women had a regular source for medical care. Two-thirds of them had been tested for HIV in the previous year. Of the five trans women who reported having HIV, all of them were Black and had been diagnosed for greater than 10 years.

Sexuality

Relationship challenges were a recurrent theme and were linked to HIV vulnerabilities. Participants described little problem finding sexual encounters but greater difficulty finding committed partners. When they found partners who accepted their gender identity, they feared being abandoned for a cisgender partner. Several participants with male partners described engaging in insertive sex and in condomless sex in order to keep their partner in the relationship.

Some participants felt that families were more likely to reject trans children than gay children. This family rejection with concomitant loss of emotional and financial support led many trans women to sex work. Sex work was able to provide money for livelihood and as well as funds for gender affirming interventions, such as hormone therapy. Street-based sex work, with its attendant risks of detention and incarceration, incurred additional vulnerabilities. One participant described being arrested while with a date who had picked her up in a stolen car. While incarcerated, she was raped by another prisoner and later learned that she had contracted HIV.

Every participant reported using condoms with male partners. Yet, it was unclear how consistently this happened. Trans sex workers asserted using condoms with all clients but were more vague about condom use with other partners. One person in particular expressed relief that she had been HIV-negative every time she was tested, even though she was aware of taking sexual risks. See Table 2 for illustrative quotes.

Other vulnerabilities: enacted stigma and violence

Experiences of enacted stigma (discrimination) and violence were pervasive. When asked directly about experiences of discrimination, 71% of respondents reported being verbally harassed, 60% reported problems getting a job, and 54% reported losing a job because of their gender. Thirty-nine per cent of all participants reported that they had been sexually assaulted, and 29% had been physically assaulted or beaten.

Racial differences in narratives of discrimination were remarkable. Employment discrimination and rejection by former friends or partners were the most common themes in the narratives of white participants. Narratives of Black participants described routine public harassment from strangers as well as police; and reports of emotional and physical abuse were common. Strategies to cope with these challenges ranged from using drugs to seeking social support. Sources of support and resilience included the trans community, accepting friends or family members, and spiritual faith.

Table 2. Illustrative quotes from IDIs with trans women.

Themes	Illustrative quotes
Relationship challenges	*It's rare that you can really get a guy to really want to stay with you, you know what I'm saying. They'll deal with you, but I mean as far as you're in a **committed relationship, no they won't**.*
	*I got involved with a guy. And he was like, 'Well, I already know what you are and who you are and I'm going to love you regardless.' And I will never find that ever again. I don't think I'll ever find a guy like him ever again. And we stayed in a relationship for eight years. He decided he wanted to get out of the relationship because **he wanted to be with a real female** so I said okay.*
Sexuality	*Then I'd go ahead and do it and **not really want to do it**, you know what I'm saying? I'm just doing it just to please them. And then, when I'm doing it, I'm not putting my heart into it. I'm, like, okay, whatever, you know? **Just so he won't go with nobody else**.*
	*… they the man and everything, you know what I'm saying, but when they're in the bedroom, sometimes the tables turn. They want to be the one, you know, **they want you to dominate them**, you know? So that ain't always true that you'll be a bottom all the time.*
	*I don't really care for me penetrating anybody or anything like that. I don't really care for all of that. But I've had boyfriends that've wanted it, so me being the lady that I am, I always would give into it, **because I don't want them to go anywhere else**. This is someone I'm dating, so I would do it. **But I really don't care for it**.*
HIV vulnerabilities	*I think it's higher because people in community, like I said earlier, some people get kicked out, some people's families disown them, they don't have anything to do. **Transitioning is expensive**. It's not free and it's not free and it's not cheap. So I think a lot of girls and lot of men, as well, they turn to **sex work**. So they're doing all this sex work and they're sleeping with these different men and women for money, so they can be able to survive, to live, to be able to transition and everything like that … And the risk of HIV and gonorrhoea is extremely high, compared to just a biological female or male who can work a regular job, who the family supports them and still loves them. **Even if they were gay biological male or gay biological females, their families still is more accepting** of that compared to gender identity.*
	*I was like oh my God you locked me up for driving on a date in a car with somebody. I didn't even know the car was stolen, you know, what I'm saying. I wouldn't have got in there. They **locked me up** for six months. And while I was in there **a guy raped me**.*
	*… They came to me like a week later and told me to come up to the infirmary and they told me that, '**The guy that did that to you, he was infected with HIV**.'*
	*Like I said, I've been transgendered for almost 11 years now, which is a really good thing to me, because I know a lot of homosexuals and transsexuals and bisexuals- just all types of people- that have contracted AIDS and HIV, and all this time I have not contracted it. I took my test and I was negative… **It's a blessing every time I go to take that test, even though I know what I do as far as sexual-wise**.*

Discussion

Using quantitative and qualitative data from one metropolitan area in the United States, we explored similarities and differences in data on HIV vulnerability among trans women compared to MSM. Intersectionality and Syndemic Theory provide useful frameworks to contextualise these findings and explore their implications for addressing HIV among trans women in Baltimore.

In the quantitative analyses, we found the prevalence of HIV to be high among both trans women (33–43%) and MSM (38%). The prevalence for each group was higher than among any other risk group in Baltimore, including injection drug users (23%) and 'high-risk' heterosexuals (6%, Flynn, 2013). Notably, in multivariable modelling that included both trans women and MSM, the strongest predictor of positive HIV status was Black race. Indeed, it is possible that the slightly higher prevalence of HIV among trans women compared to MSM in the NHBS study may have been related to the higher proportion of Black participants in the sample of trans women. The significant racial disparity in HIV suggests that experiences of race and racism intersect with homophobia and transphobia to compound existing disparities by risk group.

While almost half of MSM in the NHBS had high school or less education, a remarkable 86% and 75% of trans women in the NHBS and TSQ, respectively, had no more than a high school education. In other ways, the two groups were similar. Trans women and MSM in the NHBS reported comparable housing stability, injection drug use rates, STI diagnosis histories, and access to free condoms. These similarities may be attributable to the use of a venue-based, time-location sampling strategy that was designed to recruit MSM. These venues may cater to individuals from the same community contexts, regardless of gender identity. Trans women who frequent MSM-focused venues may also meet partners and share sexual networks with the men at these venues, leading to overlapping interpersonal risks and similar prevalence of STIs and HIV. Trans women from these venues were marginally more likely than MSM to report use of the free condoms they received. It is possible that trans women were more likely than MSM to use condoms overall. However, given ubiquitous employment discrimination against trans women (Grant et al., 2010) and the low educational attainment of trans participants, it is also possible that trans women were more likely to use free condoms due to financial constraints that limited their ability to purchase condoms or a greater need for condoms to use during sex work. The omission of questions about sexual practices and condom use at last sex among trans participants in the NHBS preclude a comparison between the two populations. However, data from the TSQ and IDIs provide some insights into trans women's sexual experiences.

Whereas most of the white trans women in the IDIs had female partners, all of the Black participants described male partners. The majority of the TSQ participants were Black and most commonly reported 'masculine men' as their sexual partners. Since HIV acquisition is much more efficient from male partners, this androphilia may account for some of the racial disparities seen among trans women. Many participants in the TSQ expressed preference for partners of the same race. Previous research has demonstrated that such assortative partnership patterns are associated with higher risk for HIV among cisgender Black men and women with male sexual partners (Adimora, Schoenbach, & Floris-Moore, 2009; Fujimoto & Williams, 2014). Also, trans women in the IDIs described perceived competition with cisgender women for partners. They noted that the desire to keep male partners compelled them to engage in unwanted sexual practices for the purposes of maintaining the relationship.

Trans women who participated in the TSQ reported a clear desire to be seen by others as women and listed multiple steps taken to express their gender to others, including the use of hormones from unlicensed providers. However, only one of the 40 participants had undergone genital reconstruction surgery. The most common reason for not having undergone desired gender affirmation interventions was the inability to afford it. As described by participants in the IDIs, sex work is a frequent source of income both to pay for gender interventions and to provide income after loss of family support. While not explicit in these narratives, sex work has also been described as a consequence of employment discrimination (Sausa, Keatley, & Operario, 2007) as well as one way that trans women may feel affirmed in their gender (Sevelius, 2013). Sex work is criminalised in the vast majority of the United States and puts trans women at risk for street violence

(Poteat et al., 2015) as well as incarceration where they face an additional risk of sexual violence from men at high risk for HIV (Beck, Berzofsky, Caspar, & Krebs, 2013; Maruschak, 2005).

Enacted stigma was frequently described by trans women during the IDIs. The private nature of interpersonal rejection and lack of job promotion salient to the narratives of white trans women stood in stark contrast to the public violence and police harassment common to the narratives of Black trans women. These racial differences in patterns of stigma and discrimination have implications for HIV vulnerability. Public incidents and police encounters place Black trans women into greater contact with the criminal justice system. Engagement with criminal justice has been associated with HIV infection (Reisner, Bailey, & Sevelius, 2014). National data suggest that one in five trans women has been in jail or prison, with the highest prevalence among Black trans women compared to other races (Reisner et al., 2014). However, published data comparing arrest or incarceration rates between MSM and trans women are lacking. While 25% of trans women in the NHBS reported a history of arrest in the prior year, the difference from the proportion of MSM arrested (16%) was not statistically significant. This lack of significance may be due to low statistical power in the small sample of trans women. Alternatively, trans women may share risk factors for arrest with MSM. During the period of data collection, most arrests in Baltimore city were linked to drug offenses (Schiraldi & Ziedenberg, 2003). Similarities in arrests between trans women and MSM in this study may have been related to similarities in patterns of drug use. The NHBS did not collect data on the reason for arrests or on the proportion of arrests that resulted in time in jail or prison. Therefore, it is possible that there were differences in incarceration despite similar rates of arrest.

Medicare is a federal health insurance programme available to people who are 65 or older and to younger people with disabilities. Therefore, it is surprising that one in five of the insured trans women in NHBS (average age 28 years) reported Medicare as their insurer, compared to 1 in 12 MSM (average age 34 years). One possible explanation is that trans people with HIV in this study had more advanced disease and qualified for disability-related Medicare on that basis. This interpretation is consistent with other research indicating significant barriers to trans women's engagement in HIV care (Sevelius, Patouhas, Keatley, & Johnson, 2014) as well as national data indicating disparities in HIV care by race, age, and gender (Hall et al., 2013). For the trans women in this study, disadvantage based on youth, Black race, feminine gender, and trans identity may intersect to form formidable barriers to early and effective HIV prevention and care.

Implications for data collection

The quantitative analysis was limited by the small number of trans participants and biased towards the null by recruitment of MSM and trans women at the similar venues. Neither the TSQ nor the 2004–2005 NHBS included questions about sexual risk behaviour or condom use among trans women, leaving important gaps in the understanding of how these may differ between MSM and trans women. Soft-tissue filler injections with loose silicone and other substances are believed to be common among trans women (Wilson, Rapues, Jin, & Raymond, 2014); however, none of the data sets asked questions about soft-tissue filler use. Data about the sexual partners of trans women were quite limited in all data sets. While the number of HIV studies among male partners of trans women is growing (Gamarel et al., 2015; Operario, Nemoto, Iwamoto, & Moore, 2011a, 2011b; Reisner et al., 2012; Wilson, Chen et al., 2014), they remain limited, leaving an important gap in our understanding of sexual networks among trans women and how these networks may impact HIV vulnerability.

These data limitations offer important lessons for future research with trans populations. The NHBS chose to include trans women in data collection, providing an important estimate of HIV prevalence among trans women in Baltimore. However, the recruitment strategies, sampling methods, and behavioural questionnaire had been designed for MSM. As a result, the number of trans participants was small and the study inadequately powered for some comparative analyses. To avoid inappropriate questions, all questions about sexual behaviour were omitted from NHBS interviews with trans women, leaving important gaps in our understanding of trans women's sexual risk factors and limiting our ability to directly compare correlates of risk between trans women and MSM. Importantly, the TSQ, designed specifically for trans participants, also did not include questions about condom use or questions about use of injectable soft-tissue fillers. Future quantitative HIV research should strive not only to include trans people but also to use sampling strategies designed to reach trans participants. These strategies should aim to achieve sample sizes large enough to power substantive quantitative analyses. Questionnaires should be developed in partnership with trans communities to ensure that all questions, including about sexual behaviour, are appropriate for trans participants and include trans-specific questions about factors such as such as hormone and silicone use.

Implications for interventions

Overall, these data paint a picture of unique and overlapping HIV vulnerabilities. HIV prevalence is remarkably high among both MSM and trans women in Baltimore. Sexual partnerships with men are likely a shared risk behaviour for both groups. However, trans women face specific vulnerabilities related to trans discrimination, sex work, and desire for gender affirmation. These factors necessitate a different approach to HIV prevention interventions among trans women, particularly Black trans women who are particularly vulnerable to HIV. In order to be relevant to the realities of trans women's lives, ideal HIV prevention efforts should affirm trans identities, address self-esteem, improve access to safe, affordable, gender affirming interventions, support resilience to racism and transphobia, and address poverty, discrimination and violence.

Syndemics of poverty, substance use, discrimination, and violence among racial, sexual, and gender minorities have been associated with increased prevalence of HIV (Oldenburg, Perez-Brumer, & Reisner, 2014; O'Leary, 2014; Operario & Nemoto, 2010). Data from our analyses support a syndemic production of HIV among trans women in Baltimore. Research to better understand how intersectional experiences of oppression (Jefferson, Neilands, & Sevelius, 2013; Operario, Reisner, Iwamoto, & Nemoto, 2014) interact to produce the syndemics that increase HIV vulnerability among trans women is critical for the development of effective interventions for this population.

Acknowledgements

The authors express our gratitude to the study participants for their willingness to share their data and their stories. The content is solely the responsibility of the authors and does not necessarily represent the official views of the NIH.

Funding

We would like to acknowledge that the NHBS data collection was supported by contracts to The Johns Hopkins University from the Maryland Department of Health and Mental Hygiene and by cooperative agreements between the Maryland Department of Health and Mental Hygiene with the Centers for Disease Control and Prevention. Additional support for this project was received from the Johns Hopkins Center for Health Disparities Solutions and the Johns Hopkins Center for Public Health and Human Rights. The analyses described here were supported by the Johns Hopkins Center for AIDS Research, an NIH-funded program, with Award Number 1P30AI094189.

References

Adimora, A. A., Schoenbach, V. J., & Floris-Moore, M. A. (2009). Ending the Epidemic of heterosexual HIV transmission among African Americans. *American Journal of Preventive Medicine*, *37*(5), 468–471. doi:10.1016/j.amepre.2009.06.020

Baral, S. D., Poteat, T., Strömdahl, S., Wirtz, A. L., Guadamuz, T. E., & Beyrer, C. (2013). Worldwide burden of HIV in transgender women: A systematic review and meta-analysis. *The Lancet Infectious Diseases*, *13*(3), 214–222. doi:10.1016/S1473-3099(12)70315-8

Beck, A., Berzofsky, M., Caspar, R., & Krebs, C. (2013). *Sexual victimization in prisons and Jails reported by inmates, 2011-12* (Report No. NCJ 241399). Washington, DC. Retrieved from http://www.bjs.gov/content/pub/pdf/svpjri1112.pdf

Bowleg, L. (2012). The problem with the phrase women and minorities: Intersectionality-an important theoretical framework for public health. *American Journal of Public Health*, *102*(7), 1267–1273. doi:10.2105/ajph.2012.300750

Crabtree, B. F., & Miller, W. L. (1999). *Doing qualitative research* (Vol. 3). Thousand Oaks, CA: Sage Publications. doi:10.1097/00006199-199507000-00011

Flynn, C. (2013, July 16). "HIV in the Baltimore-Towson Metropolitan area." Retrieved from http://www.baltimorepc.org/v2/files/pdf/BaltimoreEMA_13.ColinF.pdf

Fujimoto, K., & Williams, M. L. (2014). Racial/ethnic differences in sexual network mixing: A log-linear analysis of HIV status by partnership and sexual behavior among most at-risk MSM. *AIDS Behaviour*. doi:10.1007/s10461-014-0842-8

Gallagher, K. M., Sullivan, P. S., Lansky, A., & Onorato, I. M. (2007). Behavioral surveillance among people at risk for HIV infection in the US: The National HIV Behavioral Surveillance system. *Public Health Reports*, *122*(Suppl 1), 32–38.

Gamarel, K. E., Reisner, S. L., Darbes, L. A., Hoff, C. C., Chakravarty, D., Nemoto, T., & Operario, D. (2015). Dyadic dynamics of HIV risk among transgender women and their primary male sexual partners: The role of sexual agreement types and motivations. *AIDS Care*, 1–8. doi:10.1080/09540121.2015.1069788

German, D., Sifakis, F., Maulsby, C., Towe, V. L., Flynn, C. P., Latkin, C. A., ... Holtgrave, D. R. (2011). Persistently high prevalence and unrecognized HIV infection among men who have sex with men in Baltimore: The Besure study. *JAIDS Journal of Acquired Immune Deficiency Syndromes*, *57*(1), 77–87. doi:10.1097/QAI.0b013e318211b41e

Grant, J. M., Mottet, L. A., Tanis, J., Harrison, J., Herman, J. L., & Keisling, M. (2010). Injustice at every turn. *National Center for Transgender*, *5*, 23–23. doi:10.1016/S0016-7878(90)80026-2

Hall, H. I., Frazier, E. L., Rhodes, P., Holtgrave, D. R., Furlow-Parmley, C., Tang, T., ... Skarbinski, J. (2013). Differences in human immunodeficiency virus care and treatment among subpopulations in the United States. *JAMA Internal Medicine, 173*(14), 1337–1344. doi:10.1001/jamainternmed.2013.6841

Holden, D. (2015, January 21). "FDA's new blood donation guidelines offer little clarity for transgender people." Retrieved from http://www.buzzfeed.com/dominicholden/fda-clings-to-arbitrary-incoherent-rules-for-transgender-peo#.fh2G2ALyj3

Jefferson, K., Neilands, T. B., & Sevelius, J. (2013). Transgender women of color: Discrimination and depression symptoms. *Ethnicity and Inequalities in Health and Social Care, 6*(4), 121–136. doi:10.1108/eihsc-08-2013-0013

Maruschak, L. (2005). *HIV in prisons 2003*. Washington, DC. Retrieved from Bureau of Justice Statistics Bulletin. Publication No. NCJ 210344.

Millett, G. A., Flores, S. A., Peterson, J. L., & Bakeman, R. (2007). Explaining disparities in HIV infection among black and white men who have sex with men: A meta-analysis of HIV risk behaviors. *Aids, 21*(15), 2083–2091. doi:10.1097/QAD.0b013e3282e9a64b

Muessig, K. E., Baltierra, N. B., Pike, E. C., LeGrand, S., & Hightow-Weidman, L. B. (2014). Achieving HIV risk reduction through Healthmpowerment.org, a user-driven eHealth intervention for young black men who have sex with men and transgender women who have sex with men. *Digital Culture and Education, 6*(3), 164–182.

Oldenburg, C. E., Perez-Brumer, A. G., & Reisner, S. L. (2014). Poverty matters: Contextualizing the syndemic condition of psychological factors and newly diagnosed HIV infection in the United States. *Aids, 28*(18), 2763–2769. doi:10.1097/qad.0000000000000491

O'Leary, D. (2014). The syndemic of AIDS and STDS among MSM. *The Linacre Quarterly, 81*(1), 12–37. doi:10.1179/2050854913y.0000000015

Operario, D., & Nemoto, T. (2010). HIV in transgender communities: Syndemic dynamics and a need for multicomponent interventions. *JAIDS Journal of Acquired Immune Deficiency Syndromes, 55*(Suppl 2), S91–S93. doi:10.1097/QAI.0b013e3181fbc9ec

Operario, D., Nemoto, T., Iwamoto, M., & Moore, T. (2011a). Risk for HIV and unprotected sexual behavior in male primary partners of transgender women. *Archives of Sexual Behavior, 40*(6), 1255–1261. doi:10.1007/s10508-011-9781-x

Operario, D., Nemoto, T., Iwamoto, M., & Moore, T. (2011b). Unprotected sexual behavior and HIV risk in the context of primary partnerships for transgender women. *AIDS and Behavior, 15*(3), 674–682. doi:10.1007/s10461-010-9795-8

Operario, D. Y., Yang, M. F., Reisner, S. L.; Iwamoto, M.; Nemoto, T. (2014). Stigma and the syndemic of HIV-related health risk behaviors in a diverse sample of transgender women. *Journal of Community Psychology, 42*(5), 544–557. doi:10.1002/jcop.21636

Peacock, E., Andrinopoulos, K., & Hembling, J. (2015). Binge Drinking among Men Who Have Sex with Men and Transgender Women in San Salvador: Correlates and Sexual Health Implications. *Journal of Urban Health*. doi:10.1007/s11524-014-9930-3

Peterson, J. L., Bakeman, R., Sullivan, P., Millett, G. A., Rosenberg, E., Salazar, L., … del Rio, C. (2014). Social discrimination and resiliency are not associated with differences in prevalent HIV infection in black and white men who have sex with men. *JAIDS Journal of Acquired Immune Deficiency Syndromes, 66*(5), 538–543. doi:10.1097/qai.0000000000000203

Poteat, T., Wirtz, A. L., Radix, A., Borquez, A., Silva-Santisteban, A., Deutsch, M. B., … Operario, D. (2015). HIV risk and preventive interventions in transgender women sex workers. *Lancet, 385* (9964), 274–286. doi:10.1016/s0140-6736(14)60833-3

Reisner, S., Mimiaga, M., Bland, S. E., Driscoll, M. A., Cranston, K., & Mayer, K. H. (2012). Pathways to embodiment of HIV risk: Black men who have sex with transgender partners, Boston, Massachusetts. *AIDS Education and Prevention, 24*(1), 15–26. doi:10.1521/aeap.2012.24.1.15

Reisner, S. L., Bailey, Z., & Sevelius, J. (2014). Racial/ethnic disparities in history of incarceration, experiences of victimization, and associated health indicators among transgender women in the U.S. *Women & Health* (September), 37–41. doi:10.1080/03630242.2014.932891

Sausa, L. A., Keatley, J., & Operario, D. (2007). Perceived risks and benefits of sex work among transgender women of color in San Francisco. *Archives of Sexual Behavior, 36*(6), 768–777. doi:10.1007/s10508-007-9210-3

Schiraldi, V., & Ziedenberg, J. (2003). *Race and incarceration in Maryland*. Retrieved from http://www.justicepolicy.org/uploads/justicepolicy/documents/03-10_rep_mdraceincarceration_ac-md-rd.pdf.

Sevelius, J. M. (2013). Gender affirmation: A framework for conceptualizing risk behavior among transgender women of color. *Sex Roles, 68*(11–12), 675–689. doi:10.1007/s11199-012-0216-5

Sevelius, J. M., Patouhas, E., Keatley, J. G., & Johnson, M. O. (2014). Barriers and facilitators to engagement and retention in care among transgender women living with human immunodeficiency virus. *Annals of Behavioral Medicine, 47*(1), 5–16. doi:10.1007/s12160-013-9565-8

Singer, M. (2009). *Introduction to syndemics: A critical systems approach to public and community health*. San Francisco, CA: John Wiley & Sons.

The US food and drug administration. (2014, December 23). "Blood donations from men who have sex with other men questions and answers." Retrieved from http://www.fda.gov/BiologicsBloodVaccines/BloodBloodProducts/QuestionsaboutBlood/ucm108186.htm

Wilson, E., Rapues, J., Jin, H., & Raymond, H. F. (2014). The use and correlates of Illicit Silicone or 'fillers' in a population-based sample of transwomen, San Francisco, 2013. *The Journal of Sexual Medicine, 11*(7), 1717–1724. doi:10.1111/jsm.12558

Wilson, E. C., Chen, Y.-H., Raad, N., Raymond, H. F., Dowling, T., & McFarland, W. (2014). Who are the sexual partners of transgender individuals? Differences in demographic characteristics and risk behaviours of San Francisco HIV testing clients with transgender sexual partners compared with overall testers. *Sexual Health*. doi:10.1071/SH13202

World Health Organization. (2014). *Consolidated guidelines on HIV prevention, diagnosis, treatment and care for key populations*. Geneva: WHO Press.

Young, R. M., & Meyer, I. H. (2005). The trouble with 'MSM' and 'WSW': Erasure of the sexual-minority person in public health discourse. *American Journal of Public Health 95*(7), 1144–1149. doi:10.2105/ajph.2004.046714

Zea, M. C., Reisen, C. A., Del Rio-Gonzalez, A. M., Bianchi, F. T., Ramirez-Valles, J., & Poppen, P. J. (2015). HIV prevalence and awareness of positive serostatus among men who have sex with men and transgender women in Bogota, Colombia. *American Journal of Public Health*, e1–e8. doi:10.2105/ajph.2014.302307

Towards 'reflexive epidemiology': Conflation of cisgender male and transgender women sex workers and implications for global understandings of HIV prevalence

Amaya G. Perez-Brumer, Catherine E. Oldenburg, Sari L. Reisner, Jesse L. Clark and Richard G. Parker

ABSTRACT

The HIV epidemic has had a widespread impact on global scientific and cultural discourses related to gender, sexuality, and identity. 'Male sex workers' have been identified as a 'key population' in the global HIV epidemic; however, there are methodological and conceptual challenges for defining inclusion and exclusion of transgender women within this group. To assess these potential implications, this study employs self-critique and reflection to grapple with the empiric and conceptual implications of shifting understandings of sexuality and gender within the externally re-created etic category of 'MSM' and 'transgender women' in epidemiologic HIV research. We conducted a sensitivity analysis of our previously published meta-analysis which aimed to identify the scope of peer-reviewed articles assessing HIV prevalence among male sex workers globally between 2004 and 2013. The inclusion of four studies previously excluded due to non-differentiation of cisgender male from transgender women participants (studies from Spain, Thailand, India, and Brazil: 421 total participants) increased the overall estimate of global HIV prevalence among 'men' who engage in sex work from 10.5% (95% CI 9.4–11.5%) to 10.8% (95% CI 9.8–11.8%). The combination of social science critique with empiric epidemiologic analysis represents a first step in defining and operationalising 'reflexive epidemiology'. Grounded in the context of sex work and HIV prevention, this paper highlights the multiplicity of genders and sexualities across a range of social and cultural settings, limitations of existing categories (i.e. 'MSM', 'transgender'), and their global implications for epidemiologic estimates of HIV prevalence.

RETHINKING MSM, TRANS* AND OTHER CATEGORIES IN HIV PREVENTION

Introduction

Globally, results from meta-analyses have provided a necessary synthesis of existing empirical evidence for the identification of groups of people made vulnerable to HIV based on epidemiological trends. For example, the available literature estimates that men who have sex with men (MSM) have a 19-fold and transgender women a 49-fold increased odds of HIV infection compared to the general population (Baral et al., 2013; Beyrer et al., 2012). Additionally, female sex workers have a nearly 14-fold increased odds of HIV infection compared to women of reproductive age, and male sex workers have a nearly 21-fold increased odds of HIV infection compared to the general male population (Baral et al., 2012; Oldenburg et al., 2014). However, meta-analysis as a tool to synthesise descriptive epidemiology for key populations should be understood as a double-edged sword. On the one hand, meta-analytic methods are often considered to be at the top of the hierarchy of evidence in evidence-based medicine (Haidich, 2010), and can ground claims to support research agendas, strategic initiatives, and policies to reduce health disparities borne by key populations. Meta-analyses are particularly important for standardising characteristics that define membership within key populations that are typically excluded from routine country surveillance, despite their association with vulnerability to HIV infection. In particular, the un-reflexive exclusion of stigmatised behaviours, identities, and practices from epidemiologic estimates further promotes invisibility of key populations and makes it difficult to design effective HIV prevention programming and care.

Nonetheless, meta-analyses synthesising descriptive epidemiology carry a number of problematic implications. While meta-analyses provide standardised, globally replicable categories to better understand typologies of risk associated with epidemiological trends, such understandings become both simplified and reified in the context of meta-analyses. This is particularly problematic due to the intertwined social, biological, and behavioural drivers of the HIV epidemic and the complexity of the identities and behaviours integral to defining 'key populations' in HIV research. Furthermore, an understanding of what defines membership within a specific population is constructed through the use and re-use of common epidemiologic categories, and often reduced to a methodological description of the study's inclusion and exclusion criteria. Given the disproportionate HIV burden faced by those with alternative or non-normative genders and sexualities, critical engagement and continual reflection on the construction, use, and meanings of dominant categories in meta-analysis and quantitative research methods is imperative.

While there exists critical scholarship (primarily within the social sciences) assessing the limitations of categories based on sex and gender paradigms in existing HIV research and the subsequent impact on the production of scientific knowledge, there are few studies that pair a social science critique with empiric epidemiologic analysis to support the argument. Uniquely positioned to fill this gap and assess the potential implications of boundary construction within key population categories, here we return to our original meta-analysis (Oldenburg et al., 2014) to reframe the methodological definition of 'male sex workers', revise the population estimate of HIV prevalence, and argue for scientific reflection and reflexivity that moves beyond risk-factor ('black-box') epidemiology (Greenland, Gago-Dominguez, & Castelao, 2004). In the course of the systematic review, which informed data for our original meta-analysis, four studies were excluded due to conflated HIV prevalence among cisgender male and male-to-female (MTF) transgender women sex workers. The inclusion of these studies drove our sensitivity analysis and provided us a jumping-off point to critically engage with potential weaknesses of quantitative methods that replicate dominant classification categories related to sex and gender, and illustrate how redefining categories may impact the empirical and conceptual evidence which informs global understandings of HIV infection prevalence estimates. Building towards 'reflexive epidemiology', meaning active engagement in the complexity of categorisation, this article seeks to generate conversation and provide space for participation and reflection by researchers on the choices and implications of data coding, construction, and usage.

The legacy of categorisation of gender and sexuality in HIV epidemiology

The politics shaping scientific knowledge about HIV infection and contemporary understandings of key populations can be traced to the early years of the HIV epidemic. The acronym 'MSM' was created by activists for the purpose of drawing attention to a group in need of HIV prevention messaging and outreach: men who have sex with men who do not necessarily identify as gay (Aggleton & Parker, 2015). As the epidemic evolved so did the category, and within the epidemiology and global public health literature, MSM grew to encompass all homosexually active men (Boellstroff, 2011; Young & Meyer, 2005). In medical research, the category 'MSM' has been effective in detailing patterns of HIV and STI risk according to sexual practices that are described by biological anatomy. For that reason, 'MSM' has been important to furthering understandings of common patterns of HIV risk due to receptive anal intercourse among cisgender males, transgender women, and other individuals assigned a male sex at birth. However, scholars have argued that the construction of 'MSM' as a population category based on behaviours not only fails to account for the nuances of sexual diversities but also for the social identities critical to community organisation, thereby weakening the implications of the evidence that can be drawn from the use of this category (Boellstroff, 2011; Muñoz-Laboy, 2004; Young & Meyer, 2005). Furthermore, boundary setting around what it means to be classified as MSM may valorise one point of view while silencing others (Bowker & Star, 1999). To this point, Boellstroff calls attention to 'biological essentialism' rooted in the definition of 'man' within the MSM category (i.e. an anatomical male having sex with another anatomical male) and its direct implication for public health, principally the invisibility of transgender individuals' particular needs in early HIV epidemic response efforts (Boellstroff, 2011). Critical reflection on MSM as a category highlights how social and behavioural dimensions of gender and sexual identity are eschewed by the continued, dominant use of the term 'MSM'.

Concurrent with the struggles of identity politics and the use of 'MSM' in the late 1980s and early 1990s, 'transgender' as an identifiable category also emerged during the early years of the AIDS crisis (Stryker, 2009; Valentine, 2007). Though scholars have researched the history of 'transsexuality' (and other linguistic synonyms for gender variance) over 50 years prior to the advent of HIV and AIDS (Meyerowitz, 2009), the overlap, intersection, and conflict between HIV, MSM, and current understandings of transgender as a category have been largely overlooked. For instance, the majority of epidemiologic research interested in the incidence and prevalence of HIV and AIDS among 'MSM' has folded transgender and other gender variant populations into this initial population category of interest. As noted by Hansmann, subsuming transgender health within a larger gay and bisexual men's health agenda assumed the importance of HIV and AIDS as an urgent transgender health concern, for both transgender women and transgender men (Hanssmann, 2010). Though more recent research on transgender women who have sex with cisgender males supports this position, for transgender men there are still limited data to support such claims. Furthermore, the limited data on transgender women and the relative invisibility of transgender men have made it exceptionally difficult to highlight other pressing health problems and to develop programmes responsive to their unique needs both related to HIV infection and AIDS, and to holistic health generally.

Through the work of critical scholarship and transgender activism, conceptual and methodological conflation of MSM and transgender people, specifically transgender women, into one category in medical research and health policy is decreasing. For example, the Institute of Medicine's Report on LGBT Health (Institute of Medicine, 2011) and the World Health Organization's HIV guidelines for key populations (World Health Organization, 2014) are among a growing number of scientific publications calling for categorical distinctions between these populations. Yet, the problematic legacy of the term 'MSM' is evident. Notably, the confusion regarding the division between behavioural and social factors (e.g. sexual practices, sexual orientation and gender identity) underscores the stickiness between definitions of sex, gender, and sexuality (Epstein, 2009). Jordan-Young offers a useful metaphor of a three-ply yarn to make sense of the entanglement between sex, gender, and sexuality. This metaphor suggests that though all three are distinct and interrelated, they are also 'somewhat fuzzy around the boundaries' (Jordan-Young, 2011). Due to the importance of bodies, practices, and identities in efforts to understand the disproportionate concentration of HIV infection among MSM and transgender women, there is an urgent need to not only critically assess overlap between population categories but also to question how category construction informs empirical epidemiologic evidence.

This 'fuzziness' surrounding groupings of sexualities and gender identities can be further highlighted when considering MSM and transgender in relation to a third defining category of central interest for HIV prevention research: sex work. Sex work has been consistently associated with high HIV acquisition risks among MSM, transgender women, and cisgender women (Oldenburg et al., 2014; Operario, Soma, & Underhill, 2008). However, transgender women sex workers have been reported to have an even greater risk for HIV acquisition compared to MSM and cisgender women who engage in sex work (Operario et al., 2008). Posited reasons for their elevated risk include economic and social marginalisation resulting from a range of community and societal exclusionary practices (Infante, Sosa-Rubi, & Cuadra, 2009; Nemoto et al., 2012; Silva-Santisteban et al., 2012). The need for a person's gender to be collectively recognised has also been reported as a unique social determinant of health influencing transgender women's engagement in sex work and sexual risk behaviours further heightening HIV vulnerability (Nuttbrock et al., 2012; Reisner et al., 2009; Sevelius, 2013). These differential disparities highlighted within sex work further emphasise how attention to social processes coupled with sexuality and gender performance may provide important insights for understanding HIV vulnerability within the researcher-driven, etic category of sex worker.

In the current context of focused attention on key populations in HIV epidemiology, the definitions of and distinctions between gender identity and sexual orientation are of increasing importance. However, HIV research efforts frequently employ analytic population categories following the same logic and historical precedence of the category MSM, such as male sex worker, without giving due consideration to how the overlap and complexities of conceptual gender and sexuality distinctions and the methodological choices for analyses of data may shape findings and influence policies and programmes. For example, Oldenburg et al. (2014) reported that across 66 studies representing 28 countries, men who engaged in transactional sex practices had an almost 21-fold increased odds of elevated HIV burden compared to the general male population. However, a central question left unanswered in these epidemiologic estimates is: Who is counted, and why? According to the authors, 'in cases in which no delineation was made between reporting HIV prevalence among male and transgender male-to-female sex workers, the study was included if the majority (≥80%) of participants in the study were not transgender male-to-female' (Oldenburg et al., 2014). Justification such as this parallels rationalities employed by other meta-analyses that seek to contribute to the scientific understanding of HIV burden among key populations, but often fail to account for the potential implications of such choices.

Methods

This paper is a secondary analysis of a larger study that aimed to identify the scope of peer-reviewed published articles and generate a combined estimate of HIV prevalence among male sex workers globally between 1 January 2004 and 31 July 2013 (Oldenburg et al., 2014). The rationale for this paper is to critically examine this larger study's inclusion criteria by incorporating four studies in which no delineation was made between reported HIV prevalence among cisgender male and transgender woman sex workers, all of which were excluded from the primary meta-analysis. Here, we run sensitivity analyses by including data from the studies excluded from the original study in an updated meta-analysis. Complete methods for the original systematic review and primary meta-analysis have been previously reported (Oldenburg et al., 2014).

Systematic review

For the systematic review, the search strategy included review of seven electronic databases including PubMed, EMBASE, PsycINFO, Sociological Abstracts, POPLine, CINAHL, and Web of Science using the following search terms: 'commercial sex', 'sex work*', 'male sex worker*', 'prostitution', 'exchange sex', 'transactional sex', 'HIV', and 'men who have sex with men'. To complement a search of published manuscripts, abstract searches were also conducted from the following databases: the International AIDS Society (IAS), the American Public Health Association (APHA), the Conference on Retroviruses and Opportunistic Infections (CROI), and the International Society for Sexually Transmitted Disease Research (ISSTDR). HIV surveillance reports including demographic and health surveys (DHS) and integrated biological and behavioural surveillance (IBBS) reports were also searched. Additionally, reference lists of all included articles were reviewed for additional articles.

Meta-analysis and sensitivity analysis

Using the same meta-analytic procedures, here we conducted a sensitivity analyses by including data from the studies excluded from the original study in an updated meta-analysis. The initial meta-analysis reviewed 20,193 titles and abstracts, 547 conference abstracts, and 165 surveillance reports, 446 titles and abstracts. Of these, 89 articles, abstracts, or surveillance reports representing 34,803 individuals in 30 countries were included in the primary review. Among the remaining 89 studies that were eligible for inclusions in systematic review, however, 66 studies met the inclusion criteria for meta-analysis: containing primary, quantitative data on HIV prevalence among males (individuals assigned a male sex at birth and presently identified as a male/man) who reported exchanging any sex act for anything of value, including money, goods, or drugs. The final analysis for the original meta-analysis represented data from 28 countries and included 31,924 men who engaged in transactional sex with other men. Studies were included regardless of whether HIV status was determined by laboratory methods or via self-report. Studies published in English, Spanish, French, or Portuguese, or if enough study information was published in an English-language abstract, were included.

In the course of this systematic review which provided data for our original meta-analysis, four studies were excluded due to conflated HIV prevalence among cisgender male and MTF transgender sex workers: one abstract (Reza-Paul et al., 2008) and three peer-reviewed articles (Chariyalertsak et al., 2011; Gutiérrez et al., 2004; Reza-Paul et al., 2008; Tun, de Mello, Pinho, Chinaglia, & Diaz, 2008). In the present analysis, these four studies were included, contributing an additional 421 participants for a total analytic sample of 32,345 'men' assigned male sex at birth who engage in sex work. Sensitivity analysis used a DerSimonian-Laird random effects model (DerSimonian & Laird, 1986) to assess an overall pooled point estimate and 95% confidence interval for HIV prevalence. Pooled point estimates of HIV prevalence were calculated by country and region. A random effects model was used to account for heterogeneity of studies (Baral, Sifakis, Cleghorn, & Beyrer, 2007; DerSimonian & Laird, 1986). Random effects meta-regression was used to assess differences in HIV prevalence by definition of transactional sex. Publication bias was assessed with Egger's test (Egger, Smith, Schneider, & Minder, 1997) and Begg's test (Begg, 1994). All analyses were conducted in Stata 12.0 (StataCorp, College Station, TX).

Results

The four previously excluded studies which conflated HIV prevalence among cisgender male and MTF transgender sex workers represented data from Thailand, India, Brazil, and Spain and contributed to a total of 32,347 participants included in the analytic sample representing 70 studies and 29 countries. Table 1 shows the pooled HIV prevalence among men assigned male sex at birth who engage in transactional sex (sensitivity analysis) compared to the pooled HIV prevalence among men who engaged in transactional sex (original meta-analysis).

Compared to the meta-analysis by Oldenburg et al. (2014), results from our sensitivity analysis show that the inclusion of four previously excluded studies resulted in

Table 1. Pooled HIV prevalence among 'men' assigned male sex at birth who engage in transactional sex (sensitivity analysis) compared to the pooled HIV prevalence among men who engaged in transactional sex (original meta-analysis).

	Sensitivity analysis HIV prevalence (95% CI)	Original meta-analysis HIV prevalence (95% CI)
By country		
Brazil	13.2% (6.8–19.7%)	N/A[a]
India	14.5% (8.6–20.5%)	11.8% (6.0–17.6%)
Spain	15.7% (10.7–20.6%)	14.2% (9.6–18.8%)
Thailand	17.5% (14.1–21.0%)	17.5% (13.7–21.2%)
By regions		
Europe	11.2% 6.3–16.1%)	12.2% (6.0–17.2%)
Latin America	18.7% (15.1–22.3%)	19.3% (15.5–23.1%)
Southeast Asia	13.3% (9.8–11.8%)	12.9% (8.8–17.0%)
South Asia	2.9% (2.0–3.9%)	2.7% (1.7–3.6%)
Overall	10.8% (9.8–11.8%)	10.5% (9.4–11.5%)

[a]Country-specific prevalence data from Brazil were unavailable in original meta-analysis assessing global HIV prevalence.

an increase in the estimated global prevalence of HIV among men assigned male sex at birth who engage in sex work by 0.3%. While a 0.3% change in overall prevalence may seem unimportant, due to a seemingly small fluctuation in the HIV prevalence point estimate, it is important to underscore that a 1% increase in number of individuals led to a 3% relative increase in HIV prevalence. Additionally, the greatest percent change in point estimates reporting pooled HIV prevalence was in India, which rose by 2.7% followed by Spain, which was increased from 1.5%. Inclusion of manuscripts that collapsed MSM and transgender women into one analytic category allowed for the inclusion of country-specific prevalence data from Brazil to our global assessment of HIV prevalence. As such, this entry not only represents a change in country-level information, but additionally influenced regional and global HIV prevalence estimates. While for Thailand, the pooled HIV prevalence stayed the same, regionally, the addition of the four previously excluded studies had mixed-results (see Table 1).

Implications

This study demonstrates the utility of reflexive epidemiology to link a social science critique with empiric epidemiologic analysis in order to assess the complexities of sex, sexuality, and gender-based categories, and to understand how such categories impact global estimates of HIV prevalence. Inclusion and exclusion paradigms, though evolving, are neither simple nor without implications, and carry with them the past and ongoing presence of identity politics. These results present necessary empirical evidence to highlight two key points: (1) the implications of boundary construction around key population categories related to sex and gender, and (2) why it is important to critically reflect on who gets counted within global understandings of HIV prevalence. Our argument is not to conflate important distinctions between cisgender male and transgender women who engage in sex work and their vulnerability to HIV. Rather, this article is meant to offer a case study in reflexive epidemiology, to become a means whereby both the researcher and the reader gain a sharpened understanding of why particular conceptualisations of sexual orientation and gender identity impact medical research, and the potential for porousness and slippage between these categories if they are used uncritically.

The problem of measurement and reporting

Recognising that categories are a necessary aspect of quantitative research, these results suggest the need for more reflexive epidemiology to explore the intended and unintended effects of population category definitions regarding who gets counted and why. Learning from the troubled legacy of 'MSM', scholars have increasingly pushed back on the notion of 'transgender' as a catch-all umbrella category, and instead argue for an understanding of transgender as a dynamic and flexible collection of gender variant identities (Labuski & Keo-Meier, 2015; Singer, 2015). Though problematic for epidemiologic research, challenges to commonly used categories based-on evolving understandings of what it means to be transgender, and increased usage of the category 'transgender' within the sphere of public health research, need to be openly acknowledged. This study presents a first step in reflexive epidemiology to underscore the complexities of sex, sexuality, and gender-based categories, and how conceptualisations and operationalisation of such categories potentially impact global estimates of HIV prevalence.

There is no right way to categorically measure the entanglement between cisgender males and transgender women within HIV and AIDS research. However, when possible, more progressive research recommendations (Institute of Medicine, 2011; World Health Organization, 2014) suggest the necessary separation of gender identity and sexual orientation in both measurement and reporting. To both increase visibility and methodologically reduce the potential for misclassification, the two-step method, which asks about natal sex and current gender identity, is a recommended strategy for measurement of both natal sex and current gender identity (Reisner et al., 2014; Singer, 2015). However, these best practices are not always possible, for example, in meta-analyses where conflations or shifting definitions of population categories reported in individual studies cannot be overcome.

As in other syntheses of data collected by disparate research methodologies, nothing could be done to unravel the conflation between MSM and transgender women from the four excluded studies included in the Oldenburg et al.'s (2014) meta-analysis. As a result, efforts to apply current recommendations to previously conducted studies further excluded key vulnerabilities and obscured the complexity within these overlapping population categories. Based on available data, our current analysis highlights that the inclusion of manuscripts that collapse MSM and transgender women into one analytic category allowed for data from Brazil to be included and altered the estimate of global HIV prevalence among men assigned male sex at birth who engage in sex work. Though distinct visibility for vulnerable communities is critical to address the burden of disease among those most affected, this case study illustrates that such rationalities are also not without consequences. In other words, critical reflection of how sex and gender categories are operationalised in both measurement and reporting of HIV outcomes is essential. Meta-analysis as a tool to synthesise descriptive epidemiology for MSM and transgender women relies on the quality of data collected in individual studies. As such, in a call for more transparent quantitative research practices, there is an urgent need for researchers to clearly describe the rationalities that inform category constructions related to sex and gender, including critically reflecting on the politics that inform the selection of criteria for inclusion and exclusion.

Intersections between context and policy

Beyond influencing empiric understandings, reflexive epidemiology is needed to redirect quantitative research from a fixed understanding of risk due to behaviour (e.g. sexual practice) and/or identity (e.g. gender identity) to underscore the relationship between research and social justice. For example, the context of each of the four previously excluded studies highlights conflicting policy initiatives and social environments that may increase the vulnerability of not only transgender women, but also persons who engage in sex work and practice non-heteronormative sexual behaviours. This section focuses on linking results to existing social processes and local realities to underscore the relationship between HIV knowledge production and needed advocacy within the field of global public health.

Existing literature highlights the importance of country-level laws and policies in influencing HIV vulnerability across populations' currently delineated as 'key' (Oldenburg et al., 2016; Shannon et al., 2015). Leveraging the growing interest in structural determinants of health, quantitative research can also promote advocacy by bringing to light important omissions within legislative and policy initiatives seeking to improve the health of vulnerable populations. Though it is important to maintain a distinction between the need for research and the need for advocacy, the politics of dominant frameworks often jeopardise the meaningfulness of scientific inquiry within research related to sex and gender. This paper, for example, highlights how MSM and transgender categories are ones in which sex and gender are variables and efforts to make them seem less variable for the purposes of scholarly research: (1) reflect the institutional power of biomedicine, and (2) can make it difficult to actually capture people's lived experience. Simply put, sex and gender classifications that conflate (e.g. previously excluded studies) or distinguish are neither neutral nor without consequence. Rather, within the biomedical sciences, the power of evidence is a constitutive force shaping understandings of vulnerabilities to health and the need for political actions to ameliorate such health disparities.

Spain can be used as an example to illustrate why it is imperative for researchers to explicitly connect findings to political contexts. In Spain, there exists provisional legislation to protect the rights of those engaged in sex work, but this is explicitly designated for the protection of cisgender women *only* (ILGA, 2013; UNAIDS, 2007). Access to free medical care and legal protections for sex workers in the country is similarly limited to cisgender women. Beyond a more accurate documentation of global HIV prevalence, contextualisation of our results and assessment of why the numbers matter underscore the need for scientists to report evidence in a way that pushes the current boundaries of structural interventions to address all populations in need. The results of our study show a 1.5% increase from the reported HIV prevalence among cisgender men sex workers in Spain when including the previously omitted data that conflated cisgender men and transgender women sex workers. While this increase is vulnerable to misrepresentation when enforcing distinctions between sex and gender paradigms, it does nonetheless raise awareness in relation to both cisgender men who engage in sex work *and* transgender women – who are scarcely represented in the existing Spanish epidemiologic literature.

While, drawing attention to the contextual realities of Spain furthers the reach of our argument for reflexive epidemiology, it is only one illustration of many. Solely highlighting 'MSM' or 'transgender women' as static risk categories without taking into account the effect of unique sociocultural contexts may also erase important social and structural factors that increase HIV vulnerabilities across populations and geographic contexts and cultures. For example, co-occurring HIV epidemics have been identified not only among MSM, transgender women, and sex workers, but also injecting drug users (van Griensven et al., 2013). Counter to unitary approaches that posit one master category of analysis, the theory of intersectionality (Crenshaw, 1991) is a useful guide to highlight the various axes of race, ethnicity, gender identity, sexual orientation, economic status, ability, and education that intersect to constitute inequality and vulnerability. Quantitative adaptations of intersectionality theory are important next steps for researchers seeking to reframe and complicate the discussion of health disparities beyond limited notions of sexual orientation or gender identity as a single axis (Bauer, 2014; Bowleg, 2012).

Politics of exportation: the persistence of hegemonic understandings of sex and gender

Though not unique to meta-analyses describing HIV trends in key populations, standardised Western models of what it means to be 'MSM', 'transgender', or even 'engaged in sex work' emerge as particularly problematic when grouping data across time, varied geographic and cultural contexts, and social realities. This critique is not meant to deny the potential utility of meta-analytic techniques for describing disease burden, but rather, to challenge researchers to grapple with the complexity of gender and sexuality in order to improve measurement and reporting. Within our analysis, all countries assessed through the additional sensitivity analysis warrant further discussion to highlight the 'social imaginary' (Singer, 2015) used by public health and medical sciences to group people based on one master category.

Specific to the Indian context, scholars have highlighted that the broadness of sexualities and genders, such as *hijra*, can be at odds with rigid sex and gender categories that are linked to Western cultural norms (Asthana & Oostvogels, 2001; Lorway & Khan, 2014). Insights from ethnography by Asthana and Oostvogels of MSM and MSM 'subpopulations' suggest that the division between sexual orientation and gender identity is an artificial construct serving only the 'purpose of facilitating an understanding of the public health needs' (Asthana & Oostvogels, 2001). Contributing to this complexity, the term *kathoey*, unique to the Thai context, further underscores the spectrum of femininity as a fluid identity construct not represented by natal sex or third gender categories such as transgender (Beyrer et al., 2012; Jackson & Cook, 1999). Other examples from Latin America further problematise the application of transgender, as understood within a Global North context, to alternative gender practices elsewhere. Meanings of *travesti* in Brazil, often translated as transgender, are deeply intertwined with sexual practices and local beliefs about desire, gender, and sexuality (Kulick, 1998; Parker, 1999; Silva, 2014). As such, particularities of *hijra, kathoey, travesti*, and other terms and meanings not included here, are grounded in their own social and cultural context. These complexities have direct implications for understanding the concentration of HIV infection and best practices for prevention and care efforts. Caution should be exercised when aiming to unravel differing risks and service needs based on Western understandings of sex and gender categories.

Challenges and limitations of applying dominant biomedical categories in Western and global North countries also warrant critique. Though the problematic impact of category exportation is especially clear when looking at North/South dynamics (e.g. *hijra*, *kathoey*, *travesti*), a similar process can also be found in the extension or imposition of categories from a dominant biomedical framing to the lived experience of diverse populations and communities in the global North. For example, scholars have highlighted the relationship between gender migration and increases in medicalisation and institutionalisation of transgender and gender variant individuals in Spain over the past decade (Soley-Beltran & Coll-Planas, 2011). Paralleling similar tensions between the limitations versus utility of categorisation to gain visibility for the needs of transgender persons globally (Thompson & King, 2015), advances in medical awareness of transgender and gender variant people in Spain both allowed for greater access to medical interventions (i.e. surgeries and cross-sex hormones) while simultaneously increasing institutional control over what transgender identity means (Soley-Beltran & Coll-Planas, 2011). Though the exportation of categories from the global North to the global South is often easier to see because of both inequality in global power relations, as well as sharper cultural differences between Western and non-Western societies, as noted in the case of Spain, the same kind of process also frequently happens within Northern/Western societies. These examples underscore how without sufficient reflection on the role of researchers working within the frameworks of biomedicine and epidemiology, unequal power relations and important cultural differences can also allow dominant categories to be imposed on marginalised populations and communities.

The politics of exportation, meaning the replication of standardised Western understandings of 'key population' categories, have important implications for the translation of findings from meta-analyses into relevant policies and successful HIV prevention and promotion efforts. To be effective, translation of key findings into policies and programmes necessarily has to be sensitive to the local categories and conditions that are meaningful in terms of lived realities. However, when research outcomes and findings fail to account for emic (i.e. local) categories, it can make it almost impossible to effectively translate evidence-based science into effective practice. Meta-analyses, such as the Oldenburg et al. (2014) and the sensitivity analysis described here, are particularly salient examples of the tensions between externally created etic categories and the fluid, changing, and geographically grounded variability of emic categories. As highlighted, these critiques extend beyond meta-analytic methods to question common conceptualisations and usages of *sex*, *sexuality*, and gender-based categories in medical research. Importantly, the problems posed for translation and interpretation are not simply 'theoretical' rather, who gets counted and why affects the real lives of people on the ground. To make research *matter* in people's lives, translational efforts, such as the creation of protective legislation and/or relevant HIV prevention and promotion strategies, etc., must explicitly contended with the relationship between social processes, local realities, global inequities, and HIV vulnerability.

Limitations

There are several limitations to this critical review and sensitivity analysis that should be considered. Most importantly, the scope and generalisability of the arguments presented herein are meant to provoke thoughts related to the production of data, responsibility and reflexivity of the researcher in category construction, and potential systems-level implications of research findings. The aim of this paper was not to conduct a systematic review of all health-related scientific evidence that conflates gender and sexuality paradigms. Rather, this paper focuses on one example from prior work of some of the co-authors, and is hence a form of self-critique. Importantly, meta-analysis as a tool to synthesise descriptive epidemiology cannot overcome conflation between shifting understandings of population categories as reported in individual studies. As in the case of the Oldenburg et al. (2014) meta-analysis, nothing could have been done to unravel the conflation between MSM and transgender women as reported by the four excluded studies. However, this sensitivity analysis sheds light on the potential porousness between current understandings of sexual orientation and gender identity and illustrates how redefining categories can potentially impact empiric results.

Time is an important variable that was underdeveloped here. At different historical moments, salient categories may be very different. New categories emerge in society and in scientific discourse, just as old ones may be abandoned or re-signified. Categories that are meaningful socially may not be meaningful scientifically, and vice versa; the negotiation of meaning between society and science may be affected by a range of social and political factors. Due to rapidly evolving politics, coverage, and scientific research in and out of the HIV and AIDS context, it is imperative for future researchers to consider how definitions and the usage of categories are both the product of a particular historical time, context, and place. Our analysis has not focused on the historical changes that have taken place in important ways over the three and a half decades of the HIV epidemic. We have simply provided examples in which categories of gender and sexuality were collapsed in studies included in recent meta-analyses of the epidemiology of HIV infection, and of the ways in which failing to recognise this conflation can affect the results of these analyses. Our goal is to highlight the importance of questioning our own assumptions related to the methodological and/or conceptual choices that we make, in order to push quantitative HIV and AIDS research to more deeply engage in greater epidemiological reflexivity.

Conclusions

Through self-critique and reflection, this study grapples with both the empirical and the conceptual implications of shifting understandings of sex and gender within the externally re-created etic category of 'MSM' and 'transgender women' in epidemiologic HIV research. Empirically, our results show how the inclusion of an additional just 1% of individuals led to a disproportionate 3% relative increase in the pooled global HIV infection prevalence among men assigned male sex at birth who engage in transactional sex (sensitivity analysis) compared to the pooled HIV prevalence among men who engaged in transactional sex (original meta-analysis). Yet the implications of these results cannot be fully expressed quantitatively. Rather, the results of our sensitivity analysis provided us a jumping-off point to critically engage with the complexity, and potential implications, of sex, gender, and sexuality-based categorisation in HIV epidemiology focused on 'key populations'. Importantly, through this reflection a space emerged for active and critical reflexivity as researchers concerning the choices and consequences of data coding, construction, and usage.

RETHINKING MSM, TRANS* AND OTHER CATEGORIES IN HIV PREVENTION

The combination of social science critique with empiric epidemiologic analysis presented in this manuscript represents a first step in defining and operationalising reflexive epidemiology. The implications of our results centre on the production of knowledge about groupings of individuals (i.e. identification of key populations) and the political and structural determinants inextricably linked to HIV and AIDS research, prevention, and health promotion efforts. Though the majority of recent studies sustain a conceptual and methodological distinction between cisgender male and transgender woman sex workers, conflation of these categories is pervasive in past research and varying definitions of sex and gender paradigms today support the case for a continual re-thinking of how these categories are understood and used in HIV research. Furthermore, these results suggest not only the limitations of categories such as 'MSM' and 'transgender', but also of binary constructions of both gender and sex that render intersex and non-binary gender identities relatively invisible at this stage in HIV research and response. As such, a call for reflexive epidemiology is not to a push to specify individual characteristics with more precision, but rather to interrogate the role of the research and the researcher in the greater system (Figure 1).

Given the issues with measurement and reporting within and across populations, data transparency and sharing are imperative. Problematic issues that arose with the four case studies at the base of this critical analysis were due to how researchers chose to present HIV infection prevalence, often obscuring information on populations subsumed by larger categories. Self-critique on groupings and cleavages among sexuality and gender categories are needed to flag future work for scholars. However, self-critique is not enough. Due to the shifting dynamics of category definitions and understandings of health-related vulnerabilities intertwined in sex and gender groupings, the authors suggest that, when possible, descriptive characteristics by subpopulations on main

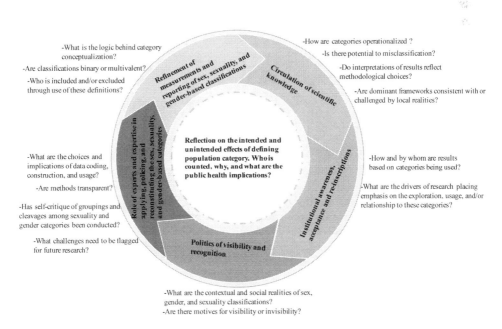

Figure 1. Model for critical engagement with 'reflexive epidemiology' to assess the complexities of sex, sexuality, and gender-based categories construction and usage within HIV epidemiology.

outcomes assessed in epidemiologic studies be included in appendices to improve future meta-analytic methods. Furthermore, availability of data and data sharing on MSM, transgender women, sex workers, and other people disproportionately burdened by HIV infection and AIDS is key in countries where country-level surveillance efforts do not report on these characteristics. Within dimensions where multiple risk factors intersect to augment vulnerability to HIV, in and across populations, the friction at the boundaries of categories necessitates further scholarly reflection. Methods seeking to assess these intersections (Bauer, 2014; Crenshaw, 1991) are an important next step in HIV epidemiologic research which seeks to identify pathways and mechanisms which contribute to HIV vulnerability.

Grounded in the context of sex work and HIV prevention, this paper highlights the multiplicity of genders and sexualities across a range of social and cultural settings, and their implications for epidemiologic estimates of HIV infection prevalence. The result is an intricate web highlighting the importance of transparency and reflexivity in category creation and application in public health and epidemiologic research. We must acknowledge that the uncritical use of unquestioned categories can not only be inaccurate, but that in some instances such inaccuracies can be oppressive and damaging to the people who are being categorised. Only by critically interrogating our use of categories will we be able to truly employ them in ways that do justice to the subjects of our research – in ways that will provide more accurate results and that will provide the basis for developing programmes and policies that will truly meet the needs of the populations that they are intended to serve. We urge researchers in the field to join us in further developing 'reflexive epidemiology' as a framework within which researchers can self-critique and engage in research transparency related to understandings of sex, sexuality, and gender. Jointly, this process will allow us to more effectively challenge and change existing practices in research and analysis that continue to marginalise and erase diverse sexual practices, sexual orientations, and gender identities in HIV and AIDS research, prevention, and health promotion efforts.

Disclosure statement

No potential conflict of interest was reported by the authors.

Funding

APB is supported by a National Institute of Child Health and Human Development T32 grant [T32HD049339; PI: Nathanson]. CEO was supported by a National Institute of Allergy and Infectious Disease T32 NRSA grant [T32AI007535; PI: Seage] and by a National Institute on Drug Abuse T32 NRSA [T32DA013911; PI: Flanigan]. SLR and JLC are partly supported by a National Institute on Mental Health R34 grant [R34MH104072; MPI: Clark, Mimiaga, Reisner].

References

Aggleton, P., & Parker, R. (2015). Moving beyond biomedicalization in the HIV response: Implications for community involvement and community leadership among men who have sex with men and transgender people. *American Journal of Public Health, 105*(8), 1552–1558. doi:10.2105/AJPH.2015.302614

Asthana, S., & Oostvogels, R. (2001). The social construction of male 'homosexuality' in India: Implications for HIV transmission and prevention. *Social Science & Medicine*, 52(5), 707–721.

Baral, S., Beyrer, C., Muessig, K., Poteat, T., Wirtz, A. L., Decker, M. R., ... Kerrigan, D. (2012). Burden of HIV among female sex workers in low-income and middle-income countries: A systematic review and meta-analysis. *The Lancet Infectious Diseases*, 12(7), 538–549. doi:10.1016/S1473-3099(12)70066-X.

Baral, S. D., Poteat, T., Strömdahl, S., Wirtz, A. L., Guadamuz, T. E., & Beyrer, C. (2013). Worldwide burden of HIV in transgender women: A systematic review and meta-analysis. *The Lancet Infectious Diseases*, 13(3), 214–222. doi:10.1016/S1473-3099(12)70315-8.

Baral, S., Sifakis, F., Cleghorn, F., & Beyrer, C. (2007). Elevated risk for HIV infection among men who have sex with men in low- and middle-income countries 2000-2006: A systematic review. *PLoS Medicine*, 4(12), e339. doi:10.1371/journal.pmed.

Bauer, G. R. (2014). Incorporating intersectionality theory into population health research methodology: Challenges and the potential to advance health equity. *Social Science & Medicine*, 110, 10–17. doi:10.1016/j.socscimed.2014.03.022.

Begg, C. B. (1994). Operating characteristics of a rank correlation test for publication bias. *Biometrics*, 50(4), 1088–1101.

Beyrer, C., Baral, S. D., van Griensven, F., Goodreau, S. M., Chariyalertsak, S., Wirtz, A. L., & Brookmeyer, R. (2012). Global epidemiology of HIV infection in men who have sex with men. *The Lancet*, 380(9839), 367–377. doi:10.1016/S0140-6736(12)60821-6.

Boellstroff, T. (2011). But do not identify as gay: A proleptic genealogy of the MSM category. *Cultural Anthropology*, 26(2), 287–312. doi:10.1111/j.1548-1360.2011.01100.x.

Bowker, G. C., & Star, S. L. (1999). *Sorting things out: Classification and Its consequences*. Cambridge, MA: MIT Press.

Bowleg, L. (2012). The problem with the phrase women and minorities: Intersectionality – An important theoretical framework for public health. *American Journal of Public Health*, 102(7), 1267–1273. doi:10.2105/AJPH.2012.300750.

Chariyalertsak, S., Kosachunhanan, N., Saokhieo, P., Songsupa, R., Wongthanee, A., Chariyalertsak, C., ... Beyrer, C. (2011). HIV incidence, risk factors, and motivation for biomedical intervention among gay, bisexual men, and transgender persons in Northern Thailand. *PLoS One*, 6(9), e24295. doi:10.1371/journal.pone.0024295.t004.

Crenshaw, K. (1991). Mapping the margins: Intersectionality, identity politics, and violence against women of color. *Stanford Law Review*, 43(6), 1241–1299. doi:10.2307/1229039.

DerSimonian, R., & Laird, N. (1986). Meta-analysis in clinical trials. *Controlled Clinical Trials*, 7, 177–188.

Egger, M., Smith, G. D., Schneider, M., & Minder, C. (1997). Bias in meta-analysis detected by a simple, graphical test. *British Medical Journal*, 315, 629–634.

Epstein, S. (2009). *Inclusion: The politics of difference in medical research*. Chicago: University of Chicago Press.

Greenland, S., Gago-Dominguez, M., & Castelao, J. E. (2004). The value of risk-factor ('Black-Box') epidemiology. *Epidemiology (Cambridge, Mass.)*, 15(5), 529–535. doi:10.1097/01.ede.0000134867.12896.23.

van Griensven, F., Thienkrua, W., McNicholl, J., Wimonsate, W., Chaikummao, S., Chonwattana, W., ... Tappero J. W. (2013). Evidence of an explosive epidemic of HIV infection in a cohort of men who have sex with men in Thailand. *AIDS (London, England)*, 27(5), 825–832. doi:10.1097/QAD.0b013e32835c546e.

Gutiérrez, M., Tajada, P., Alvarez, A., De Julián, R., Baquero, M., Soriano, V., & Holguín, A. (2004). Prevalence of HIV-1 non-B subtypes, syphilis, HTLV, and hepatitis B and C viruses among immigrant sex workers in Madrid, Spain. *Journal of Medical Virology*, 74(4), 521–527. doi:10.1002/jmv.20208.

Haidich, A. B. (2010). Meta-analysis in medical research. *Hippokratia*, 14(Suppl. 1), 29–37.

Hanssmann, C. (2010). Counting us in: Problems and opportunities in health research on transgender and gender nonconforming communities. *Seattle Journal for Social Justice*, 8(2), 541–777.

ILGA. (2013). *Annual review of the human rights situations of lesbian, gay, bisexual, trans and intersex people in Europe-2013* (pp. 1–242). International Lesbian, Gay, Bisexual, Trans & Intersex Association – Europe Region.

Infante, C., Sosa-Rubi, S., & Cuadra, S. M. (2009). Sex work in Mexico: Vulnerability of male, travesti, transgender and transsexual sex workers. *Culture, Health & Sexuality, 11*(2), 125–137. doi:10.1080/13691050802431314.

Institute of Medicine. (2011). *The health of lesbian, gay, bisexual, and transgender people: Building a foundation for better understanding.* Washington, DC: The National Academic Press.

Jackson, P. A., & Cook, N. M. (1999). *Genders and sexualities in modern Thailand.* Chiang Mai: Silkworm Books.

Jordan-Young, R. M. (2011). *Brainstorm: The flaws in the science of sex differences.* Cambridge, MA: Harvard University Press.

Kulick, D. (1998). *Travesti: Sex, gender, and culture among Brazilian transgendered prostitutes.* Chicago, IL: University of Chicago Press.

Labuski, C., & Keo-Meier, C. (2015). The (mis)measure of trans. *TSQ: Transgender Studies Quarterly, 2*(1), 13–33. doi:10.1215/23289252-2848868.

Lorway, R., & Khan, S. (2014). Reassembling epidemiology: Mapping, monitoring and making-up people in the context of HIV prevention in India. *Social Science & Medicine, 112*, 51–62. doi:10.1016/j.socscimed.2014.04.034.

Meyerowitz, J. J. (2009). *How sex changed: A history of transsexuality in the United States.* Cambridge, MA: Harvard University Press.

Muñoz-Laboy, M. A. (2004). Beyond 'MSM': Sexual desire among bisexually-active Latino men in New York city. *Sexualities, 7*(1), 55–80. doi:10.1177/1363460704040142.

Nemoto, T., Iwamoto, M., Perngparn, U., Areesantichai, C., Kamitani, E., & Sakata, M. (2012). HIV-related risk behaviors among kathoey (male-to-female transgender) sex workers in Bangkok, Thailand. *AIDS Care, 24*(2), 210–219. doi:10.1080/09540121.2011.597709.

Nuttbrock, L., Bockting, W., Rosenblum, A., Mason, M., Macri, M., & Becker, J. (2012). Gender identity conflict/affirmation and major depression across the life course of transgender women. *International Journal of Transgenderism, 13*(3), 91–103. doi:10.1080/15532739.2011.657979.

Oldenburg, C. E., Perez-Brumer, A. G., Reisner, S. L., Mattie, J., Bärnighausen, T., Mayer, K. H., & Mimiaga, M. J. (2014). Global burden of HIV among men who engage in transactional sex: A systematic review and meta-analysis. *PloS One, 9*(7), e103549. doi:10.1371/journal.pone.0103549.

Oldenburg, C. E., Perez-Brumer, A. G., Reisner, S. L., Mayer, K. H., Mimiaga, M. J., Hatzenbuehler, M. L., & Bärnighausen, T. (2016). Human rights protections and HIV prevalence among MSM who sell sex: Cross-country comparisons from a systematic review and meta-analysis. *Global Public Health,* 1–12.

Operario, D., Soma, T., & Underhill, K. (2008). Sex work and HIV status among transgender women. *JAIDS Journal of Acquired Immune Deficiency Syndromes, 48*(1), 97–103. doi:10.1097/QAI.0b013e31816e3971.

Parker, R. G. (1999). *Beneath the equator: Cultures of desire, male homosexuality, and emerging gay communities in Brazil.* New York: Routledge.

Reisner, S. L., Biello, K., Rosenberger, J. G., Austin, S. B., Haneuse, S., Perez-Brumer, A., ... Mimiaga M. J. (2014). Using a two-step method to measure transgender identity in Latin America/the Caribbean, Portugal, and Spain. *Archives of Sexual Behavior, 43*(8), 1503–1514. doi:10.1007/s10508-014-0314-2.

Reisner, S. L., Mimiaga, M. J., Bland, S., Mayer, K. H., Perkovich, B., & Safren, S. A. (2009). HIV risk and social networks among male-to-female transgender sex workers in Boston, Massachusetts. *Journal of the Association of Nurses in AIDS Care, 20*(5), 373–386.

Reza-Paul, S., Beattie, T., Pasha, A., Venugopal, M. S., Ramesh, B. M., Jinendra, M., Moses, S. (2008). High HIV prevalence among male sex workers in Mysore, India-need for integrating care and support with prevention. *AIDS 2008-VXII International AIDS Conference: Abstract No.THPE0304.*

Sevelius, J. M. (2013). Gender affirmation: A framework for conceptualizing risk behavior among transgender women of color. *Sex Roles*, *68*(11–12), 675–689. doi:10.1007/s11199-012-0216-5.

Shannon, K., Strathdee, S. A., Goldenberg, S. M., Duff, P., Mwangi, P., Rusakova, M., … Boily M.-C. (2015). Global epidemiology of HIV among female sex workers: Influence of structural determinants. *The Lancet*, *385*(9962), 55–71. doi:10.1016/S0140-6736(14)60931-4.

Silva, M. L. E. (2014). Queer sex vignettes from a Brazilian favela: An ethnographic striptease. *Ethnography*. doi:10.1177/1466138114534335

Silva-Santisteban, A., Raymond, H. F., Salazar, X., Villayzan, J., Leon, S., McFarland, W., & Caceres, C. F. (2012). Understanding the HIV/AIDS epidemic in transgender women of Lima, Peru: Results from a sero-epidemiologic study using respondent driven sampling. *AIDS and Behavior*, *16*(4), 872–881. doi:10.1007/s10461-011-0053-5

Singer, T. B. (2015). The profusion of things: The 'transgender matrix' and demographic imaginaries in US public health. *TSQ: Transgender Studies Quarterly*, *2*(1), 58–76. doi:10.1215/23289252-2848886.

Soley-Beltran, P., & Coll-Planas, G. (2011). 'Having words for everything'. Institutionalizing gender migration in Spain (1998-2008). *Sexualities*, *14*(3), 334–353. doi:10.1177/1363460711400811.

Stryker, S. (2009). *Transgender history*. Berkeley, CA: Seal Press.

Thompson, H., & King, L. (2015). Who counts as 'transgender?' Epidemiological methods and a critical intervention. *TSQ: Transgender Studies Quarterly*, *2*(1), 148–159. doi:10.1215/23289252-2848913.

Tun, W., de Mello, M., Pinho, A., Chinaglia, M., & Diaz, J. (2008). Sexual risk behaviours and HIV seroprevalence among male sex workers who have sex with men and non-sex workers in Campinas, Brazil. *Sexually Transmitted Infections*, *84*(6), 455–457. doi:10.1136/sti.2008.031336.

Valentine, D. (2007). *Imagining transgender: An ethnography of a category*. Durham: Duke University Press.

World Health Organization. (2014). *Values and preferences of key populations: Consolidated report*. Retrieved from http://apps.who.int/iris/bitstream/10665/128258/1/WHO_HIV_2014.11_eng.pdf

Young, R. M., & Meyer, I. H. (2005). The trouble with 'MSM' and 'WSW': Erasure of the sexual-minority person in public health discourse. *American Journal of Public Health*, *95*(7), 1144–1149. doi:10.2105/AJPH.2004.046714.

A global research synthesis of HIV and STI biobehavioural risks in female-to-male transgender adults

Sari L. Reisner and Gabriel R. Murchison

ABSTRACT
There is a growing interest in HIV infection and sexually transmitted infection (STI) disease burden and risk among transgender people globally; however, the majority of work has been conducted with male-to-female transgender populations. This research synthesis comprehensively reviews HIV and STI research in female-to-male (FTM) transgender adults. A paucity of research exists about HIV and STIs in FTMs. Only 25 peer-reviewed papers (18 quantitative, 7 qualitative) and 11 'grey literature' reports were identified, most in the US or Canada, that include data identifying HIV and STI risks in FTMs (five with fully laboratory-confirmed HIV and/or STIs, and five with partial laboratory confirmation). Little is known about the sexual and drug use risk behaviours contributing to HIV and STIs in FTMs. Future directions are suggested, including the need for routine surveillance and monitoring of HIV and STIs globally by transgender identity, more standardised sexual risk assessment measures, targeted data collection in lower- and middle-income countries, and explicit consideration of the rationale for inclusion/exclusion of FTMs in category-based prevention approaches with MSM and transgender people. Implications for research, policy, programming, and interventions are discussed, including the need to address diverse sexual identities, attractions, and behaviours and engage local FTM communities.

Overview

There is a growing interest in HIV infection and sexually transmitted infection (STI) disease burden and risk among transgender people globally, but the majority of work has considered only male-to-female (MTF) transgender people (Baral et al., 2013; Herbst et al., 2008). This research synthesis focuses on HIV and STIs among female-to-male (FTM) transgender people. We begin with a review of transgender terminology, briefly consider the diagnostic history of transgenderism and its consequences for sexual health research, and comprehensively and critically review the research literature on HIV and STIs in FTMs globally. We then highlight gaps, opportunities, and future directions. FTMs' diverse sexual attractions, behaviours, and identities are underscored as key to understanding their HIV and STI risk, underscoring the need for gender-affirmative risk assessments that attend to the specific bioanatomies of physical bodies. Findings from this review can be used to inform future research, policy, programming, and interventions in FTM sexual health.

Transgender identity and sexuality

The term 'transgender' describes people who do not identify with the sex category assigned to them at birth, or whose gender identity or behaviour falls outside of gender norms (Currah & Minter, 2000). *Trans masculine* describes people assigned a female sex at birth who identify on the masculine continuum – as male, men, FTM, transgender men, trans men, men of transgender experience, or affirmed men; or genderqueer (neither male nor female), bi-gender or pangender (both male and female), androgynous, butch, boi, aggressive, and other diverse gender identities and expressions not typically expected of female-assigned sex people. Trans masculine communities are heterogeneous, and not all trans masculine people are stereotypically 'masculine' in their interests or gender presentation. In order to be concise, this review uses 'FTM' as shorthand for transgender men and other trans masculine people, but it is important to note that not all members of the aforementioned groups identify with the 'FTM' label.

'Gender dysphoria' refers to discomfort with the gender that one was assigned at birth (Bockting, 2015). Transgender people use a range of strategies to lessen feelings of gender dysphoria and affirm their gender identities. Gender affirmation can be thought of as having three primary dimensions: (1) social elements, such as adopting a name and pronouns that align with one's gender identity; (2) medical elements, such as masculinising hormones and/or surgeries; and (3) legal elements, such as changing one's legal name or gender designation. The process of making gender-affirming changes is known as 'gender transition', or simply 'transition'. A gender affirmation process may include any combination of social, medical, and/or legal changes, depending on individual desires, regional law and policy, financial means, life circumstances, and local norms.

It is now clear that transgender people have diverse sexual orientations, identities, and behaviours, and can be sexually attracted to people of any gender (Grant et al., 2011; Kuper, Nussbaum, & Mustanski, 2012). Until recently, however, the study of sexual behaviour (and therefore sexual risk) in FTMs has been limited by a narrow schema of transgenderism within psychiatry and other disciplines. In the popular and professional conception of transgenderism that developed in North America and Western Europe beginning in the mid-twentieth century, 'true transsexuals' (who would now be called 'transgender') invariably wished to embody the conventional physiology, appearance, and behaviours of the 'opposite sex'. Those not expected to be gender-conforming in their new sex were denied medical treatment (Meyerowitz, 2004). As a result of these restrictions, transgender communities learned to present themselves to physicians and psychologists as preparing to become traditionally masculine men or traditionally feminine women. Sexual orientation was a crucial part of this gender performance, since people taking on a male gender were expected to be exclusively attracted to females. As a result, many patients concealed non-heterosexual attractions from the professionals treating them, reinforcing the perception that nearly all 'transsexuals' were straight

(Meyerowitz, 2004). As late as 2013, the American Psychiatric Association (APA) held that 'virtually all [FTMs] will receive the same specifier – Sexually Attracted to Females – although there are exceptional cases involving [FTMs] who are Sexually Attracted to Males' (American Psychiatric Association, 2000).

The APA's stance was reflective of, and influential towards, research in transgender sexual health. As a result of the presumption that FTMs were sexually active almost exclusively with non-transgender women, many researchers have assumed that they are at low risk for HIV and STIs (Kenagy & Hsieh, 2005). More recently, sexual health and sexuality research has documented diverse sexualities and sexual practices among FTMs. Indeed, recent data suggest that FTMs in North America are much less likely to be heterosexual (i.e. attracted primarily to women) than non-transgender men (Grant et al., 2011). Furthermore, even straight-identified FTMs' sexual practices may put them at risk for HIV and STIs. For instance, they may partner with transgender women, and engage in similar HIV risk behaviours as non-transgender heterosexual couples. They may, like some non-transgender men, identify as straight but nonetheless engage in sex with other men. And certain sexual practices with non-transgender women also carry risks, including HPV exposure – particularly concerning among FTMs, given reduced rates of cervical cancer screening in this group (Peitzmeier, Khullar, Reisner, & Potter, 2014). It is therefore essential that assessment of sexual behaviour in FTMs be attentive to the myriad of gender identities in FTMs themselves as well as the heterogeneity of their sexual partners, while also attending to the specificity of physical bodies engaged in sexual behaviours. There is a diverse range of bioanatomies potentially represented among FTMs and their partners during sexual encounters (e.g. surgically unaltered bodies, bodies that have been altered to various degrees depending on individual desires and access to medical technologies). Addressing this diversity is important for determining prevention and care needs, as well as HIV and STI sexual risk. This review captures the current empirical knowledge on how sexual identity and behaviour among FTMs produce unique HIV and STI biobehavioural risk patterns in this population.

Literature review of HIV and STI risk in FTMs

Review methodology

Peer-reviewed articles published before 1 August 2014 were collected from PubMed, Embase, Ovid, PsycINFO, CINAHL PLUS, Web of Science, Sociological Abstracts, and Medadvocates. The review included peer-reviewed articles and grey literature reports that presented FTM-specific data on sexual risk behaviour, HIV status, or STI infection. It included both qualitative and quantitative studies.

Articles and citations were downloaded from the databases and organised using citation management software (QUOSA, EndNote X5, and Zotero). In order to ensure that this review was as broad as possible, search terms included MeSH terms for 'transgender' cross-referenced with terms for 'health' and 'HIV'. We also included a range of terms similar to transgender, such as 'FTM', 'trans man', and 'transman'. Searches for peer-reviewed papers were limited to material published in English. Additional data sources, including the International AIDS Society, the World Professional Association for

Transgender Health, and the National Library of Medicine's Meeting Abstracts, were searched for 'grey literature' material.

Results of review

We identified 25 peer-reviewed papers (18 of which included quantitative data and 7 qualitative data). Two of the qualitative studies lack a direct focus on sexual health, but include content relevant to sexual risk behaviour. Eleven 'grey literature' sources were identified (7 posters and abstracts, 3 needs assessments, and 1 additional dataset). Overall, 81% of the included literature is quantitative or mixed-methods, and 19% is qualitative.

Table 1 outlines the existing quantitative research. Ten studies had laboratory-confirmed HIV serostatus, documenting 0% (in six studies), 2.2%, 3%, and 4.3% (1 of 23) HIV seropositivity among FTMs.[1] Most studies found self-reported HIV prevalence between 0% and 10%, and self-reported unknown HIV serostatus from 5% to 57%. In comparison, the adult (ages 13+ years) HIV prevalence for the US, where the majority of the studies were conducted, is approximately 0.7% in males and 0.2% in females (Centers for Disease Control and Prevention, 2012). However, HIV prevalence is estimated to be over 15% among US MSM (Beyrer et al., 2012), and even higher (16–68%) among MTF transgender women (Baral et al., 2013; Herbst et al., 2008).

One study had laboratory-confirmed STI screening data for FTMs, revealing a 5% prevalence of Chlamydia. Lifetime self-reported STI history across samples was between 6% and 47%. Across studies, 7–69% of FTMs engaged in fluid-exchange genital-genital sexual risk behaviours; this excludes Kenagy (2002) where 91% engaged in 'high risk' sexual behaviour because the author included unprotected oral sex with female partners. Several studies documented behaviours that may contribute to HIV risk, including sex work, unprotected anal or vaginal sex with male casual partners, low utilisation of STI screening and other sexual health preventive services, and high prevalence of psychological distress and substance use.

Insight into motivations for sexual risk behaviour was provided by seven qualitative studies. Table 2 summarises the results of the seven qualitative studies, all peer-reviewed, that addressed sexual risk behaviour among FTMs. These studies offer valuable insight into the psychosocial and sociocultural context of FTMs' sexual risk behaviours. The most detailed accounts have focused on 'TMSM', that is, FTMs who have sex with men.[2] According to this literature, many post-transition TMSM describe gay identities or sex with men as a source of validation for their male identities (Bockting, Benner, & Coleman, 2009; Hein & Kirk, 1999; Williams, Weinberg, & Rosenberger, 2013). However, acceptance from male partners is at times uncertain or tenuous, and FTMs sometimes make riskier sexual choices, like agreeing to sex without a barrier, in order to avoid rejection (Clements, Kitano, Wilkinson, & Marx, 1999; Reisner, Perkovich, & Mimiaga, 2010; Rowniak & Chesla, 2013). Some non-transgender men may even attempt to sexually manipulate or coerce FTMs by questioning their gender (Reisner et al., 2010; Rowniak & Chesla, 2013).

The qualitative literature reveals that some TMSM engage in risk behaviours as they explore a new sexual identity, or integrate into a new community or sexual subculture, during or after gender transition. Some FTMs describe a phase of post-transition sexual experimentation, which may involve incidental or intentional risk-taking behaviour (Clements et al., 1999). FTMs who join gay men's communities may be particularly

Table 1. Summary of FTM sexual behaviours and sexual risk indicators across studies.

Study (year)	Location, sampling, design	Number of participants	Socio-demographics	Sexual behaviours	Sexual risk behaviours	HIV/STI
Reisner, White, Mayer, and Mimiaga (2014)	Boston, MA; urban community health centre (July 2007–Dec 2007); retrospective chart review	23 FTM	• Mean age 31.6 • 52.2% white, 13.0% black, 21.7% Asian/Pacific Islander/Native Hawaiian • 26.1% ≤ high school diploma • 34.8% private insurance • 56.5% bisexual, 8.7% gay, 4.3% straight, 30.4% unknown • 21.7% lifetime suicide attempt • 47.8% on hormones	Past three months sexual partners: 30.4% females, 30.4% males, 34.8% both	26.1% sexual risk behaviour in past three months ('i.e. sex with a male without a condom, condom breakage, and anonymous sex partners')	4.3% HIV positive (one case)
Horvath, Iantaffi, Swinburne-Romine, and Bockting (2014)	US national; convenience sample; cross-sectional survey	523 FTM (43% of total sample of N = 1229)	• Mean age 26.2 • 77% white, 1% Hispanic/Latino • 13% ≤ high school diploma • 42% income < 2x the 2003 HHS poverty guidelines • 25% rural • 35% lifetime suicide attempt	8% married or civil union	Past three months unprotected penis-anus or penis-vagina sex: 11% with primary partner, 6% with other partner, 16% with any partner	• 0.4% HIV positive (one case; self-report) • No information on STIs

Bauer, Redman, Bradley, and Scheim (2013)	Canada; respondent-driven sampling; cross-sectional survey	173 gay, bisexual, or MSM FTM (a subset of the 227 FTM in Bauer et al., 2012)	• 16.9% history of gender-related physical or sexual assault • 36.1% history of gender-related harassment or threats	• 45% in monogamous relationship, 18% in open or polyamorous relationship, 12.3% single and dating, 24.6% single and not dating • Past year sex partners: 17.9% 0, 45.4% 1, 22.7% 2–4, 14.1% 5+ • Past year: 65.4% received oral sex, 67.2% gave oral sex, 34.2% receptive anal, 29.0% insertive anal, 67.1% receptive genital, 56.6% insertive genital	• Past year fluid-exposed sex: 0.1% receptive anal, 0.0% insertive anal, 9.5% receptive genital, 0.8% insertive genital • 17.5% no past-year HIV risk sexual behaviour, 73.3% low/moderate risk, 9.2% high risk • 15.8% lifetime sex work/exchange sex	• 21.0% past-year HIV testing, 36.3% over one year ago, 42.7% never
Olson, Clark, Schrager, Simons, and Belzer (2013)	Los Angeles; urban teaching hospital pediatric transgender programme; baseline data from prospective study (survey and chart review)	35 FTM (50% of total sample of N = 70)	• Total sample 51.5% white, 28.8% Latino/a, 10.6% African American. No data on FTM group alone. • Age range 12–24 • All prior to hormone therapy initiation	No data	6% history of transactional sex	No data
Patrascioiu et al. (2013)	Catalonia; chart review	92 FTM (39% of total sample of N = 234)	No data	No data	No data	HIV prevalence 2.2%
Rodolico, Helien, Nagelberg, Rey, and Levalle (2012)	Argentina; clinic-based cross-sectional survey	18 FTM (25% of total sample of N = 71)	No data	• 34% practice genital sex • 34% practice oral sex • Anal sex not recorded • 34% sexual activity in past month • 50% relationship satisfaction	23% 'use condoms'	No HIV or STI data

(Continued)

Table 1. Continued.

Study (year)	Location, sampling, design	Number of participants	Socio-demographics	Sexual behaviours	Sexual risk behaviours	HIV/STI
Bauer et al. (2012)	Canada; respondent-driven sampling; cross-sectional survey	227 FTM spectrum (52.4% of total sample of N = 433)	• 70% non-aboriginal white, 25% non-aboriginal racialised, 6% aboriginal • 35% < high school diploma • 52% earn < $15,000 annually • 25% completed medical transition	• 12% 5+ sex partners in past year • Sex partners include: 10% trans men, 21% non-trans men, 7% trans women, 44% non-trans women, 14% genderqueer • 28% receptive partner in anal sex • 57% receptive partner in genital sex • 15% ever sex work	• 7% high risk = receptive genital sex with flesh genitals (no prostheses or toys) and fluid exposure [0% high risk receptive anal, 0% high risk insertive anal] • 69% low/moderate risk • 25% no risk (no past-year sex partners) • 42% sex while drunk or high in past year	• 0.6% HIV positive • 23% HIV serostatus unknown
Butt, Mena, and Muzny (2011)	US; literature review of HIV risk behaviours and prevalence	Not applicable	Not applicable	No data	No data	HIV prevalence rates between 0% and 2% among FTMs, except for 10% positive finding in Stephens, Bernstein, and Philip (2011)
Pell, Prone, and Vlahakis (2011)	Sydney, Australia; private urban clinic with sexual health focus; retrospective chart review	17 FTM (10.8% of total sample N = 158)	• Mean age 34.4; range 21.5–56.9 • 82.3% Australian-born • 91.7% employed • 13.3% history of IVDU • 93% on hormone therapy • 23.6% surgery	No data	0% history of sex work	0% HIV positive
Grant et al. (2011)	US national; electronic survey and site-specific paper-and-pen surveys; convenience sample	1776 FTM (28% of total sample N = 6346)	• 46% queer, 25% heterosexual, 13% gay/same-gender loving, 13% bisexual, 2% other, 2% asexual • 42% underemployed • 19% uninsured	7% history of sex work	No data on sexual risk behaviours	0.48% HIV incidence (not analysed by sexual orientation)

Stephens et al. (2011)	San Francisco, CA; San Francisco City STI Clinic (Jan 2006–Dec 2009); retrospective chart review	69 FTM patient visits (not unique cases: 16 patients had at least 4 visits)	• Mean age 31.5, median 28 • 77% White • No data on SES or health insurance	• 49% unprotected sex in past 3 months • Median number of 4.5 (SD = 3) non-trans male partners in past 3 months • 23% transactional sex ever	• 10% HIV positive • 4% HIV unknown • Diagnosis at visit: 3.7% rectal GC, 4.9% pharyngeal GC, 11.1% rectal CL, 4.2% pharyngeal CL, 2.4% urogenital CL, 2.4% syphilis morbidity, 4.2% syphilis titer, 2.9% HIV
Chen, McFarland, Thompson, and Raymond (2011)	San Francisco, CA; STI clinic sample; cross-sectional HIV testing data (HIV test sites funded by the SF DPH)	59 FTM	• Median age 27 (18–54) • 73% White non-Hispanic • 45% no health insurance • No data on SES	• Sex partners by gender in past 12 months: 61% male, 63% female, 47% transgender • Sexual behaviours with male sex partners in past 12 months: 51% receptive vaginal sex, 19% insertive anal, 39% receptive anal	• 63% unprotected receptive sex (vaginal or anal) in past 12 months • 10% any unprotected sex (vaginal or anal) with known HIV-positive person in past 12 mo • 32% unprotected anal sex since last HIV test
Rowniak, Chesla, Rose, and Holzemer (2011)	San Francisco, CA; convenience sample; semi-structured qualitative interviews	17 FTM (eligibility: age 21+, identify as FTM, on Testosterone hormone therapy for > 1 year, understand English)	• Median age 36 (range 23–64) • 10 participants white • No data on SES or health insurance • 0% had bottom surgery	• 82% (n = 14) reported having gay men as sexual partners and self-identified as gay, bisexual, or queer • 5 engaged in sex work	• 0% HIV-positive (lab-confirmed) • STI history past 12 months: 2% Gonorrhea, 5% Chlamydia, 2% syphilis
Johnson, Radix, Santos Ramos, Mayer, and Mukerjee (2010)	New York, NY; urban community health centre	77% FTM clients	No data	• Only 3 participants reported 'always using condoms' for intercourse (type of sex not specified) • 2 in serodiscordant relationship with non-trans male • 40% high risk activity, such as unprotected anal or vaginal intercourse, with men	• 1 participant HIV positive (self-reported) • No information on STIs
Reisner et al. (2010)	New England; convenience sample; cross-sectional, mixed-methods design	16 FTM who reported sex with non-trans men	• Mean age 33 • 88% white • 38% earned < $11,999 per year • 31% ≤ high school diploma • 25% no health insurance	• Gender of sexual partners past 12 mo: 100% non-trans males, 69% non-trans females, 56% FTM/trans men, 13% MTF/trans women • 44% sex work ever • 19% Sex work past 12 months	• No HIV cases among the 40% of clients tested • No information on STIs • 0% HIV seropositive (self-report) • 38% STI history (lifetime)
				• 44% unprotected vaginal sex with non-trans male • 25% unprotected vaginal or anal sex with non-trans female • 19% unprotected vaginal or anal sex with transgender • Unprotected vaginal sex with mean of 4.0 (SD 9.0) non-trans male sex partners	

(Continued)

Table 1. Continued.

Study (year)	Location, sampling, design	Number of participants	Socio-demographics	Sexual behaviours	Sexual risk behaviours	HIV/STI
Sevelius (2009)	U.S. national sample; convenience sample; cross-sectional	45 FTM	• Age 18–60 • 82% white • 10% ≤ high school diploma • 24% no health insurance	• Median # non-trans male partners in past year = 3 • 84% oral sex • 69% receptive vaginal sex • 60% anal sex	• 91% any unprotected oral sex past year with non-trans male • 69% any unprotected receptive vaginal sex in past year with non-trans male • 60% any unprotected anal sex in past year with non-trans male	• 2.2% HIV • 47% lifetime STI diagnosis
Adams et al. (2008)	Online survey and qualitative interviews with bisexual-, gay-, or queer-identified trans men in Ontario	15 FTM for quantitative online survey; 6 FTM for qualitative interviews	• 33% income under $20,000 • 93% white • 93% queer, 47% bisexual, 40% gay (multiple responses possible) • 53% university degree	• 73% receptive anal sex with non-trans men; • 60% receptive frontal sex with non-trans men • 87% perform oral sex with non-trans men • ≥53% fisting • ≥60% rimming • ≥73% sex with trans men • ≥53% BDSM	• 47% always use condom for frontal sex with non-trans men; 40% most of the time; 7% rarely use • 80% always use condom for anal sex with non-trans men; 13% most of the time • 60% use condom 'sometimes' or less for oral sex on non-trans men	0% HIV positive
Schulden et al. (2008)	CBOs in Miami Beach FL, New York City, and San Francisco, CA; convenience sample; cross-sectional survey and HIV testing	42 FTM (7% of the total sample of N = 601)	81% racial/ethnic minority (52% non-Hispanic Black, 17% Hispanic)	24% sex work past year	• 36% unprotected receptive vaginal sex in past year • 29% unprotected receptive anal sex in past year	0% HIV positive (lab-confirmed)
Herbst et al. (2008)	Meta-analysis 29 studies (1990–2004); 15 studies included MTF and FTM transgender people	5 studies	No data	• 31% sex work • 34% 2+ partners in past 6 months	• High risk sex behaviour in prior 3 months (91%–93%) but behaviour not specified • 7% UVS, 4% UAS • 22% Genital-genital contact	• 0%–3% HIV prevalence (5 studies) • No studies of HIV incidence • 6–7% STI prevalence (lifetime) (2 studies)
Lobato et al. (2007)	Porto Alegre, Brazil; teaching hospital transgender programme; clinic-based descriptive cross-sectional survey	16 FTM (11.6% of total sample N = 138)	• 87.5% less than high school • 18.7% history of sexual abuse • 43.8% psychoactive substance use • 6.3% history of suicide attempt	Mean age at first intercourse 16.18 years	0% history of sex work	0% prevalence of HIV syphilis, gonorrhea, and chlamydia

Study	Setting/Sampling	Sample	Demographics	Sexual Behavior	HIV/STI Status
Myers, Remis, and Husbands (2007)	Ontario; venue-based cross-sectional survey of MSM (primarily non-trans)	22 FTM (0.9% of total sample N = 2438)	• Mean age 31.8 • 18% high school or less • 59% income less than $40,000 • 85% white • 20% lifetime IV drug use	No data	• 33% (4 of 12 with data) unprotected receptive anal sex with casual partner or regular partner of unknown/positive status in previous six months	• 0% of 17 previously tested self-reported positive • 0% positive of 14 tested in study
Xavier, Hannold, Bradford, and Simmons (2007)	Virginia; convenience sample; cross-section survey	121 FTM (35% of total sample N = 350)	Median age 28 (18–64)	• 94 sexually active FTMs in past 6 mo • 18% non-trans men • 82% non-trans women • 11% trans men • 3% trans women	• 71 FTMs with primary partners: 51% unprotected sex • 15 FTMs with other partners: 47% unprotected sex	• 0% HIV positive (self-report) • 5% HIV unknown • 25% never tested for HIV
Kenagy (2005)	Greater Philadelphia area; convenience sample using snowball sampling; 2 surveys	69 FTM (37.9% of original sample of N = 182)	• Mean age 29.4 • 27% white (42% Black, 10% multiracial, 8% biracial, 10% Hispanic, 3% other) • 54% ≤ high school diploma • No data on health insurance	No data	• 59% unprotected sexual activity (mostly oral sex) in past 12 mo • Racial differences in unprotected sexual activity: 74% FTM of color vs 22% of white FTMs (p < .001) • 7% unprotected vaginal-penile intercourse with no condom • 6% unprotected anal-penile intercourse • 28% sex while drunk or high • 9% sex with HIV-positive partner	• 0% HIV positive • 8% HIV status unknown • No information on STIs
Kenagy and Hsieh (2005)	Philadelphia, PA and Chicago, IL; 2 needs assessments	62 FTM (34% of the original sample of N = 192)	• Mean age 26.8 • 35% White, 33% Black, 32% other • 54% high school or less	No data	• 71% no protection used during last time having sex • 81% high risk sexual activities in past 3 months: ["High risk" = vagina-penis, anal-penis, oral-penis, oral-vagina, oral-anal sex, or sex with someone known to be HIV positive without using a condom or a latex barrier]	No data

(Continued)

Table 1. Continued.

Study (year)	Location, sampling, design	Number of participants	Socio-demographics	Sexual behaviours	Sexual risk behaviours	HIV/STI
Sperber, Landers, and Lawrence (2005)	Boston, MA; RDS, convenience sample; focus groups	17 FTM (50% of the original sample of $N = 34$)	• Mean age 27.9 • 88% white, 6% Latino, 6% other • 41% bisexual, 29% straight, 18% gay, 6% queer, 6% none • 6% uninsured	No data	No data	No data
Bockting, Robinson, Forberg, and Scheltema (2005)	Minnesota; pilot evaluation of transgender sexual health intervention	34 FTM (19% of total sample $N = 181$)	No data	• 61% had primary partner (67% non-trans female, 10% non-trans male, 24% transgender) • 68% attracted to women only, 15% attracted to men only, 18% attracted to both, 29% attracted to trans persons	• 9% report difficulty controlling sexual behaviour • 56% unprotected oral sex • No significant difference from MTF group on rates of unprotected anal or vaginal intercourse (27% in total sample)	Not reported separately for FTM group
Xavier, Bobbin, Singer, and Budd (2005)	Washington, D.C.; cross-sectional convenience/snowball sample	60 FTM and female-assigned gender-variant people (24% of total sample of $N = 248$)	• Median age 26 • 12% identified as man; 38% woman; 45% transgender • 75% African American; 12% white • 43% of adults high school or less • 23% unemployed • 26% income under $15,000 • 12% using hormones	27% gay; 45% lesbian; 11% bisexual	• 53% unprotected oral sex in past year • 50% unprotected genital sex in past year • 20% sex while inebriated in past year • 10% unprotected anal sex in past year • 0% unprotected sex with known HIV+ person in past year	3% HIV positive
Gross and Davis (2004)	Los Angeles, CA; cross-sectional survey	30 FTM (46% of total sample of $N = 65$)	No data	No data	• 'High rates' of sex while intoxicated • Lower rates of condom use than MTF group	No data

Kenagy (2002)	Philadelphia, PA; convenience sample; mixed-methods	32 FTM (39.5% of the original sample of N = 81)	• Mean age 26.4 • 60% Black, 13% multiracial, 13% biracial, 13% other (Hispanic and white) • Highest grade attended: Mean 12.1 grade	No data	91% engaged in 'high risk' sexual activity (defined as vagina-penis, anal-penis, oral-penis, oral-vagina, oral-anal, or vagina-vagina sex without a condom or dental dam)	• 0% HIV positive (self-report) • 57% never had HIV test • 6% STI history • 66% never tested for STDs
Clements-Nolle, Marx, Guzman, and Katz (2001)	San Francisco, CA; RDS, targeted/purposive sampling; cross-sectional survey and HIV testing	123 FTM (23.9% of total sample N = 515)	• Median age 36 (range 19–61) • 67% White, 10% Black, 11% Latino, 7% API, 4% Native American • 4% less than high school diploma • 41% no health insurance	31% sex work ever	• Unprotected receptive anal sex: 27% with male, 6% with transgender • Unprotected vaginal sex: 63% with male, 25% with transgender	• 2% HIV positive (lab-confirmed) • No data on STIs

Table 2. Summary of qualitative study content

Williams et al. (2013)	Interviews with 25 FTMs in San Francisco. Discusses gay trans men, sexual identity as 'bottom' (receptive partner), and sex with men as an affirmation of masculinity, which other studies have linked to sexual risk behaviour Reisner, White et al. (2014); Rowniak and Chesla (2013). Considers role of anatomy, and hormonal and surgical interventions, in sexual behaviour
Rowniak and Chesla (2013)	Interviews with 17 FTMs in San Francisco. 10 participants identified as gay, and none as heterosexual. One participant became HIV positive shortly after gender transition. Another recalled undertaking risky behaviour in an effort to fit in with other gay men, many of whom had HIV. Others described trans men who have acquired HIV at male sex venues, and explained that some non-trans men 'take advantage' of FTM partners for barrier-free sex
Kosenko (2011)	Semi-structured interviews with transgender adults in the US, including 15 FTMs, mostly 'mid-transition'. Participants described a lack of safer-sex education targeting lesbian communities, in which they had participated before transition. They also described a lack of confidence navigating sexual situations as gay males, absence of FTM-specific sexual health information, and the effect of hormone therapy on sex drive
Bockting et al. (2009)	Interviews and psychological assessments with 25 FTMs attracted to men (60% self-described gay, 32% bisexual, and 8% queer) in the US and Canada. FTM participants were more likely to be bisexual than non-transgender controls, were comfortable with their sexual orientation and gender identity, and were similar to controls in sexual satisfaction and self-esteem
Namaste (1999)	Interviews with 5 FTMs in Quebec, and a discussion group at an FTM conference in Boston. FTMs reported not considering themselves at risk for HIV, and participants cited 'low self-esteem' as contributing to sexual risk behaviour
Hein and Kirk (1999)	Description of an HIV risk reduction group intervention for Boston-area TMSM. The intervention focused on mutual support and strategising for the challenges the participants encountered in sexual interactions with non-trans men. Participants reported strong motivation to remain HIV negative
Clements et al. (1999)	Focus groups with MTF and FTM residents of San Francisco. Participants reported that 'low self-esteem' was a primary reason for sexual risk-taking, and that affirmation via sex with non-trans partners motivated sexual risk behaviour. For FTM participants, trying unprotected sex was sometimes part of a gender exploration process, body dissociation made it more difficult to practice barrier use, and sex drive changes related to hormone use increased sexual risk-taking

sensitive to norms around HIV infection. In communities where HIV-positive status is perceived as normative, FTMs may feel that seroconversion will increase their sense of belonging, and may conceal their HIV-negative status to avoid rejection by HIV-positive partners (Rowniak & Chesla, 2013). In contrast, in communities where HIV-positive status is stigmatised, FTMs may be motivated to avoid HIV infection (Hein & Kirk, 1999), but HIV-positive FTMs may feel doubly marginalised.

Qualitative research has focused on TMSM because they are expected to engage in the highest-risk behaviours, such as anal-penile and vaginal-penile intercourse, more frequently than FTMs who are not sexually active with men. While this attention may be warranted, it should not be to the exclusion of non-MSM FTMs. Some of the TMSM findings can be generalised: the 'gender role trigger', for instance, may contribute to coercion by partners of any gender. The 'gender role trigger' refers to engaging in behaviours that are consistent with gender role-based expectations and that validate or affirm a current male gender identity, even when such behaviours may place individuals at risk for HIV or STIs. Other dynamics may vary by sexual identity and partner choice. Future research should explore risks specific to FTMs of other sexual identities, including those who have sex with transgender women.

Gaps and opportunities

There are notable gaps in the epidemiologic literature on HIV and STI risk in FTMs. The most glaring gap is the dearth of research assessing HIV and STIs in this population, and the sexual and drug using behaviours that may render FTMs vulnerable to HIV and STIs. Who are FTMs having sex with? What kinds of sex are FTMs having – prevalence of receptive and/or insertive anal and/or vaginal sex? What are the patterns of sexual partnerships, number of main and casual sexual partners, and sexual network configurations that render FTMs as a population at-risk? Is substance use a salient risk factor in sexual encounters? Are there differences in risk between FTMs who have not surgically altered their bodies and those who have? What factors promote resilience in this community, leading to positive sexual health outcomes for FTMs? There are many questions that remain unanswered and represent opportunities for future research.

Existing studies enrol small sample sizes and rely on convenience samples, limiting generalisable prevalence estimates of HIV and STIs. Also lacking are HIV and STI incidence data. Few have used laboratory-confirmed HIV or STI results. Data on HPV infection is particularly limited. There are no studies using longitudinal cohort designs to examine sexual behaviour over time. There are few epidemiologic studies of FTM sexual risk outside the US or Canada, and data from lower- and middle-income countries are particularly sparse. Existing research is also limited by inconsistent and imprecise measurement of HIV/STI risk behaviours. Studies rarely separate vaginal and anal sex, do not examine risk by sex partner gender, and differ in timeframes of risk assessment.

Investigation of biomedical and behavioural interventions appropriate for FTM populations has been limited. We were unable to identify any data about biomedical prevention strategies such as microbicides or HIV pre-exposure prophylaxis (PrEP) in FTMs. FTMs are typically excluded from drug efficacy trials, even those that include transgender women (MTFs). When they are enrolled, FTMs have not been recruited or analysed separately. For instance, NEXT-PrEP, a safety and tolerability study of a PrEP regimen, treated FTM participants as 'female' Failure to set FTM-specific recruitment targets or document their transgender status has made it impossible to assess drug safety, acceptability, or efficacy within this group. There are also no published efficacy trials of behavioural interventions to reduce HIV and STI risk among FTMs in particular.

Addressing HIV and STI risk among FTMs also requires research into their sexual and social contexts. Little is known about FTMs' partners and sexual networks, and this information is particularly crucial in preventing HIV 'bridging' with MSM communities. Social and structural factors influencing FTMs remain under-investigated, and data are lacking about how FTM identities are conceptualised and enacted in non-Western contexts.

Recommendations for HIV and STI research in FTMs

Below we offer several recommendations to guide future research efforts based on this synthesis of current research.

Recommendation 1: routinely collect transgender status information in health surveillance

Capturing transgender identity in health surveillance systems will be essential to understanding HIV and STI prevalence for these populations. At present, most systems do not identify transgender respondents, and transgender status has been inconsistently measured and operationalised. 'Two-question' measures, which assess current gender identity separately from assigned sex at birth, appear to be the most reliable and valid approach, and have been cognitively tested with transgender and non-transgender participants in the US (Reisner, Conron, et al., 2014; Tate, Ledbetter, & Youssef, 2012). Standardised transgender status measures should be added to venue-based and regional HIV and STI surveillance programmes, and FTM- and MTF-specific results should be routinely reported. Efforts should be made to develop survey items that can assess transgender identity in a range of languages, cultural contexts, and geographic areas.

Recommendation 2: validate and standardise sexual risk behaviour assessments

Across HIV and STI research in FTMs, sexual risk behaviours are inconsistently measured and operationalised. This weakness must be addressed with the development of validated and standardised sexual risk assessments, acceptable and cognitively tested with transgender and non-transgender populations alike. Such assessments should ask about specific sexual risk behaviours with male, female, and transgender sexual partners, capturing both the participants' and sexual partners' anatomy and their gender identities. These questions will help to elucidate HIV and STI risk within groups, as well as 'bridging' between groups.

Recommendation 3: elucidate sex and gender pathways

Sex and gender are recognised globally as core social determinants of health and wellbeing across a wide variety of geographic settings and contexts (World Health Organization, 2008). *Sex* refers to biological differences among male, female, and intersex people, such as genetics, hormones, secondary sex characteristics, and anatomy. *Gender* typically refers to 'cultural meanings of patterns of behaviour, experience, and personality that are labelled masculine or feminine' (Institute of Medicine, 2011). Gender is a multidimensional construct that is culturally dependent, and includes gender *identity* (internal sense of being male, female, or another gender), gender *behaviours* (how a person expresses their gender identity through appearance and mannerisms), and gender *beliefs* (cognitive beliefs about gender, gender role conformity, and gender socialisation) (Krieger, 2003). Research in FTM health should consider each gender-related dimension's role in HIV and STI risk – alongside biological sex-linked pathways potentiating HIV infection and STIs.

Recommendation 4: account for a range of gender identities

People who transition from 'female to male' vary in their self-described gender identities. Some understand themselves as fully male, while others see themselves as some combination of male and female, or as another gender altogether. Those who identify as neither fully male nor fully female can be described as 'non-binary'. Gender identity may be context-dependent, may manifest differently across cultures and geographies, and may shift over time.

Non-binary gender identities can introduce challenges to sexuality, since partners may not understand a non-binary gender identity or be willing to affirm it. However, these identities may also result from a reflective process that leads to a more secure sense of self. Bockting et al. (2009) found that for 20% of FTMs in their sample, a binary male identity at the time of transition eventually gave way to a non-binary identity. This shift was not associated with regrets about transition; rather, non-binary identity reflected the perspectives on gender that participants developed through their transition experiences, including a rejection of conventional beliefs about what it means to be male or female. Future research should acknowledge the range of gender identities in FTMs and consider both the potential challenges and protective effects of non-binary identity for sexual health.

Recommendation 5: consider social, medical, and legal gender affirmation

For FTMs, medical gender affirmation often includes cross-sex hormone therapy with testosterone, which deepens the voice, causes growth of body and facial hair, redistributes body fat to a more masculine appearance, and causes the menstrual cycle to end. Surgical interventions may include genital reconstructive surgery, mastectomy (known as chest reconstruction or 'top surgery'), and/or hysterectomy and oophorectomy. Only a minority of FTMs access genital surgeries (e.g. metoidioplasty or phalloplasty), due to a combination of costs, outcomes, complication rates, and personal preference (Grant et al., 2011). However, testosterone therapy induces clitoral growth, which many FTMs find desirable. FTMs often describe their body parts using terms that correspond with their gender identity (e.g. penis or micro-phallus) rather than anatomical sex (i.e. clitoris) and may refer to vaginal sex as 'frontal sex' (Adams et al., 2008). Anatomical changes that may accompany testosterone therapy or hysterectomy, such as vaginal dryness, can increase the risk of HIV and STI transmission (Sevelius, Scheim, & Giambrone, 2010), and more research is needed to understand the biological impact of hormone therapy on per-act probability risk of HIV and STI transmission.

Gender affirmation may affect the available pool of sexual partners, choice of sexual partners, sexual behaviours, and levels of sexual comfort and safety. 'Passing' – being seen or recognised by others as the desired or identified gender – is often an outcome of medical gender affirmation, and can create both sexual opportunities and risks. Adams et al. (2008) found, for instance, that TMSM who 'passed' as male had greater access to MSM sexual networks. However, they had to contend with assumptions that they were non-transgender and had penises, forcing them to either disclose their transgender status to interested partners, facing potential rejection, or conceal their bioanatomical differences. Increased 'passing' and concurrent social acceptance might increase self-esteem, potentially reducing sexual risk behaviour (Rosario, Schrimshaw, & Hunter, 2006), but could also heighten risk by increasing the number of available partners. Research should account for 'passing' or 'recognition' as a key outcome of gender affirmation, with multiple possible effects on sexual risk.

Recommendation 6: foreground diversity of sexual attractions, behaviours, and identities

FTMs' sexual behaviours may include vaginal and/or anal sex with non-transgender women, non-transgender men, and other transgender people (Bauer, Travers, Scanlon, & Coleman, 2012; Bockting et al., 2009). Sexual attractions and behaviours may change over the course of gender transition. For instance, 40% of 605 FTMs recruited online from 19 different countries (83% US) reported a shift in sexual orientation during gender transition, most commonly from attraction to women only to attraction to both women and men (Meier, Pardo, Labuski, & Babcock, 2013). Post-transition FTMs' male partners are typically gay, bisexual, or queer men, rather than straight-identified men, and sex with MSM may expose FTMs to the high prevalence of HIV and STIs in these communities.

Like non-transgender people, transgender people describe their sexual identities using varying terms, which convey not only the genders of their sexual partners but also subcultural affiliations. 'Queer', for instance, is the most commonly endorsed sexual identity among FTMs in a Western context (Meier et al., 2013; Reisner, Gamarel, Dunham, Hopwood, & Hwahng, 2013). 'Queer' was originally a derogatory slur used against LGBT people, but has been reclaimed since the early 1990s, particularly by those who reject distinct sexual identities. Communities that form around queer identity (as contrasted with lesbian, gay, or bisexual identity) have historically been more likely to embrace openly transgender people, though this is not universally true (Stryker, 2008).

Transgender men may also participate in communities of gay-identified men, distinct from (though sometimes overlapping with) queer-identified communities. FTMs face prejudice within gay men's communities, but recent developments – including reports from the qualitative literature on TMSM (Adams et al., 2008; Bockting et al., 2009; Williams et al., 2013), and increased production of 'gay FTM' pornography featuring encounters between transgender and non-transgender men – suggest that gay FTMs are more visible than ever before. Psychosocial dynamics, particularly stigma and efforts to avoid rejection, can put FTMs in gay communities at heightened risk for unsafe sexual encounters (Rowniak & Chesla, 2013). Nonetheless, for some FTMs, gay identity is crucial in developing a secure sexual and social identity (Bockting et al., 2009; Hein & Kirk, 1999; Williams et al., 2013).

Research should explore the variety of sexual subcultures that FTMs participate in, which may predict sexual practices (including safer-sex practices), degrees of stigmatisation or affirmation within sexual networks, and HIV and STI prevalence among partners. Measuring sexual identity – which may include 'straight', 'gay', 'bisexual', 'queer', or other labels – can help to capture this variability. It is not known whether North American and Western European FTMs' tendency towards non-heterosexual identities and behaviours extends to other cultural contexts; more information is needed on FTMs' sexual attractions, behaviours, and identities in different languages, contexts, and geographic regions.

Recommendation 7: integrate health and human rights perspectives

Identifying the cultural context and consequences of pathologisation is an important step towards human rights for FTMs globally. Social exclusion and repressive (or insufficiently supportive) environments contribute to stigma in health care settings, limit access to health and HIV services, and restrict materials and publications relating to sexual health. The need for protection from non-consensual interventions (such as reparative or conversion therapy, or even 'corrective' rape intended to suppress gender-variant identities) is particularly urgent. Sexual health risks in FTMs may be heightened by discrimination in other aspects of life, including employment, housing, and education, that produces social and economic insecurity. For instance, the results of this review suggest that sex work and transactional sex are not unusual among FTMs (Herbst et al., 2008; Reisner et al., 2010; Schulden et al., 2008), representing one path by which economic marginalisation can put FTMs at heightened risk for HIV and STIs. Special attention should be paid to the sexual health needs of FTMs in lower- and middle-income countries, a topic on which additional data is sorely needed.

Recommendation 8: engage FTM communities

Involving FTM communities – research 'with' not 'on' FTMs – is essential to creating responsive, culturally competent public health research and advocacy efforts. The principles of community-based participatory research (CBPR) represent one potentially valuable framework for research and interventions with FTMs (Leung, Yen, & Minkler, 2004). This approach is consistent with depathologisation and human rights perspectives used to advance transgender health research and advocacy in global contexts (International Stop Trans Pathologization Campaign, 2012). Community engagement also ensures that research centres the needs and preferences of local FTMs. Given the extreme variation and rapid evolution of FTM identities and norms, this specificity and local engagement of community is indispensable.

Conclusion: the way forward

There is a paucity of data on HIV infection and STIs in FTMs, making it difficult to assess HIV and STI risk in this population. The general lack of awareness about transgender people, and FTMs specifically, exacerbates the problem leaving a large scientific gap. There is inadequate research to assess or determine the nature or level of risk in this population, including the sexual and drug using behaviours rendering FTMs vulnerable to HIV and STIs. Research and interventions with sexual minority populations (e.g. MSM) should be expected to justify their exclusion or inclusion of FTMs to ensure scientific accountability. Studies of MSM should seriously consider including and documenting TMSM sexual risk, and should offer a rationale for any decision to exclude them. Research and interventions with MTFs should consider the needs of local FTMs, and determine whether their work may be of value to this population, particularly in light of shared challenges like sex work and limited health care access. Furthermore, FTM communities worldwide need research, policy, and programming designed for their unique sexual health needs. These projects must consider the diverse sexual identities, attractions, and behaviours in this subpopulation, and should engage local FTM communities in needs assessment, decision-making, and implementation of public health research, policy, and programming.

Disclosure statement

No potential conflict of interest was reported by the authors.

Funding

Reisner's effort for this publication was partly supported by The National Institute of Mental Health (NIMH) of the National Institutes of Health under award number R34MH104072 (MPI: Clark,

Mimiaga, Reisner). The content is solely the responsibility of the authors and does not necessarily represent the official views of the National Institutes of Health.

Notes

1. Stephens et al. (2011) reported 10% pre-existing and 2.9% new HIV diagnoses, but data were reported on the basis of clinic visits, such that some individuals were counted more than once.
2. 'TMSM' refers to 'trans men who have sex with men,' in keeping with the use of 'MSM' to refer to 'men who have sex with men' (Reisner et al., 2010).

References

Adams, A., Lundie, M., Marshall, Z., Pires, R., Scanlon, K., Meir Scheim, A. I., & Smith, T. (2008). Getting primed: Informing HIV prevention with Gay/Bi/Queer Trans Men in Ontario. Retrieved from http://www.actoronto.org/research.nsf/pages/gettingprimed

American Psychiatric Association. (2000). *Diagnostic and statistical manual of mental disorders* (4th ed., text rev.). Washington, DC: Author.

Baral, S. D., Poteat, T., Stromdahl, S., Wirtz, A. L., Guadamuz, T. E., & Beyrer, C. (2013). Worldwide burden of HIV in transgender women: A systematic review and meta-analysis. *Lancet Infectious Diseases, 13*(3), 214–222. doi:10.1016/s1473-3099(12)70315-8

Bauer, G. R., Redman, N., Bradley, K., & Scheim, A. I. (2013). Sexual health of trans men who are gay, bisexual, or who have sex with men: Results from Ontario, Canada. *International Journal of Transgenderism, 14*(2), 66–74. doi:10.1080/15532739.2013.791650

Bauer, G. R., Travers, R., Scanlon, K., & Coleman, T. A. (2012). High heterogeneity of HIV-related sexual risk among transgender people in Ontario, Canada: A province-wide respondent-driven sampling survey. *BMC Public Health, 12*, 292. doi:10.1186/1471-2458-12-292

Beyrer, C., Baral, S. D., van Griensven, F., Goodreau, S. M., Chariyalertsak, S., Wirtz, A. L., & Brookmeyer, R. (2012). Global epidemiology of HIV infection in men who have sex with men. *Lancet, 380*(9839), 367–377. doi:10.1016/S0140-6736(12)60821-6

Bockting, W. O. (2015). Gender dysphoria. In P. Whelehan, & A. Bolin (Eds.), *The international encyclopedia of human sexuality* (1st ed., pp. 449–450). West Sussex: John Wiley & Sons Ltd. doi:10.1002/9781118896877.wbiehs175

Bockting, W. O., Benner, A., & Coleman, E. (2009). Gay and bisexual identity development among female-to-male transsexuals in North America: Emergence of a transgender sexuality. *Archives of Sexual Behavior, 38*, 688–701. doi:10.1007/s10508-009-9489-3

Bockting, W. O., Robinson, B. E., Forberg, J., & Scheltema, K. (2005). Evaluation of a sexual health approach to reducing HIV/STD risk in the transgender community. *AIDS Care, 17*(3), 289–303. doi:10.1080/09540120412331299825

Butt, S., Mena, L., & Muzny, C. (2011). Transgenders and HIV: A literature review of HIV risk behaviours and prevalence rates. *Sexually Transmitted Infections, 87*, A248. doi:10.1136/sextrans-2011-050108.351

Centers for Disease Control and Prevention. (2012). Monitoring selected national HIV prevention and care objectives by using HIV surveillance data—United States and 6 US dependent areas—2010. *HIV Surveillance Supplemental Report, 17*(3). Retrieved from http://www.cdc.gov/hiv/library/reports/surveillance/2010/surveillance_report_vol_17_no_3.html

Chen, S., McFarland, W., Thompson, H. M., & Raymond, H. F. (2011). Transmen in San Francisco: What do we know from HIV test site data? *AIDS and Behavior, 15*(3), 659–662. doi:10.1007/s10461-010-9859-9

Clements, K., Kitano, K., Wilkinson, W., & Marx, R. (1999). HIV prevention and health service needs of the transgender community in San Francisco. *International Journal of Transgenderism, 3*, 1–2. Retrieved from http://web.archive.org/web/20070513053216/http://www.symposion.com/ijt/hiv_risk/clements.htm

Clements-Nolle, K., Marx, R., Guzman, R., & Katz, M. (2001). HIV prevalence, risk behaviors, health care use, and mental health status of transgender persons: Implications for public health intervention. *American Journal of Public Health*, *91*(6), 915–921. doi:10.2105/AJPH.91.6.915

Currah, P., & Minter, S. P. (2000). *Transgender equality: A handbook for activists and policymakers*. Retrieved from National LGBTQ Task Force website: http://www.thetaskforce.org/static_html/downloads/reports/reports/TransgenderEquality.pdf

Grant, J. M., Mottet, L. A., Tanis, J., Harrison, J., Herman, J., & Keisling, M. (2011). *Injustice at every turn: A report of the national transgender discrimination survey*. Retrieved from National LGBTQ Task Force website: http://www.thetaskforce.org/static_html/downloads/reports/reports/ntds_full.pdf

Gross, J., & Davis, M. (2004). Female-to-male transgenders and HIV risk behaviors in Los Angeles, California. Paper presented at the XV International AIDS Conference, Bangkok. Abstract retrieved from https://www.iasociety.org/Abstracts/A2171264.aspx

Hein, D., & Kirk, M. (1999). Education and soul-searching: The enterprise HIV prevention group. *International Journal of Transgenderism*, *3*, 1. Retrieved from http://web.archive.org/web/20070708145630/http://www.symposion.com/ijt/hiv_risk/hein.htm

Herbst, J. H., Jacobs, E. D., Finlayson, T. J., McKleroy, V. S., Neumann, M. S., & Crepaz, N. (2008). Estimating HIV prevalence and risk behaviors of transgender persons in the United States: A systematic review. *AIDS and Behavior*, *12*(1), 1–17. doi:10.1007/s10461-007-9299-3

Horvath, K. J., Iantaffi, A., Swinburne-Romine, R., & Bockting, W. (2014). A comparison of mental health, substance use, and sexual risk behaviors between rural and non-rural transgender persons. *Journal of Homosexuality*, *61*(8), 1117–1130. doi:10.1080/00918369.2014.872502

Institute of Medicine. (2011). *The health of lesbian, gay, bisexual, and transgender people: Building a foundation for better understanding*. Retrieved from https://iom.nationalacademies.org/Reports/2011/The-Health-of-Lesbian-Gay-Bisexual-and-Transgender-People.aspx

International Stop Trans Pathologization Campaign. (2012). Reflections on the ICD revision process from a depathologization and human rights perspective. Retrieved from http://www.stp2012.info/STP2012_Reflections_ICD.pdf

Johnson, J., Radix, A., Santos Ramos, J., Mayer, G., & Mukerjee, R. (2010). If you've got it, check it: Establishing a sexual health clinic for transgender clients at a New York City community health center. Paper presented at the XVIII International AIDS Conference, Vienna. Abstract retrieved from https://www.aids2014.org/Abstracts/A200736134.aspx

Kenagy, G. P. (2002). HIV among transgendered people. *AIDS Care*, *14*(1), 127–134. doi:10.1080/09540120220098008

Kenagy, G. P. (2005). Transgender health: Findings from two needs assessment studies in Philadelphia. *Health & Social Work*, *30*(1), 19–26. doi:10.1093/hsw/30.1.19

Kenagy, G. P., & Hsieh, C. M. (2005). The risk less known: Female-to-male transgender persons' vulnerability to HIV infection. *AIDS Care*, *17*(2), 195–207. doi:10.1080/19540120512331325680

Kosenko, K. A. (2011). Contextual influences on sexual risk-taking in the transgender community. *Journal of Sex Research*, *48*, 285. doi:10.1080/00224491003721686

Krieger, N. (2003). Genders, sexes, and health: What are the connections—And why does it matter? *International Journal of Epidemiology*, *32*(4), 652–657. doi:10.1093/ije/dyg156

Kuper, L. E., Nussbaum, R., & Mustanski, B. (2012). Exploring the diversity of gender and sexual orientation identities in an online sample of transgender individuals. *Journal of Sex Research*, *49*(2/3), 244–254. doi:10.1080/00224499.2011.596954

Leung, M. W., Yen, I. H., & Minkler, M. (2004). Community based participatory research: A promising approach for increasing epidemiology's relevance in the 21st century. *International Journal of Epidemiology*, *33*(3), 499–506. doi:10.1093/ije/dyh010

Lobato, M. I., Koff, W. J., Schestatsky, S. S., Chaves, C. P. V., Petry, A., Crestana, T., ... Henriques, A. A. (2007). Clinical characteristics, psychiatric comorbidities and sociodemographic profile of transsexual patients from an outpatient clinic in Brazil. *International Journal of Transgenderism*, *10*(2), 69–77. doi:10.1080/15532730802175148

Meier, S. C., Pardo, S. T., Labuski, C., & Babcock, J. (2013). Measures of clinical health among female-to-male transgender persons as a function of sexual orientation. *Archives of Sexual Behavior*, *42*(3), 463–474.

Meyerowitz, J. J. (2004). *How sex changed: A history of transsexuality in the United States*. Cambridge, MA: Harvard University Press.

Myers, T., Remis, R., & Husbands, W. (2007). *Technical report—Lambda survey: M-Track Ontario second generation surveillance*. Retrieved from http://www.catie.ca/en/resources/technical-report-lambda-survey-m-track-ontario-second-generation-surveillance

Namaste, V. K. (1999). HIV/AIDS and female-to-male transsexuals and transvestites: Results from a needs assessment in Québec. *International Journal of Transgenderism*, *3*, 1. Retrieved from http://web.archive.org/web/20081206173303/http://www.symposion.com/ijt/hiv_risk/namaste.htm

Olson, J., Clark, L., Schrager, S., Simons, L., & Belzer, M. (2013). Baseline characteristics of transgender youth naïve to cross-sex hormone therapy. *Journal of Adolescent Health*, *52*, S35–S36. doi:10.1016/j.jadohealth.2012.10.086

Patrascioiu, I., Lopez, C. Q., Porta, M. M., Velazquez, G. B. A., Hanzu, F. A., Gomez-Gil, E., ... Rabinovich, I. H. (2013). Characteristics of the HIV positive transgender population of Catalonia. Paper presented at the 15th European Congress of Endocrinology, Copenhagen. Abstract retrieved from http://www.endocrine-abstracts.org/ea/0032/ea0032p341.htm

Peitzmeier, S. M., Khullar, K., Reisner, S. L., & Potter, J. (2014). Pap test use is lower among female-to-male patients than non-transgender women. *American Journal of Preventive Medicine*, *47*(6), 808–812. doi:10.1016/j.amepre.2014.07.031

Pell, C., Prone, I., & Vlahakis, E. (2011, June). *A clinical audit of female to male (FTM) transgender patients attending Taylor Square Private Clinic (TSPC) in Sydney, Australia, Aiming to Improve Quality of Care*. Poster presented at the 20th World Congress of Sexual Health, Glasgow. Poster retrieved from http://f1000research.com/posters/1934

Reisner, S. L., Conron, K. J., Tardiff, L. A., Jarvi, S., Gordon, A. R., & Austin, S. B. (2014). Monitoring the health of transgender and other gender minority populations: Validity of natal sex and gender identity survey items in a US national cohort of young adults. *BMC Public Health*, *14*(1), 1224. doi:10.1186/1471-2458-14-1224

Reisner, S. L., Gamarel, K. E., Dunham, E., Hopwood, R., & Hwahng, S. (2013). Female-to-male transmasculine adult health: A mixed-methods community-based needs assessment. *Journal of the American Psychiatric Nurses Association*, *19*(5), 293–303. doi:10.1177/1078390313500693

Reisner, S. L., Perkovich, B., & Mimiaga, M. J. (2010). A mixed methods study of the sexual health needs of New England transmen who have sex with nontransgender men. *AIDS Patient Care and STDs*, *24*(8), 501–513. doi:10.1089/apc.2010.0059

Reisner, S. L., White, J. M., Mayer, K. H., & Mimiaga, M. J. (2014). Sexual risk behaviors and psychosocial health concerns of female-to-male transgender men screening for STDs at an urban community health center. *AIDS Care*, *26*(7), 857–864. doi:10.1080/09540121.2013.855701

Rodolico, M. D. C., Helien, A., Nagelberg, A., Rey, H., & Levalle, O. (2012). Sexual habits and hormonal treatment in transsexual patients. *Journal of Sexual Medicine*, *9*, 84. doi:10.1111/j.1743-6109.2012.02643.x

Rosario, M., Schrimshaw, E. W., & Hunter, J. (2006). A model of sexual risk behaviors among young gay and bisexual men: Longitudinal associations of mental health, substance abuse, sexual abuse, and the coming-out process. *AIDS Education and Prevention*, *18*(5), 444–460. doi:10.1521/aeap.2006.18.5.444

Rowniak, S., & Chesla, C. (2013). Coming out for a third time: Transmen, sexual orientation, and identity. *Archives of Sexual Behavior*, *42*(3), 449–461. doi:10.1007/s10508-012-0036-2

Rowniak, S., Chesla, C., Rose, C. D., & Holzemer, W. L. (2011). Transmen: The HIV risk of gay identity. *AIDS Education and Prevention*, *23*(6), 508–520. doi:10.1521/aeap.2011.23.6.508

Schulden, J. D., Song, B., Barros, A., Mares-DelGrasso, A., Martin, C. W., Ramirez, R., ... Heffelfinger, J. D. (2008). Rapid HIV testing in transgender communities by community-based organizations in three cities. *Public Health Reports*, *123*(Suppl. 3), 101–114. Retrieved from http://www.publichealthreports.org/

Sevelius, J. (2009). "There's no pamphlet for the kind of sex I have": HIV-related risk factors and protective behaviors among transgender men who have sex with nontransgender men. *Journal of the Association of Nurses in AIDS Care, 20*(5), 398–410. doi:10.1016/j.jana.2009.06.001

Sevelius, J., Scheim, A., & Giambrone, B. (2010). What are transgender men's HIV prevention needs? [Fact sheet]. Retrieved from UCSF Center for AIDS Prevention Studies website: http://caps.ucsf.edu/factsheets/transgender-men/

Sperber, J., Landers, L., & Lawrence, S. (2005). Access to health care for transgender persons: Results of a needs assessment in Boston. *International Journal of Transgenderism., 8*(2/3), 75–91. doi:10.1300/J485v08n02_08

Stephens, S. C., Bernstein, K. T., & Philip, S. S. (2011). Male to female and female to male transgender persons have different sexual risk behaviors yet similar rates of STDs and HIV. *AIDS and Behavior, 15*(3), 683–686. doi:10.1007/s10461-010-9773-1

Stryker, S. (2008). *Transgender history*. Berkeley, CA: Seal Press.

Tate, C. C., Ledbetter, J. N., & Youssef, C. P. (2012). A two-question method for assessing gender categories in the social and medical sciences. *The Journal of Sex Research, 50*(8), 767–776. doi:10.1080/00224499.2012.690110

Williams, C. J., Weinberg, M. S., & Rosenberger, J. G. (2013). Trans men: Embodiments, identities, and sexualities. *Sociological Forum, 28*(4), 719–741. doi:10.1111/socf.12056

World Health Organization, Commission on Social Determinants of Health. (2008). Closing the gap in a generation: Health equity through action on the social determinants of health. Retrieved from http://apps.who.int/iris/bitstream/10665/43943/1/9789241563703_eng.pdf

Xavier, J. M., Bobbin, M., Singer, B., & Budd, E. (2005). A needs assessment of transgendered people of color living in Washington, DC. *International Journal of Transgenderism, 8*(2–3), 31–47. doi:10.1300/J485v08n02_04

Xavier, J. M., Hannold, J. A., Bradford, J., & Simmons, R. (2007). The health, health-related needs, and lifecourse experiences of transgender Virginians. Retrieved from Virginia Department of Health website: http://www.vdh.state.va.us/epidemiology/DiseasePrevention/documents/pdf/THISFINALREPORTVol1.pdf

'Men who use the Internet to seek sex with men': Rethinking sexuality in the transnational context of HIV prevention

R. Souleymanov and Y.-T. Huang

ABSTRACT
MISM (i.e. men who use the Internet to seek sex with men) has emerged in public health literature as a population in need of HIV prevention. In this paper, we argue for the importance of rethinking the dominant notions of the MISM category to uncover its ethnocentric and heteronormative bias. To accomplish this, we conducted a historical, epistemological and transnational analysis of social sciences and health research literature ($n = 146$) published on MISM between 2000 and 2014. We critically unravel the normative underpinnings of 'westernised' knowledge upon which the MISM category is based. We argue that the essentialist approach of Western scholarship can homogenise MISM by narrowly referring to behavioural aspects of sexuality, thereby rendering multiple sexualities/desires invisible. Furthermore, we argue that a Eurocentric bias, which underlies the MISM category, may hinder our awareness of the transnational dynamics of sexual minority communities, identities, histories and cultures. We propose the conceptualisation of MISM as hybrid cultural subjects that go beyond transnational and social boundaries, and generate conclusions about the future of the MISM category for HIV prevention and health promotion.

Men who use the Internet to seek sex with men (MISM)[1] is one of the latest epidemiological risk categories making its way into HIV prevention discourse. This category revolves around one of the latest innovations in online technologies (wireless Internet and smartphone applications) that utilise global positioning systems, allowing MISM in major urban centres around the world to find partners for social or sexual encounters (Blackwell, Birnholtz, & Abbott, 2015).

While researchers are still trying to understand the complex link between Internet use and new cases of HIV infections among MISM (Grov, Breslow, Newcomb, Rosenberger, & Bauermeister, 2014), the Internet has become a platform to target these men and carry out HIV prevention programmes globally (Saxton, Dickson, & Hughes, 2013; Zou et al., 2013). As a result, MISM has emerged in public health literature as a category of people in need of HIV prevention. The way the term MISM is becoming legitimised (particularly, in North American scholarship) seems to suggest that researchers hold the idea of MISM as a stable category, which explains many sexual behaviours, desires or identities, regardless of context, place and history.

Most research on how MISM find and interact with sexual partners online has been conducted in the Global North (primarily in the U.S.A), with an inclination towards a Western, biomedical/essentialist view of sexuality. The inscription of sexuality in a biomedical paradigm initially began in Europe (mostly in Germany), after the Second World War shifted to the U.S.A, and later extended globally (Corrêa, de la Dehesa, & Parker, 2014). Essentialist perspectives homogenise MISM by narrowly referring to behavioural aspects of sexuality. Researchers in Latin American (Corrêa et al., 2014) and African contexts (Heloo, 2010), however, have noted that concepts of sexuality may involve different processes of negotiating identities, desires and behaviours, therefore complicating HIV interventions when they are applied in a global context. By limiting HIV prevention to the dominant, essentialist, and Western conceptualisation of sexuality, efforts may not target hard to reach populations and marginalised groups who may also be in need of public health interventions.

Some researchers began to call for a critically attuned, transnational analysis of this phenomenon (Race, 2014), suggesting that the roles that socio-economic and political disparities between industrialised and industrialising nations play in men's use of the Internet for sex warrants a unique investigation (Grov et al., 2014). We build on this call by arguing that the Eurocentric bias of Western scholarship underlying the MISM category may hinder our awareness of the transnational dynamics of sexual minority communities, identities, histories and cultures. Parker (2009) eloquently reminds researchers that sexuality categories used to describe sexual lives through the language of Western disciplines may be far from universal, and indeed may be a poor representation of sexual experiences and possibilities in various social and cultural contexts. Thus, the Western bias implicit in the MISM category can perpetuate 'epistemic violence'[2] (Spivak, 2005), thereby rendering 'the other' ways of knowing and being invisible and silenced.

This paper is an attempt to destabilise this ethnocentric, colonial, heteronormative and essentialist category before it crystallises in public health discourse. The predominant notion of the MISM category has to do with biological males being 'homosexually' active, but the complex nature of their sexual activity is under-analysed, and rarely located in socio-cultural or temporal contexts.

The critique of the MISM category entails pragmatic implications. When Rosser and Horvath (2007) applied the category of MISM and generated conclusions for Internet-based HIV prevention for gay men, they encountered issues in using the MISM category. They asked whether online HIV interventions should attempt to target all people who fall under MISM, or specific subgroups of MISM that are more at risk (Rosser & Horvath, 2007). This circumstance highlighted that the category itself may not accurately capture people in relation to their HIV risks. Our paper articulates the issue brought up by Rosser and Horvath (2007) from a different vantage point; that is, how operationalisation of the MISM category forces people in the Global South to prove their sexualities in terms and language originating from the Global North (in particular North American scholarship), and underestimates the structural risk factors that position marginalised people in proximity to HIV.

In this paper, we outline a transnational review of the MISM category relative to its epistemological analysis. Our analysis elucidates the limited scope of this category in research and its implications for HIV prevention. We followed Michel Foucault's (1976) epistemological approach to unsettle and destabilise taken-for-granted assumptions on this emerging category in public health research, which may engender the epistemic violence committed against non-Western sexual minority communities, identities and cultures. We argue that a critical engagement with epistemological and transnational discursive lenses concerning sexual minority populations is essential in order to extend respect to this group in a globalised context, and give some voice to sexualities that have been discursively marginalised.

Methodology

We approach research on MISM as discursive formations, and focus on the way social power, dominance and inequality are enacted, as well as discursively reproduced and resisted by text. Discourses comprise a system of thoughts that operate to legitimise a specific mode of knowledge, thereby constructing social institutions and people's daily practices (Rogers, Malancharuvil-Berkes, Mosley, Hui, & Joseph, 2005). Rooted in both poststructuralist and postmodernist approaches that challenge the positivist claim of fixed and final knowledge, critical discourse analysis (CDA) is aimed to interrogate hegemonic discourses that are constructed to manipulate our recognition of what deserves the status of truth (Agger, 1991). CDA suggests an analytical focus on how the form and content of language play out in producing a set of ideologies and power dynamics (Fairclough, 1992).

Our analysis utilises CDA with the intention of elucidating the way in which privileged systems are constructed and reproduced (Gee, 2011; van Dijk, 2008). In the process of CDA, text will be approached as a discursive artefact that acts to produce power relations (Rogers et al., 2005). In addition to identifying discourses, motifs and narratives running through a text (Gee, 2011), our analysis seeks to discern what opinions have been included or represented and what have been excluded or obscured when the category of MISM is deployed in the literature. We then pose the following questions:

(1) How are the discourses on MISM represented in literature through behavioural/essentialist terms that disregard the cultural and contextual components of the meaning of sexuality?
(2) How the deployment of discourses on MISM in literature may be linked to a grand discourse on the sexuality of men having sex with men in contemporary Western society, which subsequently organises HIV prevention and the treatment of health issues in a transnational context?

Study retrieval and selection

The analysed materials included studies published between 2000 and 2014 (since the first mention of men using Internet to seek sex with other men) from the following databases: (1) ProQuest; (2) Ovid; (3) PubMed; and (4) Google Scholar. For the current study, all databases were investigated over a 15-year period (2000–2014).

The key search terms for the current study were 'gay', 'bisexual', 'homosexual', 'MSM', 'MISM', 'Men', 'Internet', 'Online', 'Web', 'App', 'Sex', 'Cruising', 'Dating' and 'Hookup'. For the purposes of this review, full-length, empirically based and theoretical research articles and reports focusing on MISM were included in this study. Our inclusion criteria were: (1) studies published between 2000 and 2014; (2) English language articles from national and international peer-reviewed or scholarly journals dedicated to health, medicine, public health, social sciences and interdisciplinary research; and (3) articles on MISM (i.e. studies on men who use the Internet to seek social and sexual relationships with other men, including, gay, queer, bisexual, homosexual, cis- or transgender men and sexual minority populations from all geographic locations).

Results

A total of 314 references were retrieved from the initial search. We excluded 162 publications because they did not meet one or more of the three inclusion criteria. Following this, we excluded 12 duplicates and 4 studies, which were not published in English. In the end, we identified 146 publications as potentially relevant for analysis.

In this section, we identify multiple discourses on MISM; unravel the normative underpinnings of MISM as a homogeneous object of HIV and STI prevention; point out the ethnocentricism and heteronormativity implicit in this nomenclature; and explore the construction of MISM as risky subjectivities.

'MISM' as a stable, homogeneous and essentialising replacement for sexuality

Under this theme, we found that the epistemological frameworks primarily used among researchers (e.g. essentialism), and the methodologies for data analysis (e.g. quantitative) complicate exploration of the social and cultural aspects of sexuality. Textually, references to MISM in the academic discourse on HIV and STI connote a unifying meaning, even though semantically the term is deployed in different forms: 'MISM' (Rosser et al., 2011), 'Internet-Using MSM' (Wilkerson, Smolenski, Horvath, Danilenko, & Rosser, 2010), 'MSM who use Internet for social and sexual networking' (Zou et al., 2013) and 'MSM app users' (Lehmiller & Ioerger, 2014).

While the meaning of 'what' or 'who' is the population of interest is left largely to the readers' interpretation, the essentialist approach prevalent in Western scholarship homogenises MISM by referring to the behavioural aspects of sexuality, such as 'sexual risk behaviors' (Young, Szekeres, & Coates, 2013), 'engaging in unprotected anal sex' (White, Mimiaga, Reisner, & Mayer, 2012) and 'sexual risk-taking' (Adam, Murphy, & de Wit, 2011). While some studies attended to the diverse backgrounds of MISM (Mustanski, Lyons, & Garcia, 2011; Young et al., 2013), the majority of studies conducted in the Western context promoted essentialist notions of sexuality. Epistemologically, essentialism allows for a discursive link to be established between MISM, STI risk and online technologies through cause-and-effect analyses that cement the idea that MISM is a population at increased risk for HIV and STIs (Liau, Millett, & Marks, 2006).

Few studies (Brown, Maycock, & Burns, 2005; Davis, Hart, Bolding, Sherr, & Elford, 2006; Dowsett, 2015; Race, 2014) utilised non-essentialising epistemological standpoints (e.g. critical theory, social constructionism, interpretative phenomenology, poststructuralism), taking into account the different ways in which men reflexively manage aspects of their sexuality online. This non-essentialising scholarship complemented dominant, behavioural constructions of this category.

'MISM' as an object of intervention for HIV and STI prevention

Under this theme, we uncover the social practice of Western scholarship to form intervention objects for public health needs. We explore how MISM discourses identified in the literature move beyond a cause-and-effect motif to become established as an object of intervention through HIV programmatic discourses. Studies were primarily conducted in the U.S.A, with the exception of two studies, one conducted in China and another in New Zealand.

A number of studies ($n = 12$) that we reviewed treat online technologies as something finite, tangible and homogeneous, yet suggest that websites and apps catering to sexual networking for MISM should consider aggressively increasing their focus towards HIV prevention messages and interventions (e.g. Levine & Klausner, 2005). Some studies also alluded to the importance of collaboration between public health institutions and commercial businesses that own these online technologies.

Researchers also emphasised multiple prevention strategies for MISM, including programmes that take into account men's perception of using condoms and pre/post exposure prophylaxis (PrEP and PEP) (Bauermeister, Carballo-Diéguez, Ventuneac, & Dolezal, 2009); behavioural surveillance of MISM (Saxton et al., 2013); culturally competent online HIV outreach (Rhodes et al., 2011); strategies that increase men's consumption of sexual health information (Wilkerson et al., 2010); web-based informational programmes about PrEP (Krakower et al., 2012); and the promotion of change in individual knowledge, motivations and community norms (Hirshfield et al., 2012).

Deployment of western sexualities in a transnational context

In this section, we examined studies conducted in East/Southeast Asia, Middle East and South America. We focused on the use of sexuality labels when discourses on MISM are evoked. We found a particular ethnocentric bias, where the majority of examined studies utilised Western labels to describe MISM and disregarded the cultural and contextual components of the meaning of sexuality.

Within these studies, we identified a common pattern of referring to sexuality notions behaviourally. Wei and colleagues (2012) looked at HIV disclosure and sexual risk behaviours among an online sample of 'HIV-positive MSM' ($n = 416$) in nine different countries in East and Southeast Asia. Zou and colleagues (2013) reported data on 'MSM who use the Internet for social and sexual networking' living in Beijing and Urumqi. While, the majority of people in Urumqi are Chinese Muslims, the scholars rendered invisible the cultural and contextual components of their sexuality.

In some cases, researchers conflated identities and behaviours, but allowed participants to self-identify. For instance, Ko and colleagues (2012) conducted an online behavioural survey with Taiwanese men ($n = 1316$) to estimate the prevalence of online sex-seeking. While they refer to all participants in their study as 'MSM', 94.4% of participants in their study also self-identified as 'homosexual'. Other studies take a slightly different approach to the classification of sexuality. Blas, Menacho, Alva, Cabello, and Orellana (2013) conducted a grounded theory study with 22 men in Peru, and their sexualities were classified as the following: 'closeted gay-identified MSM', 'out-of-the-closet gay-identified MSM' and 'self-identified heterosexual MSM'.

Even in a transnational context, some studies omit to provide social and contextual information on the sexuality of participants. Importantly, it is not even clear what type of sex is being sought online. For instance, Matarelli (2013) studied 86 Middle Eastern men who resided in 16 different countries in the Middle East and used the Internet to sex-seek. They simply refer to all participants in their study as 'MSM'.

Heteronormativity and social exclusion: 'MISM' as risky subjectivities

This theme illustrates how scientific discourses on MISM shape and reinforce the identities of these men as a site of omnipresent risk that needs to be regulated. Unintentionally, some studies may perpetuate heteronormativity by promoting discourses on medicalisation and the stigmatisation of deviance among these men. Discourses on medicalisation are perpetuated in a plethora of studies that position MISM in proximity to HIV and STIs (e.g. Adam et al., 2011; Liau et al., 2006). Likewise, discourses on the stigmatisation of deviance may be promoted via research that positions the behaviours of MISM as problematic (e.g. Klein, 2009). Studies may conceal a raft of unproblematised assumptions that focus on sexuality through a medicalised, psychologised lens is sufficient and ethical, or that MISM are reckless risk-takers.

Linguistically, enacting the subjectivities of MISM as a site of risk in public health research is instrumental to the maintenance of heteronormativity and social exclusion. For instance, Ybarra and Bull (2007) found that 'MSM' have been overwhelmingly the most common target group for Internet-based outreach globally. Few studies have paid attention to sex-seeking among other populations (e.g. women). Furthermore, when other populations (e.g. men who have sex with women) are mentioned, studies typically assumed a comparative approach and naturalised only heterosexual peoples' use of Internet for sex. Many scholars also suggest that 'MSM' are more likely to seek sex online and exhibit risky behaviours compared to 'non-MSM' (Bull, McFarlane, & Rietmeijer, 2001; Malu, Challenor, Theobald, & Barton, 2004). Therefore, what can be observed is that within discourses on online technologies, queer sexualities remain embedded inside the larger heteronormative system, which links them to disciplinary, patriarchal and hegemonic discourses of risk, abnormality and ill-health, while rendering non-queer sexualities intact.

Discussion

This work argues for revisiting sexuality discourses on MISM in order to encourage public health researchers to become aware of how the Western colonial legacy and epistemological standpoints are associated with the reproduction and recasting of the practices of biopolitics through the global 'deployment of sexuality discourses' (Foucault, 1976). We encourage public health professionals to take a critical stance on the social practices of research that perpetuate epistemic violence (Spivak, 2005).

The first important finding is that researchers primarily utilised the essentialist paradigm, and considered that this population of men along with the online technologies they use can be understood and captured categorically or behaviourally through objective processes and using the proper analytical tools (e.g. correlational, chi-square, multivariable analyses). The act of essentialising people's sexualities assumes that people who fall into a MISM category share common cultures, history or demographics, therefore, either stereotyping people or assuming uniformity where it might not exist.

These research practices missed important opportunities to collect and provide information about the complexity of the processes of identification, and reduced MISM to mere biological sex without attention to inter- and intra-group differences. Importantly, this essentialised discourse leads to examination only at the level of behaviour. While this may yield fruitful information, it may inevitably translate to challenges in understanding the underlying structural factors that facilitate the adoption of risky behaviours. One implication of essentialisation manifests itself at the level of public health services. By reducing MISM to mere biology or behaviour, public health researchers fail to collect contextual data and cultural factors that could be important in making interventions effective. If collected, such contextual data, for example, may improve the engagement of men through the use of culturally relevant language in prevention programmes and their retention of preventative information. If 'MISM' is used cross-culturally, without making specific references to culture or social context, funders and policy-makers may then recommend services (e.g. online HIV prevention, sexual health outreach through smartphones) that may not be culturally sensitive. Consequently, essentialisation and the separation of complex realities into specific categories curtails our understanding of the nuances of HIV transmission, and therefore how best to act upon them.

In the context of local and global HIV prevention with MISM, Western sexuality notions operationalised via behavioural terms took preference over sexual identities or socio-culturally relevant sexuality notions. While the development of the MISM category within public health, with its legitimate interest in behaviour is understandable and may generate important knowledge, the limitations of the behavioural category remain. For example, the category quickly moves from behaviour to blurred ideas of sexual attraction and, in a number of cases, even to a subject identity. Public health researchers are not asking questions about the motivations and contexts that facilitate men adopting high-risk behaviours, such as unprotected sexual relations. Furthermore, the focus on behaviour neglects some of the larger, structural, political and socio-economic factors that need to be addressed when considering disease transmission in the Global South. HIV prevention messages that seek to modify the behaviour of individuals neglect broader political, economic and social factors that explain how and why individuals and certain populations entirely are vulnerable to infectious disease. Consequently, public health education that limits itself to matters of behaviour misses a crucial opportunity to influence policy and social context in order to change structural factors (e.g. criminalisation laws, social determinants of health, institutional arrangements) that facilitate the transmission of infectious disease.

MISM as a category is homogeneous and reductionist, and it is not clear how MISM equates being gay in a socio-behavioural context. Contextually, the formation and perpetuation of MISM as a stable and homogenous object is dependent on the greater public health discourse at a knowledge translation level. Data generated from the studies we reviewed came from surveys, which require clean categories for analysis. With the exception of a few publications, the research studies rendered the social and cultural aspects of sexuality invisible, and only few studies allowed participants to identify their sexuality. Dowsett (2015) already highlighted the limitation of online technologies to obviate any need for sexual orientation and identities, and suggested instead that these technologies constitute sexuality as a new binary where one is either '0-1-I fuck or I don't fuck. Nothing else matters' (p. 536).

Second, a vast number of studies that we reviewed put forth MISM as a target of HIV and STI prevention. Contextually, the identification of MISM as a population of men in need of HIV prevention is linked to the contemporary social practice of Western public health scholarship to form intervention objects for public health needs. For instance, we have already observed how sexuality labels come together in the case of MSM because of HIV/AIDS. In their critique of the term MSM, Young and Meyer (2005) argued that the use of reductive labels with marginalised populations is unethical, instead proposing that researchers should aim for a deeper understanding of the meaning of sexuality.

Given the need for a stable object that everyone can agree and intervene upon, HIV prevention efforts became organised around a common understanding of the MISM category. Some scholars' very prudent analysis suggests that some form of risk categorisation may be essential for HIV surveillance, policies or prevention programmes (Aggleton, Bell, & Kelly-Hanku, 2014). Nevertheless, given that few HIV interventions today are population-wide, public health professionals should be aware of the implications of intervention strategies when employing the concept of MISM. Developing biomedical interventions such as condoms, vaccines, PreP and microbicides may require not only knowledge about behaviour but also an understanding of the socio-cultural nuances of sexuality, which current research renders unimportant. Such nuances might inform us of the ways these men are considered an at-risk population, or render others vulnerable to HIV/STI infections.

MISM as a category is also based on 'westernised' knowledge. Studies conducted in countries in East Asia, the Middle East and South America primarily utilised Western labels (e.g. 'online sex-seeking MSM'), importing notions about sexuality in particular from North American scholarship. Henrickson (2007) highlights that while the Internet allows sexual minority populations to experiment and formulate their identities in a global context, we will face challenges as long as English remains the prevailing language of the Internet. Likewise, given that access to technologies is a privilege, when MISM is applied in a Global South context, it may be primarily representing higher-class sexual minority men.

Western discourses on MISM deal with HIV/STI prevention efforts that link multiple regions under the same category and language. Contextually, the rhetorical and political pull to have a coherent category of MISM may be tied to the demands and allocations of global public health funding (e.g. significant funding by US institutions). For example, US-funded global initiatives such as 'prevention with positives' have become an integral part of HIV prevention globally. This rhetoric, for instance, is reflected in research on HIV-positive MISM in China (Wei, Lim, Guadamuz, & Koe, 2012). Likewise, MISM as a category stands not only at the juncture of public health needs and individual agency but also consumerism and neoliberalism. This juncture is shown through connotations derived from studies, which were suggestive of the importance of collaboration between health institutions and US commercial businesses for the creation of effective interventions.

Similar to Parker's (2009) argument, Huang and colleagues (2014) bring to the attention of public health researchers that Western concepts of sexual desires, identities, orientations, self-labeling, processes of negotiating femininity, masculinity and thirdness, sexual disclosure or simply 'feeling different' (p. 649) may hold different values and meanings in different contexts. HIV prevention studies may yield different results among a group of men who are perceived by researchers to hold similar characteristics to men in Western countries (Huang et al., 2014).

Global public health researchers may need to consider the tensions in which MISM as a sexuality category clashes with: (1) dominant Western categories of the biological male, homosexual, bisexual, transgender, transsexual, femme, butch, queer, etc.; (2) non-Western conceptualisations of sexualities; (3) cultural conceptualisations of sexuality which depend on sexual positioning during intercourse (e.g. penetrated, penetrative, non-penetrative, versatile); (4) socio-cultural conceptualisations of desiring men in a homosocial context, such as seeking friends, building socio-sexual capital or social support networks (as in the case of countries where sexual behaviour between people of the same sex is prohibited by law); and importantly, (5) relational factors influencing the sexual behaviour of these men.

Among the key issues which require attention is a greater sensitivity to the diverse range of men who comprise the MISM category, and the need for more accurate descriptions of sexuality as complex, multiple, fluid and embedded in social and economic contexts (Huang & Souleymanov, 2016). The concept of hybridity (Bhabha, 1994) can be informative in explaining the circulation of discourses on MISM in the globalised plane. Acknowledgement of the hybridised, transnational nature of sexuality and online technologies steers us away from problematic binaries (i.e. Western vs. non-Western, or global vs. local) that have until now framed our notions of sexuality. Through this framework, it is feasible that some western risk categories may co-exist with non-western notions of sexuality.

Finally, using an epistemological argument, we suggested that through the representation of MISM as a site of risk public health research is instrumental in the maintenance of heteronormativity, social exclusion and construction of the 'otherness' of the disreputable population. Chambon's (2013) argument on the legacy of 'othering' on the basis of the classification and categorisation practice is relevant to our understanding of epistemic violence. The existing literature illustrates that the division between normative (i.e. heterosexual) and non-normative sexualities (i.e. MISM, MSM) is a consequence of forces governing the production of true discourses on sex (Foucault, 1976) and patriarchal hegemony. The unintended effect is that these discourses can also precipitate sexual, and AIDS-related stigma because they position sex-seeking and queer people in general as problems that need to be fixed. Foucault's notion of bio-politics (Foucault, 1978) shows that deployment of the term MISM consolidates a disciplinary discourse on sexual activities among queer people, leading to the re-medicalisation of sexuality and the stigmatisation of deviance.

While we have argued for the importance of unsettling dominant discourses on MISM, in doing this we have had to contend with the limitations of our paper, which stem from: (1) our purposive sampling methodology, which is not meant to be an exhaustive review of the literature; (2) the paper's orientation towards critical theory, which may render other theoretical perspectives unrepresented; and (3) the framing of online technologies as finite, and homogeneous. Public health researchers should consider the implications of the fact that the Internet and online apps are starting to offer new spaces for queer actors to explore and re-define sexualities in a transnational context. Insights contained in this paper may take on different meanings and lend themselves to different interpretations when online technologies are gazed at through a historical lens. Nevertheless, even with these limitations, our paper builds on several insights. As we move forward, we propose the following questions for global public health researchers to consider:

(1) How do the essentialist notions of MISM hinder effective programmes, initiatives and recognition of the structural drivers of HIV?
(2) To what degree does the public health field perpetuate epistemic violence through institutionalising dominant discourses of MISM or adopt knowledge that is reflexive of the transnational dynamics of sexual minority communities, identities and cultures?
(3) What challenges do public health researchers, policy-makers and funders face regarding the conceptualisation of MISM as a hybrid cultural subject that goes beyond transnational and social boundaries and incorporates the intertwining of non-Western and Western identities, communities and the meshing of cultures, values and desires?

Implications and recommendations

We recommend that the tendency towards ethnocentric and essentialist bias in sexuality categories should be addressed in the production and mobilisation of reflexive public health knowledge that counters dominant, essentialist discourses on MISM. Corrêa et al. (2014) suggest that instead of essentialising sexuality and gender to a mere biological level in order to capture more precisely the relationship between biology, context and culture, public health research must be complexified. In particular, researchers should no longer simply adopt the values of a single culture (e.g. Western, North American) but instead must work out values in the midst of complexity and diversity. Bringing this reflexive process into public health practice will have an effect on cross-cultural sensitivity in public health programming and research endeavours.

Furthermore, we encourage public health professionals to: (1) adopt procedures that recognise the wide variability of experiences and presentations of sexual minority populations who seek sex online; (2) establish channels of communication with communities participating in research in order to familiarise oneself with the backgrounds and values of research participants; (3) provide opportunities for participants to describe how they experience their cultural backgrounds and sexual identities; (4) emphasise the strengths of sexual minority cultures when discussing their differences in relation to heterosexual populations; (5) explore relational factors that influence these men to seek risky sex online; and (6) make use of indigenous, critical and emancipatory methodologies (e.g. ethnography, critical theory) to improve cross-cultural sensitivity. Such reflexivity may challenge the values of public health practitioners and promote the development of anti-oppressive public health practices.

Before the category of MISM crystallises, there should be an attempt by public health researchers and investment from funders to move beyond quantitative methodologies. Additionally, there should be a call for the critique of hierarchies between western and non-western knowledge systems, and a greater awareness of the transnational dynamics of sexual minority communities, identities, histories and cultures. Reflexivity, as a tool, should be put forward to encourage researchers to stand in a self-critical position to raise questions about how knowledge in public health is produced and how relations of power are exercised through the process of knowledge production (D'Cruz, Gillingham, & Melendez, 2007). Reflexivity may prevent epistemic violence and uncover the potential for social justice. Social justice in a globalised world can be achieved by adopting a commitment to practices that 'create spaces within the culture of domination' (hooks, 2004, pp. 155–156) and bring back into existence previously subjugated knowledge(s). This effort will give voice to sexual minority communities and populations whose ways of knowing and being have been situated outside the boundaries of mainstream society.

Notes

1. 'MISM' is used as an acronym in this paper, primarily for the sake of convenience. The use of the essentialist term MISM in this article is not meant to imply the appropriateness of applying this construct to people in non-Westernised cultures. We also acknowledge that different authors utilised a variety of sexuality labels: 'MISM', 'Internet-Using MSM', 'MSM who use Internet for social and sexual networking' and 'MSM app users' among many others.
2. Epistemology is the theory of knowledge, which attempts to answer questions about what should count as legitimate knowledge, and what approaches are appropriate for gaining this knowledge. Epistemic violence, according to Spivak (2005), refers to a discursive act of disqualifying the knowledge and voices of a marginalised group within Western context.

Disclosure statement

No potential conflict of interest was reported by the authors.

References

Adam, P. C. G., Murphy, D. A., & de Wit, J. B. F. (2011). When do online sexual fantasies become reality? The contribution of erotic chatting via the Internet to sexual risk-taking in gay and other men who have sex with men. *Health Education Research, 26*, 506–515. doi:10.1093/her/cyq085

Agger, B. (1991). Critical theory, poststructuralism, postmodernism: Their sociological relevance. *Annual Review of Sociology, 17*, 105–131. Retrieved from http://www.jstor.org/stable/2083337.

Aggleton, P., Bell, S. A., & Kelly-Hanku, A. (2014). 'Mobile men with money': HIV prevention and the erasure of difference. *Global Public Health, 9*, 257–270. doi:10.1080/17441692.2014.889736

Bauermeister, J. A., Carballo-Diéguez, A., Ventuneac, A., & Dolezal, C. (2009). Assessing motivations to engage in intentional condomless anal intercourse in HIV-risk contexts ('Bareback Sex') among men who have sex with men. *AIDS Education and Prevention, 21*, 156–168. doi:10.1521/aeap.2009.21.2.156

Bhabha, H. (1994). *The location of culture*. New York, NY: Routledge.

Blackwell, C., Birnholtz, J., & Abbott, C. (2015). Seeing and being seen: Co-situation and impression formation using Grindr, a location-aware gay dating app. *New Media & Society, 17*, 1117–1136. doi:10.1177/1461444814521595

Blas, M. M., Menacho, L. A., Alva, I. E., Cabello, R., & Orellana, E. R. (2013). Motivating men who have sex with men to get tested for HIV through the Internet and mobile phones: A qualitative study. *PloS One*, *8*. doi:10.1371/journal.pone.0054012

Brown, G., Maycock, B., & Burns, S. (2005). Your picture is your bait: Use and meaning of cyberspace among gay men. *The Journal of Sex Research*, *42*, 63–73. Retrieved from http://www.ncbi.nlm.nih.gov/pubmed/15795806.

Bull, S. S., McFarlane, M., & Rietmeijer, C. A. (2001). HIV and sexually transmitted infection risk behaviors among men seeking sex with men on-line. *American Journal of Public Health*, *91*, 988–989. doi:10.2105/AJPH.91.6.988

Chambon, A. (2013). Recognising the other, understanding the other: A brief history of social work and Otherness. *Nordic Social Work Research*, *3*, 120–129. doi:10.1080/2156857X.2013.835137

Corrêa, S., de la Dehesa, R., & Parker, R. (2014). Science, technology and sexuality: Biopolitics, medicalization, and resistance. In S. Corrêa, R. de la Dehesa, & R. Parker (Eds.), *Sexuality and politics: Regional dialogues from the Global South* (pp. 69–92). Rio de Janeiro: Sexuality Policy Watch. Retrieved from www.sxpolitics.org/sexuality-and-politics/volume2.html.

Davis, M., Hart, G., Bolding, G., Sherr, L., & Elford, J. (2006). Sex and the Internet: Gay men, risk reduction and serostatus. *Culture, Health & Sexuality*, *8*, 161–174. doi:10.1080/13691050500526126

D'Cruz, H., Gillingham, P., & Melendez, S. (2007). Reflexivity, its meanings and relevance for social work: A critical review of the literature. *British Journal of Social Work*, *37*, 73–90. doi:10.1093/bjsw/bcl001

van Dijk, T. A. (2008). Critical discourse analysis. In D. Schiffrin, D. Tannen, & H. E. Hamilton (Eds.), *The handbook of discourse analysis*. (pp. 349–371). Oxford: Blackwell.

Dowsett, G. W. (2015). 'And next, just for your enjoyment!': Sex, technology and the constitution of desire. *Culture, Health & Sexuality*, *17*, 527–539. doi:10.1080/13691058.2014.961170

Fairclough, N. (1992). Discourse and text: Linguistic and intertextual analysis within discourse analysis. *Discourse & Society*, *3*, 193–217. doi:10.1177/0957926592003002004

Foucault, M. (1976). *The history of sexuality, Volume 1: An Introduction*. London: Allen Lane.

Foucault, M. (1978). *The birth of biopolitics: Lectures at the Collège de France, 1978–1979*. New York, NY: Palgrave Macmillan.

Gee, P. J. (2011). *Discourse analysis: An introduction to theory and method*. New York, NY: Routledge.

Grov, C., Breslow, A. S., Newcomb, M. E., Rosenberger, J. G., & Bauermeister, J. A. (2014). Gay and bisexual men's use of the Internet: Research from the 1990s through 2013. *The Journal of Sex Research*, *51*, 390–409. doi:10.1080/00224499.2013.871626

Heloo, B. (2010). Sexuality, HIV and AIDS: Putting prevention in the hand of women issues, challenges and the way forward. Paper presented at the African Regional Dialogues on Sexuality and Geopolitics, Lagos, Nigeria, October 5–6.

Henrickson, M. (2007). Reaching out, hooking up: Lavender netlife in a New Zealand study. *Sexuality Research & Social Policy*, *4*, 38–49. Retrieved from http://link.springer.com/article/10.1525%2Fsrsp.2007.4.2.38#/page-1.

Hirshfield, S., Chiasson, M. A., Joseph, H., Scheinmann, R., Johnson, W. D., Remien, R. H., ... Margolis, A. D. (2012). An online randomized controlled trial evaluating HIV prevention digital media interventions for men who have sex with men. *PloS One*, *7*, e46252. doi:10.1371/journal.pone.0046252

hooks, b. (2004). Choosing the margin as a space of radical openness. In S. Harding (Ed.), *The feminist standpoint theory reader: Intellectual and practical controversies* (pp. 153–160). London: Routledge.

Huang, L., Nehl, E. J., Lin, L., Meng, G., Liu, Q., Ross, M. W., & Wong, F. Y. (2014). Sociodemographic and sexual behavior characteristics of an online MSM sample in Guangdong, China. *AIDS Care*, *26*, 648–652. doi:dx.doi.org/10.1080/09540121.2013.844760

Huang, Y., & Souleymanov, R. (2016). Rethinking epistemological debates and transnationalism of sexuality between the west and Taiwan: Implications for social workers. *British Journal of Social Work*, *46*, 98–114. doi:10.1093/bjsw/bcu067

Klein, H. (2009). Sexual orientation, drug use preference during sex, and HIV risk practices and preferences among men who specifically seek unprotected sex partners via the Internet. *International Journal of Environmental Research and Public Health, 6*, 1620–1632. doi:10.3390/ijerph6051620

Ko, N.-Y., Koe, S., Lee, H.-C., Yen, C.-F., Ko, W.-C., & Hsu, S.-T. (2012). Online sex seeking, substance use, and risky behaviors in Taiwan: Results from the 2010 Asia Internet MSM sex survey. *Archives of Sexual Behavior, 41*, 1273–1282. doi:10.1007/s10508-012-9908-8

Krakower, D. S., Mimiaga, M. J., Rosenberger, J. G., Novak, D. S., Mitty, J. A., White, J. M., & Mayer, K. H. (2012). Limited awareness and low immediate uptake of pre exposure prophylaxis among men who have sex with men using an Internet social networking site. *PloS One, 7*, e33119. doi:10.1371/journal.pone.0033119

Lehmiller, J. J., & Ioerger, M. (2014). Social networking smartphone applications and sexual health outcomes among men who have sex with men. *PloS One, 9*, e86603. doi:10.1371/journal.pone.0086603

Levine, D., & Klausner, J. D. (2005). Lessons learned from tobacco control: A proposal for public health policy initiatives to reduce the consequences of high-risk sexual behavior among men who have sex with men and use the Internet. *Sexuality Research and Social Policy, 2*, 51–58. doi:10.1525/srsp.2005.2.1.51

Liau, A., Millett, G., & Marks, G. (2006). Meta-analytic examination of online sex seeking and sexual risk behavior among men who have sex with men. *Sexually Transmitted Diseases, 33*, 576–584. doi:10.1097/01.olq.0000204710.35332.c5

Malu, M. K., Challenor, R., Theobald, N., & Barton, S. E. (2004). Seeking and engaging in Internet sex: A survey of patients attending genitourinary medicine clinics in Plymouth and in London. *International Journal of STD & AIDS, 15*, 720–724. doi:10.1258/0956462042395230

Matarelli, S. A. (2013). Sexual sensation seeking and Internet sex-seeking of Middle Eastern men who have sex with men. *Archives of Sexual Behavior, 42*, 1285–1297. doi:10.1007/s10508-013-0073-5

Mustanski, B., Lyons, T., & Garcia, S. C. (2011). Internet use and sexual health of young men who have sex with men: A mixed-methods study. *Archives of Sexual Behavior, 40*, 289–300. doi:10.1007/s10508-009-9596-1

Parker, R. (2009). Sexuality, culture and society: Shifting paradigms in sexuality research. *Culture, Health & Sexuality, 11*, 251–266. doi:10.1080/13691050701606941

Race, K. (2014). Speculative pragmatism and intimate arrangements: Online hook-up devices in gay life. *Culture, Health & Sexuality, 3*, 1–16. doi:10.1080/13691058.2014.930181

Rhodes, S. D., Vissman, A. T., Stowers, J., Miller, C., McCoy, T. P., Hergenrather, K. C., ... Eng, E. (2011). A CBPR partnership increases HIV testing among men who have sex with men (MSM): Outcome findings from a pilot test of the CyBER/testing Internet intervention. *Health Education & Behavior, 38*, 311–320. doi:10.1177/1090198110379572

Rogers, R., Malancharuvil-Berkes, E., Mosley, M., Hui, D., & Joseph, G. O. G. (2005). Critical discourse analysis in education: A review of the literature. *Review of Educational Research, 75*, 365–416. doi:10.3102/00346543075003365

Rosser, B. R. S., & Horvath, K. (2007). Ethical issue in Internet-based HIV primary prevention research. In S. Loue & E. C. Pike (Eds.), *Case studies in ethics and HIV research* (pp. 95–102). Cleveland, OH: Springer.

Rosser, B. R. S., Wilkerson, J. M., Smolenski, D. J., Oakes, J. M., Konstan, J., Horvath, K. J., ... Morgan, R. (2011). The future of Internet-based HIV prevention: A report on key findings from the Men's INTernet (MINTS-I, II) sex studies. *AIDS and Behavior, 15*, 91–100. doi:10.1007/s10461-011-9910-5

Saxton, P., Dickson, N., & Hughes, A. (2013). Who is omitted from repeated offline HIV behavioural surveillance among MSM? Implications for interpreting trends. *AIDS and Behavior, 17*, 3133–3144. doi:10.1007/s10461-013-0485-1

Spivak, G. C. (2005). Scattered speculations on the subaltern and the popular. *Postcolonial Studies: Culture, Politics, Economy, 8*, 475–486. doi:10.1080/13688790500375132

Wei, C., Lim, S. H., Guadamuz, T. E., & Koe, S. (2012). HIV disclosure and sexual transmission behaviors among an Internet sample of HIV-positive men who have sex with men in Asia: Implications for prevention with positives. *AIDS and Behavior*, *16*, 1970–1978. doi:10.1007/s10461-011-0105-x

White, J. M., Mimiaga, M. J., Reisner, S. L., & Mayer, K. H. (2012). HIV sexual risk behavior among black men who meet other men on the Internet for sex. *Journal of Urban Health*, *90*, 464–481. doi:10.1007/s11524-012-9701-y

Wilkerson, J. M., Smolenski, D. J., Horvath, K. J., Danilenko, G. P., & Rosser, B. R. S. (2010). Online and offline sexual health-seeking patterns of HIV-negative men who have sex with men. *AIDS and Behavior*, *14*, 1362–1370. doi:10.1007/s10461-010-9794-9

Ybarra, M. L., & Bull, S. S. (2007). Current trends in Internet-and cell phone-based HIV prevention and intervention programs. *Current HIV/AIDS Reports*, *4*, 201–207. doi:10.1007/s11904-007-0029-2

Young, R. M., & Meyer, I. H. (2005). The trouble with 'MSM' and 'WSW': Erasure of the sexual-minority person in public health discourse. *American Journal of Public Health*, *95*, 1144–1149.

Young, S. D., Szekeres, G., & Coates, T. (2013). The relationship between online social networking and sexual risk behaviors among men who have sex with men (MSM). *Plos One*, *8*(5), e62271. doi:10.1371/journal.pone.0062271

Zou, H., Wu, Z., Yu, J., Li, M., Ablimit, M., Li, F., & Poundstone, K. (2013). Internet facilitated, voluntary counseling and testing (VCT) clinic-based HIV testing among men who have sex with men in China. *PloS One*, *8*, e51919. doi:10.1371/journal.pone.0051919

From marginal to marginalised: The inclusion of men who have sex with men in global and national AIDS programmes and policy

Tara McKay[ID]

ABSTRACT

In the last decade, gay men and other men who have sex with men (msm) have come to the fore of global policy debates about AIDS prevention. In stark contrast to programmes and policy during the first two decades of the epidemic, which largely excluded msm outside of the Western countries, the Joint United Nations Programme on HIV/AIDS now identifies gay men and other msm as 'marginalized but not marginal' to the global response. Drawing on archival data and five waves of United Nations Country Progress Reports on HIV/AIDS (2001–2012), this paper examines the productive power of international organisations in the development and diffusion of the msm category, and considers how international organisations have shaped the interpretation of msm in national policies and programmes. These data show that the increasing separation of sexual identity and sexual behaviour at the global level helped to construct notions of risk and disease that were sufficiently broad to accommodate the diverse interests of global policy-makers, activists, and governments. However, as various international and national actors have attempted to develop prevention programmes for msm, the failure of the msm category to map onto lived experience is increasingly apparent.

Introduction

Categorisation and enumeration of HIV infections and sexual behaviours are among the primary ways that researchers, policy-makers, and international organisations 'see' AIDS (Biruk, 2012). The epidemic and responses to it are ripe with categories, typologies, and classification systems: epidemic patterns, transmission routes, risk groups, and behaviours. These categories are, in part, an attempt to regularise information, to allow comparisons across time and space, and, hopefully, to direct limited resources to where they are most needed. However, AIDS cases, risk groups, and sexual behaviours are not just out there waiting to be counted, categorised, and measured. At the most basic level, what we know about AIDS – in the form of statistics on prevalence and incidence, and even routes of transmission – is strongly influenced by where, among whom and how hard governments, researchers, and clinicians look for the disease (Biehl, 2007; Buckley, 2008; Treichler, 1999).

International organisations also play a substantial role in this process by directing attention and resources to some issues and not others. As political scientist Martha Finnemore (1999) writes, international organisations have immense productive power as they 'define shared international tasks (like "development"), create and define new categories of actors (like "refugee"), create new interests for actors (like "promoting human rights"), and transfer models of political organisation around the world (like markets and democracy)' (p. 669). Thus, an organisation's adoption of 'development' or 'refugee' or, in our case for this special issue, gay men or 'men who have sex with men' (msm) [1] as specific categories of concern signals a need for policies to address such issues or populations. These signals have been shown to reconfigure the policy preferences and activities of governments (Hafner-Burton & Tsutsui, 2005), NGOs on the ground (Watkins, Swidler, & Hannan, 2012), and other donor organisations (Shiffman, 2006). Yet, few studies have examined the organisational factors that shape the articulation of new categories or the downstream effects of changes in the way that an organisation conceptualises categories over time.

This paper examines the productive power of international organisations in the early development and diffusion of a category of individuals that came to be called 'msm' in global AIDS programmes and policy using archival data from World Health Organization's (WHO) Global Programme on AIDS (GPA) and its successor, the Joint United Nations Programme on HIV/AIDS (UNAIDS). While other work has considered the emergence and consequences of employing the category of msm in community-led prevention efforts, research, and public health (Aggleton & Parker, 2015; Boellstorff, 2011; Young & Meyer, 2005), this study aims to capture how msm have been understood and employed by international organisations, especially during the early years of the epidemic before the msm category had solidified. Using data from biennial UN Country Progress Reports, I extend this historical analysis to capture the ways that the institutional response to AIDS has shaped the interpretation and inclusion of msm in national policies and programmes. Ultimately, I demonstrate that the inclusion of gay men and other msm is intertwined with the emergence and expansion of the msm category, which creates opportunities for inclusion in policy at the same time that it complicates data collection and prevention activities on the ground. In the next section I introduce the data in more detail, followed by an historical analysis of how the category of msm emerged and was employed within the institutional contexts of the GPA and UNAIDS.

Data

This paper draws on two primary sources of data in order to examine the construction and downstream effects of early global policies targeting gay men and other msm. First, I employ archival data from WHO, GPA, and UNAIDS to examine how international organisations have conceptualised and navigated barriers to recognition of homosexual, gay and bisexual, and msm as a global AIDS priority. In the archival data, I pay particular attention to the various annual reports produced by WHO, GPA, and UNAIDS, including their global strategies, budget reports, and planning projects. I also examine reports from stakeholder meetings, commissioned research and literature reviews, and consensus statements and policy recommendations specifically concerning homosexual or gay men, bisexual men, and other msm. These texts provide insight on the public face of GPA and UNAIDS as well as on internal discussions that resulted – or failed to result – in policy recommendations regarding gay and bisexual men and other msm through the mid-2000s. I supplement archival data with insights from key informant interviews collected for a larger project on the inclusion of msm in global AIDS policy. Additionally, beginning in the mid- and late-2000s, several new organisations, including two of the largest funders of HIV prevention and treatment, the Global Fund to Fight HIV, TB, and Malaria (Global Fund) and the US President's Emergency Plan For AIDS Relief (PEPFAR), frequently worked in concert with UNAIDS and explicitly identified msm as a priority in their HIV policies and programmes. Thus, their conceptions and utilisation of the msm category are discussed briefly towards the end of paper; however the analysis focuses on the effects of early efforts to establish gay men and other msm as a priority before msm was a widely adopted category of concern.

Second, I draw on five waves of HIV/AIDS UNGASS Country Progress Reports ($N = 728$) to examine the downstream effects of early global policies targeting gay men and other msm. In 2001 the UN General Assembly convened a Special Session on HIV/AIDS (UNGASS). At this special session, 189 UN member countries recognised and agreed to meet specific goals for the provision of HIV prevention and treatment and agreed to prepare a follow-up report documenting the country's progress towards these goals in 2003 and 2006. Continued biennial follow-up reports were agreed to at the second UNGASS meeting in 2006. From 2003 to 2012, 196 out of 201 recognised countries and territories submitted at least one report. The mean number of reports submitted per country was 3.6.

For each report, governments were requested to supply data on specific indicators requested by UNAIDS and to write a narrative report describing the status of the epidemic and the national response. I coded report narratives to reflect the inclusion of gay men and other msm in national HIV prevention programmes and policy. The coding categories differentiate between countries that explicitly identify msm as a programming priority and those that do not as well as the extent to which the country engages msm along two dimensions: epidemiological surveillance activities and prevention programmes. Countries were grouped into three categories: (1) no acknowledgement of msm as an HIV programming concern and no reported surveillance or prevention targeting msm; (2) acknowledgement of msm as HIV programming concern, a small number (e.g. one or two) of prevention programmes targeting subpopulations of msm may be in planning phase or only serving a single municipality, and national surveillance activities of msm are passive, geographically limited or in planning phase; and (3) acknowledgement of msm as HIV programming concern, an active surveillance programme that regularly (e.g. at least every three years) collects prevalence data among msm, and state-sponsored prevention programmes targeting msm are in place beyond pilot stage and available in more than one municipality or subnational unit of administration. The three categories can generally be conceived as composing an ordinal scale from 1 'No prioritisation', to 2 'Weak prioritisation', to 3 'Strong prioritisation'. For further discussion of coding and examples from the Country Progress Reports, see Appendix A in online supplemental material.

In the next section, I turn to the historical analysis of the construction and institutionalisation of early global policies targeting gay men and other msm.

An epidemic divided

In 1985 WHO drafted the first global strategy for the prevention and control of AIDS and in February, 1987, established the Special Programme on AIDS – renamed the GPA in 1988 – under the leadership of Dr. Jonathan Mann. As part of its mandate, GPA was to direct a 'coherent and rational plan for prevention and control of AIDS' and provide technical and financial assistance to countries for developing a comprehensive national AIDS programme for the provision of information and education, health and social services, humane care, and epidemic monitoring (GPA, 1988b, p. 6). In its first year of operation, GPA had a substantial influence on the global response, providing technical, and financial assistance to over 130 countries for the development of national AIDS programmes. Over the next four years, the programme quickly became the largest programme at WHO in terms of both total staff and budget (Gibbons, 1990; GPA, 1997).

In contrast to this massive and rapid response, GPA directed limited attention to homosexual and bisexual men in global AIDS prevention and policy. Under GPA leadership, no guidelines for the development of surveillance or prevention programmes targeting gay, bisexual, or other msm were developed by WHO. As I demonstrate below, the organisational structure and ideology of GPA should have facilitated the inclusion of gay and bisexual men in the global response. Yet, throughout the late 1980s, GPA's emphasis on distinct 'patterns' of transmission to differentiate sexual transmission among homosexual and bisexual men in developed countries from sexual transmission among heterosexual men and women in developing – especially African – contexts created a substantial barrier to recognising the potential for same-sex sexual transmission in developing contexts. The decision-making structure of GPA and growing tensions between GPA, WHO leadership, and member states during the early 1990s further contributed to GPA's indifference to mounting evidence of the importance of same-sex sexual transmission to HIV epidemics in developing countries and the need to extend surveillance and prevention to address new infections among gay men and other msm. Facing a crisis of authority, GPA actively avoided the inclusion of homosexual and bisexual men in global and national policy recommendations due to concerns about 'cultural sensitivity' and to promote government commitment to other programmes.

Notably, several aspects of the organisation and structure of GPA should have facilitated the inclusion of gay and bisexual men in the global response. First, in order to facilitate a rapid response to new information and bypass political and ideological opposition from states, GPA had been specifically designed to have substantial autonomy over organisational policies and practices during its first few years, especially in the areas of human rights and NGO participation. Respect for the human rights of individuals and groups affected by HIV and AIDS, including gay men, was deemed 'vital' to the success the national implementation of the global strategy (GPA, 1988a), a point which Mann underscored frequently in his reports to the World Health Assembly, the UN General Assembly, and at the International AIDS Conferences (Mann, 1988). Additionally, GPA sought to support civil society responses to local epidemics, especially in country contexts where political will to address AIDS was weak. To accomplish this, GPA invited the International

Lesbian and Gay Association and other human rights and AIDS NGOs to participate in the various HIV/AIDS conferences organised by WHO and sponsored the first international meeting of AIDS Service Organisations held in Vienna in 1989. GPA also commissioned research on structural impediments to NGO development and functioning at the country level and rerouted funds directly to NGOs, including lesbian and gay organisations, instead of passing them through government programmes where they 'risked becoming hostage to national and local politics' (Mann & Kay, 1991, p. S227).

Despite political barriers to doing so, GPA's Social and Behavioural Research Unit also worked to expand research on sexual behaviour (Carballo, 1990; Carballo, Cleland, Carael, & Albrecht, 1989). A substantial amount of this research was devoted to measuring HIV-related knowledge, attitudes, and behaviour among heterosexual populations in developing contexts (Cleland & Ferry, 1995). However, the unit also maintained an independent interest in expanding research on homosexuality, bisexuality, and HIV/AIDS around the world. In May 1989, GPA held the first international consultation on HIV prevention among gay, bisexual, and other msm with presentations by researchers and prevention workers from developed and developing countries (Dowsett, 1989; Parker, Guimarães, & Struchiner, 1989). From this meeting, GPA developed an ambitious research programme to examine how gay men and their communities were responding to the epidemic by adopting safer sex practices. The WHO Homosexual Response Studies, as they were called, integrated and in some cases funded a set of national studies carried out in seven countries, including five developed countries – the United Kingdom, Austria, the Netherlands, Greece, Israel – and two developing countries – Costa Rica and Brazil. A key element in these studies was the use of a common study design and survey instrument with 'common reference to the physical aspects of sexual behaviour' that would facilitate comparisons across national contexts with 'different cultural manifestations of homosexual behaviour' (Coxon et al., 1990, p. 62). The studies also included qualitative and ethnographic research on cultural variation and local community responses to the epidemic (Parker & Carballo, 1990; Parker et al., 1989; Parker, Herdt, & Carballo, 1991). As a group, the studies found a promising decrease in receptive anal sex with casual partners and an increase in condom use among gay and bisexual men across the study sites (GPA, 1992a, p. 47).

Notably, this work served as an impetus for emerging discussions around sexual categories through the researchers' attention to the social contexts in which sexual behaviour occurs and their insistence on the need for better qualitative data on variations in sexual behaviour, meanings, and identity (Coxon & Carballo, 1989; Coxon et al., 1990; Parker & Carballo, 1990; Parker et al., 1991). Elements of the Homosexual Response Studies are documented in the early social science literature on HIV/AIDS, discussed in detail in GPA's 1991 Progress Report (GPA, 1992a, pp. 47–49), and were presented at the 1993 International AIDS Conference (Coxon, 1993). However, as many of those involved in this work lament, GPA never published a formal report of the proceedings of the 1989 consultation or on the results of the commissioned research despite repeated promises to do so (Interview, 18 Nov 2014; see also Parker, Khan, & Aggleton, 1998, p. 334). GPA's failure to publish a report on the proceedings of the consultation on HIV prevention among gay and bisexual men stands out against the 67 other policy-related consultations conducted by GPA from 1986 to 1989 on a range of issues, including several where data were scant or the proposed solutions were politically fraught, such as the imposition of bans on international travel of HIV positive individuals, requirements for the notification of sexual partners, prevention in prisons, and the presence of HIV positive individuals in sports. Researchers present at the time attribute GPA's failure to publish the proceedings to the highly controversial and politicised nature of discussions around homosexual behaviour and gay communities at the time (Interview, 18 Nov 2014; see also Parker et al., 1998, p. 334; Boellstorff, 2011, p. 292).

In December 1992, GPA held a second informal stakeholder on HIV among 'behaviourally bisexual men'[2] (GPA, 1992b). Like other GPA stakeholder meetings, the objectives of the meeting on bisexuality and HIV were to take stock of existing research and identify examples of successful prevention activities in order to provide policy guidance. The research presented at the meeting drew on experiences from both developed and developing countries, including portraits of HIV infection and prevention activities targeting behaviourally bisexual men in Australia, Brazil, Costa Rica, India, Nigeria, Singapore, the United States, and the United Kingdom. Throughout the meeting, the emerging tension between sexual identity and sexual behaviour was apparent as researchers voiced concerns that sexual behaviour among bisexual men – defined as 'men who have had partners of both sexes over a recent period of time (in the last five years or less)' – may not 'coincide entirely with … sexual preference or bisexual identity' (GPA, 1992b, p. 2). Further, participants agreed that men who were active in a gay community were likely to be quite different from men who do not identify as homosexual and therefore were not reached through 'gay channels', such as men who engage in same-sex sex in public venues or single-sex contexts, men who are in primary relationships with women, and young men who are engaged in prostitution (GPA, 1992b, pp. 2, 9). Researchers were particularly concerned with the likelihood of underestimating both same-sex sexual behaviours due to underreporting caused by prevailing social and cultural attitudes and by the exclusion of homosexual and bisexual men in sentinel surveillance of antenatal clinics, a primary mode of data collection in many developing contexts. The consensus from the consultation on bisexual behaviour was that 'the contribution of bisexual behaviour to HIV transmission is certain to be greater than the existing data indicate' (GPA, 1992b, p. 3) given nonmarginal rates of sex with male and female partners among msm in contexts with available data and that an effective global response to AIDS would require a range of targeted, community-based interventions for and by msm. At the same time, the report published on the meeting provides rather weak guidance to future policy and programmes on the need to incorporate behaviourally bisexual men:

> [I]t remains difficult to assess the full public health implications of bisexual practices and specifically, the extent to which these practices contribute to HIV transmission in different regions and contexts. This reflects limitations in existing behavioural and epidemiological studies, which either do not look at homosexual practices at all or, when they do, aggregate men who have sex with men into a single risk category. (GPA, 1992b, pp. 9–10)

This ambivalent conclusion provides insight into one of the key organisational elements that impeded GPA from developing programmes and policy targeting homosexual and bisexual in the global response. The decision-making structure of GPA, which relied heavily on small groups of experts who could be mobilised on short notice to produce a rapid response to new information or events that could be widely disseminated (Mann & Kay, 1991, p. S224), was particularly problematic for policy issues where consensus was not easily established given a lack of research. In the late 1980s and early 1990s, this was decidedly the case for recommendations for preventing HIV among homosexual and bisexual men. Two years prior to the stakeholder meeting on HIV among behaviourally bisexual men, GPA commissioned a review of research on this topic, which similarly found a lack of information to be a key problem for making authoritative policy recommendations:

> [O]ur knowledge bisexual behaviour in relation to HIV transmission is very limited... Overall, available evidence derives from somewhat disparate and isolated studies which have not arisen from any unified set of concerns or research agenda. It is therefore difficult to build up any authoritative picture of bisexual behaviour and inferences about its role in HIV transmission must at present be tentative. (Boulton & Weatherburn, 1990)

In the absence of data to empirically justify a policy position, GPA continued to make no specific recommendations regarding the inclusion of homosexual or bisexual men in AIDS programmes and policy.[3]

Instead, in the 1992 *Global AIDS Strategy*, WHO used vague, coded language in policy recommendations, such as the need to provide 'frank messages about sexual transmission' (WHO, 1992, p. 7), and fell back on its widely disseminated conceptions of the epidemic that emphasised a divide between North America, Europe, and Australia from developing contexts, especially sub-Saharan Africa (Chin & Mann, 1988; Chin, Sato, & Mann, 1990; Mann, Chin, Piot, & Quinn, 1988). While brief attention is paid to legal and other barriers 'that would hinder people from receiving and acting on prevention messages (e.g. the enforcement of laws against mutually voluntary sexual activity between adult males)' (11), the prevention concerns of msm are otherwise unaddressed in the 1992 *Strategy*.

WHO and GPA's persistent assertion of an epidemic divide is a prominent feature of several early documents disseminated by WHO and is present in GPA's (then the Control Programme on AIDS) first global strategy for HIV prevention, which reads:

> Two 'classic' epidemiological patterns have been recognized in the developed and developing world. In the developed world, transmission is most important among male homosexuals and bisexuals and intravenous drug users ... In parts of the developing world (e.g., Africa), heterosexual transmission dominates the epidemiological scene. (CPA, 1986, p. 3)

In the 1992 *Strategy*, consideration of homosexual transmission is further minimised and presented as perhaps no longer even relevant in Western contexts. In the update on the status of the epidemic, it reads:

> Although the first reported cases were among homosexual men in a few industrialized countries, it soon became clear that this was an epidemic of much greater scope ... In the world as a whole, heterosexual intercourse has rapidly become the dominant mode of transmission of the virus ... Homosexual transmission, on the other hand, has remained significant in North America, Australasia and northern Europe, although even in these areas heterosexual transmission is showing the fastest rate of increase. (6)

GPA's presentation of a 'classic' division of prevention needs in the West from prevention needs in developing contexts and minimisation of the importance of same-sex sexual transmission in both developed and developing contexts and has had durable, long-term effects on prevention. As Esacove (2010) demonstrates of Malawi, AIDS programming in sub-Saharan Africa has consistently promoted heteronormative and 'modern' (read: Western) understandings of sex and relationships, emphasising condom use for penile-vaginal sex, monogamy, gender equality within loving sexual partnerships, and, at their most prescriptive, abstinence in the absence of marriage. Such programming has left little room to discuss diversity of sexual desire and behaviour and still less room for same-sex sexualities in countries like Malawi.

GPA's reification of an epidemic divide that refuted the presence of gay men and other msm in developing contexts was grounded in an interpretation of epidemiological data – data that were increasingly recognised as inadequate in its own stakeholder consultations – that highlighted the importance of heterosexual transmission in developing contexts; however, the epidemic divide also served another purpose. Outside of the consensus meeting, GPA faced substantial hurdles in disseminating programme priorities to individual countries due to a lack of enforcement power. While GPA had a clear mandate to establish a *unified* international response, this mandate was in tension with the necessity to respect state sovereignty. The primacy of national integrity and decision-making within WHO ensured that each country remained free to 'develop its own detailed programme' (GPA, 1988b, p. 3) – or not. As such, national AIDS strategies could deviate dramatically from GPA policy recommendations and had substantial latitude to avoid socially or politically contentious groups or behaviours such as homosexuals and same-sex sex. Throughout the late 1980s, a handful of countries, including a few African countries believed to have very high rates of HIV infection, refused to establish a national AIDS strategy all together. Thus, GPA's emphasis on the divided epidemic and use of vague language that grouped *all* sexual transmission of HIV in the same policy recommendation served as a means to ensure government commitment to other programmes by dropping explicit references to sexual behaviours and marginalised groups. Later, as tensions emerged between GPA, member states, and the WHO Regional Directors and Director-General (Godlee, 1994; Orkin, 1990), GPA increasingly tempered its demands on national AIDS programmes despite GPA's growing awareness of the importance of same-sex sexual transmission to HIV epidemics in developing countries, especially emerging Asian epidemics.

In sum, although several organisational factors ought to have facilitated the inclusion of gay men and other msm in the global response to AIDS, including the independent research interests of the Social and Behavioural Research Unit, GPA ultimately avoided taking a formal policy stance on HIV prevention among homosexual and behaviourally bisexual men throughout the late 1980s and early 1990s. They did so despite increasing awareness of high rates of infection among these groups around the world. As demonstrated above, this failure reflects barriers posed by both the organisational structure of GPA and the strategies GPA adopted to promote government commitment to other AIDS programmes.

From marginal to marginalised

As donors became increasingly dissatisfied with WHO management over the early 1990s (Center for Global Development, 2009), international funding for GPA declined in 1991 for the first time since the programme's inception (GPA, 1992a, pp. 15–16). The US, GPA's largest donor, moved away from multilateral support towards administration of its own bilateral aid programmes. Meanwhile, both WHO and GPA had lost their leadership role in health and AIDS policy due to increasing competition from other organisations, especially the World Bank, UNDP and UNICEF, which established their own AIDS policies and programmes. In 1994, the six UN organisations comprising the GPA Management Committee agreed to dismantle GPA and replace it with a new organisation, the UNAIDS. The formal objectives of UNAIDS were largely similar to the GPA: to provide global leadership in response to the HIV/AIDS epidemic, toward the end of achieving global consensus on policy and programmatic approaches. Like GPA, UNAIDS was also tasked with strengthening the capacity of national governments to develop and implement comprehensive national strategies for monitoring, care, and prevention.

In contrast to GPA, however, the UNAIDS Secretariat made early moves to incorporate gay men and other msm into the global policy response. The programme's first operations report in 1995 states that 'worldwide, most infections are transmitted heterosexually, though sex between men continues to be major route of HIV spread' and insisted that 'gay men living in a community where their sexual orientation is stigmatised' were a key driver of the global epidemic because of their lack of access to 'life-saving information about safer sex' (ECOSOC, 1995, pp. 5–6). Attention to gay men and other msm continued as the programme was scaled up. In 1998, UNAIDS developed and disseminated the first technical guidelines on *AIDS and Men who have Sex with Men* which attempted to deconstruct the developed/developing divide present in HIV prevention and policy by arguing that:

> Worldwide, 5–10% of all HIV cases are due to sexual transmission between men ... *In all countries*, though, the likely extent of male-to-male sex is probably underestimated. Governments, nongovernmental organizations (NGOs) and the private sector must accept its presence and take it fully into account in AIDS prevention work. The attitude that has prevailed in some places–that 'these things don't exist (or hardly exist) in our society, so we don't need to take any action' – is both wrong and dangerous, since it is likely to ignore a significant (even if relatively small) part of the overall epidemic. (emphasis added; UNAIDS, 1998, p. 4)

Employing an inclusive understanding of msm, the 1998 UNAIDS technical guidance aimed to demonstrate the universality of same-sex sex by delineating the various populations and places where governments, NGOs, donors, and researchers might find sub groups of msm including gay-identified men and bisexually-identified men, as well as other msm who do not identify as gay for to cultural or other reasons, such as male sex workers and men having sex with other men in institutional settings (e.g. prisons). The msm category was highly mutable at this time. By 2000, when UNAIDS reissued an updated version of *AIDS and Men who have Sex with Men* (UNAIDS, 2000), the category of msm expanded to include 'transgender MSM' (p. 3). Drawing on this broad understanding of msm, UNAIDS repeatedly recommended expanding efforts to address HIV among msm 'in all countries' in policy guidelines, including the 1999 UNAIDS Report (UNAIDS, 1999), the 2001 Global Strategy Framework on HIV/AIDS (UNAIDS, 2001b) and the United Nations System Strategic Plan adopted in the same year (UN, 2001b).

However, like GPA, UNAIDS conducted its work in an inherent state of tension. On the one hand, UNAIDS was tasked with promoting global consensus on policy and programmatic approaches, while on the other hand the organisation was to respect the decisions of national policy-makers. Like most other UN bodies with the exception of the Security Council, UNAIDS had limited power to locally enforce the policies it recommended. Thus, the official position of UNAIDS on national AIDS programmes was that 'there can be *no universally valid blueprint for tackling HIV/AIDS*' (emphasis added). Rather, national AIDS programmes continued to be responsible for identifying the mode(s) of HIV transmission most relevant in the area(s) in which they conduct treatment and prevention activities and would 'need to select ... a 'package' of strategies, interventions and activities that is *best suited to its local context*, and then tailor the approaches to the needs of individuals and communities' (emphasis added, ECOSOC, 1995, para 46). While this approach was intended to promote strategies targeting local needs and concerns, in effect it created substantial latitude for national programmes to dismiss, ignore, or work around UNAIDS policy recommendations, especially those concerning populations of msm.

Dissenting states also continued to wield substantial power over the content of global AIDS policy within the broader forum of the United Nations, as demonstrated by the outcome of the 2001 United Nations General Assembly Special Session on HIV/AIDS. In 2001, the UN General Assembly convened the first ever Special Session on HIV/AIDS and establish a global agenda, the *Declaration of Commitment on HIV/AIDS* that would be adopted by all states. Among the key concerns raised at the Special Session and highlighted in the *Declaration* were the gross inequalities limiting access to treatment in the global South, the need to mainstream HIV concerns into development, poverty, and security sectors, the mobilisation of new funding resources, and the continued need for prevention activities to ensure the health and human rights of vulnerable groups.

But countries disagreed on who these vulnerable groups were and what should be done to protect them. While country delegations unanimously supported the explicit inclusion of women and children as vulnerable groups in the *Declaration*, other more stigmatised groups, such as msm, sex workers, and injection drug users were excluded from the final document. Whereas the proposed text of the *Declaration* drafted by UNAIDS Secretariat staff explicitly included the need for prevention efforts to 'target other vulnerable populations, including sex workers, drug users and men who have sex with men' (UNAIDS, 2001a, p. 5); the final *Declaration* ratified by the UN General Assembly includes no mention of gay men or other msm. Rather, the final text includes a vague and muddled prevention target 'to reduce HIV incidence for those *identifiable groups*, within *particular local contexts*, which currently have high or increasing rates of HIV infection, or which *available public health information* indicates are at the highest risk of new infection' (emphasis added; UN, 2001a, p. 7). This language ensured that states were free to continue to disregard HIV among populations of msm so long as they did not make an effort to identify or initiate surveillance among these groups.

Nonetheless, the *Declaration* encouraged a 'comprehensive approach to prevention' that included the expansion of human rights and prevention efforts among populations 'at greatest risk of and most vulnerable to new infection as indicated by such factors as ... sexual practices' (UN, 2001a, p. 10). While this language did not specifically identify gay men or msm, it remained open to interpretation, establishing enough latitude for other organisations such as the WHO to argue for the development of interventions targeting msm as a priority in follow-up reports to the UNGASS meeting (WHO, 2002). Further, the *Declaration* established universal targets for scaling up prevention and reducing infections that were endorsed by all 189 member countries. Countries were, for the first time, required to report on their progress on a number of issues including surveillance infrastructure, access to prevention and HIV testing as well as progress on enacting legal protections to prohibit discrimination of people with HIV/AIDS and vulnerable groups. The *Declaration* also established a standardised set of indicators so that efforts to increase the quantity and quality of services could be compared across states. Through these changes, countries became more accountable than ever to UNAIDS, the UN system, and their constituents. Two years later, in 2003, UNAIDS used the data from the first Country Progress Reports on the targets outlined in the 2001 *Declaration* to highlight the continued absence of msm to country-level surveillance, research, and prevention activities 'even when evidence points to the prominence of this mode of transmission in the epidemic' (UNAIDS, 2003, p. 5). By mid-2005, the UNAIDS Programme Coordinating Board contested the refusal of some countries to address HIV among msm for cultural or political reasons and recommended that 'issues such as men who have sex with men, drug use, sex work, gender vulnerability, and prison populations must be incorporated into prevention plans in all regions' (emphasis added, PCB, 2005).

The inclusion of msm in national aids programmes

By establishing standard indicators through which sex among men became visible and actionable, UNAIDS contributed to the rapid inclusion of msm into national AIDS programmes and policy in the mid- and late-2000s. Based on County Progress Reports submitted to UNAIDS per the 2001 *Declaration* and subsequent reaffirmations of

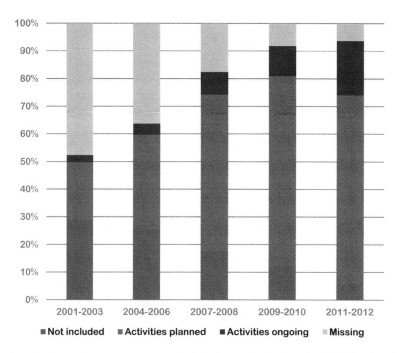

Figure 1. Percent of countries where msm are included as a priority in national AIDS policy, by level of inclusion and year.

commitment to HIV/AIDS, the number of countries that did not include msm in their national AIDS prevention programmes (no prioritisation) decreased from 29% to 6% between 2001 and 2012 (see Figure 1), while the percentage of countries that identified msm as a concern (weak prioritisation) and the percentage of countries with ongoing, widespread surveillance and prevention activities (strong prioritisation) targeting msm grew from 21% to 69% and 3% to 20%, respectively.[4]

Table 1 presents the probability that a country changed its level of prioritisation of msm for all countries and territories that submitted at least two reports from 2003 to 2012. Countries that changed status generally proceeded in an orderly fashion from no inclusion of msm to weak prioritisation of msm to strong prioritisation of msm. Slightly less than half (46%) of countries that did not prioritise msm in their first report (time t) showed evidence of weak prioritisation in a subsequent report (time $t + 1$). Occasionally, countries explicitly stated that a transition had occurred, as in the case of Tuvalu in 2012, which notes that:

> [I]n the 2010 UNGASS report men to men sex (MSM) was not identified as a risk population. In 2011, anecdotal evidence suggests that MSM is becoming prevalent. At this stage there has been no specific programmes [sic] targeted at this population. (Government of Tuvalu, 2012, p. 9)

Movement from weak to strong prioritisation was substantially more limited; only 12% of countries initially classified as weakly prioritising msm exhibited strong prioritisation in a subsequent report. Thus, while nearly all countries now identify a *need* to conduct surveillance and prevention activities, few countries are engaged in widespread surveillance and prevention activities include and target msm.

Due to changes in funding resources and/or social or political changes within countries over time, a small number of countries ($N = 5$) regressed from strong prioritisation to weak prioritisation or from weak prioritisation to no prioritisation. Romania serves as an example of a reversal. In the 2012 report the government notes that:

> [A]ccess to harm reduction programmes for groups vulnerable to HIV infection diminished, in 2011 more than half of the service providers closed their operations due to lack of funds and no future prospects for reopening the following period of time. Despite consistent advocacy efforts to MoH [Ministry of Health], no funds were allocated for prevention programmes for vulnerable groups, in the context of HIV increase [sic] among IDUs and MSMs. (Government of Romania, 2012, p. 7)

This event is foreshadowed in Romania's 2010 report, which states that:

Table 1. Transition probability matrix for prioritisation of HIV among msm for all countries.

Prioritisation (t)		1 N	1 (%)	2 N	2 (%)	3 N	3 (%)	Total N	Total (%)
(1)	No prioritisation	67	(54)	56	(46)	0	(0)	123	(100)
(2)	Weak prioritisation	3	(1)	243	(87)	35	(12)	281	(100)
(3)	Strong prioritisation	0	(0)	2	(2)	78	(98)	80	(100)
Total		70	(15)	301	(62)	113	(23)	484	(100)

Note: Countries that did not submit any report and countries that only submitted one report are excluded from the matrix.
Source: UNGASS Country Progress Reports on HIV/AIDS.

[w]hile the HIV/AIDS treatment is one of the key success stories of Romania in HIV field [sic], the achievements recorded in prevention field are very fragile, because most of the HIV prevention programmes are funded exclusively from international grants and they have limited financial support from Romanian governmental authorities. (Government of Romania, 2010, p. 9)

msm and its discontents

The discrepancy between countries' recognition of the need to target msm and actual practice can be explained in part by the very ambiguity of the msm category. For UNAIDS, the ambiguity of the msm category was an asset in getting national AIDS programmes to incorporate msm into national AIDS programmes. However, for HIV policy and prevention programmes this ambiguity creates several practical concerns. As new national and international actors have joined discussions around HIV prevention and policy targeting msm, understandings of who constitutes msm and ideas about what should be done to reduce HIV infection among msm are increasingly called into question. The American Foundation for AIDS Research (amfAR) and the Naz Foundation International have been particularly outspoken about how the flexibility of the msm category is precisely what makes it inadequate for use in community-based prevention programmes (e.g. see amfAR, 2006, p. 1; Khan, 1997, pp. 114–115).

Moreover, the flexibility of the msm category complicates the collection and comparison of epidemiological data on HIV. In UNGASS Country Progress Reports, countries occasionally disaggregate the msm category in order to precisely convey information about HIV prevalence and risk that varies across subgroups of msm. The 2012 Country Progress Report submitted by Bangladesh is notable for its discussion of findings from a 2011 surveillance study:

[N]one of the MSM or MSW [male sex workers] tested was positive for HIV. Among the transgendered community (*hijra*) the HIV prevalence was 1%... Though there were no changes in the rates of active syphilis in MSM, MSW and *hijra*, large proportions of MSM and MSW, report STI symptoms (MSW more than MSM), as well as multiple sex partners (including women), group sex (often associated with violence and without condoms) and very low condom use with all types of partners. MSMs are highly networked, so if HIV were to emerge, it could spread very rapidly in this population. (Government of Bangladesh, 2012, p. 6)

More often, however, if countries report any data, they report whatever data they have and use those data as a placeholder for all msm, obscuring the specific needs and contexts of subgroups of msm. When traced back to the original studies or reports, these data commonly reflect more visible gay-identified men or men surveyed at a gay venue, where HIV prevalence may be substantially higher or lower than HIV prevalence among other msm depending on the specific context. For example, in Malawi, HIV prevalence among msm is reported as 21.4% in the country's 2012 Progress Report (Government of Malawi, 2012, p. 4). Malawi does not conduct surveillance of HIV infection among msm; this figure comes from a small snowball study conducted in 2007 of predominantly gay-identified men and bisexually-identified men in one urban centre and surrounding areas (Baral et al., 2009). These data likely overestimate HIV prevalence among msm in Malawi for several reasons, including the recruitment of men from the networks of men served by human rights and HIV/AIDS community-based organisations and the study's focus on men living in urban centres and living in the Southern region, where HIV prevalence is highest among the general population (NSO, 2011). A later study begun in 2011 by the same research group, which expanded the study to include greater geographical variation in networks of msm (e.g. multiple sites in urban and peri-urban areas in the North, Central, and Southern regions) and is reported on in Malawi's 2015 Progress Report (Government of Malawi, 2015, p. 24), suggests the 2007 study may overestimate HIV prevalence among msm in the Southern Region by almost 10% when data are properly weighted (Wirtz et al., 2013). The second study estimates HIV prevalence at 12.5% among Malawian msm living in the Southern Region, which is more in line with estimated HIV prevalence of 11% among Malawian men aged 15–49 living in the Southern region in 2010 DHS data (NSO, 2011). Discrepancies such as these suggest that gay- and bisexually identified men, especially men living in the South, may be at higher risk of HIV infection compared with nongay identified Malawian msm overall.

Malawi is not alone in its reliance on small, isolated studies of subpopulations of msm to develop a picture of the HIV prevalence and prevention needs among msm. The 2012 report submitted by Afghanistan (Islamic Republic of Afghanistan, 2012) reports data from a 2009 study focused on sexual exploitation among msm, especially 'male juvenile sexual exploitation' using data from a sample of 50 adult msm and 36 'male juveniles incarcerated in juvenile rehabilitation homes, along with staff at these homes, as well as working street males accessing Aschiana working street males centres' (Khan, 2009, p. 15). Due to the nonrepresentative sampling, the authors of the study explicitly note that, 'the study is limited and biased (25)' and is not intended to represent the behaviours or needs of all msm in Afghanistan. Yet, these data on incarcerated young men and men engaged in sex work are intertwined with the data on 'adult MSM' in the country's Progress Report. This is explained as the result of no other data being available, a common statement found in reports for countries where a research team only recently made inroads but the government has yet to established routine surveillance practices. While use of nonrepresentative data is understandable in the absence of more comprehensive information, inadequate attention has been paid to how these kinds of data limitations shape our understanding of HIV incidence and prevalence, sexual behaviours, condom use, testing behaviours, number and kind of sexual partners, and knowledge of HIV among diverse groups of msm.[5]

The inclusion of msm into donor programmes and policies

In addition to providing a basis for the inclusion of msm into national AIDS policies and programmes, UNAIDS also worked with other donors to promote new funding streams for research on msm at the local, national, and regional levels. Like governments and local prevention efforts, these donors struggle with how to understand and engage the flexibility of the msm category. One of the first organisations to establish a programmatic response[6] to HIV specifically among msm was the American Foundation for AIDS Research (amfAR), a private foundation that has been engaged in research on HIV since 1985. Following their mobilisation of research and outreach among msm in Asia in 2005 and 2006, amfAR established *The MSM Initiative* in 2007, a programme that aimed to support grassroots HIV prevention, care, and advocacy for msm around the world. Between 2007 and 2011, *The MSM Initiative* provided more than $2.5 million in small grants for research, prevention, and advocacy work with msm in low- and middle-income countries (amfAR, 2011). Throughout much of its work in this area, amfAR is notable for its attention to the ways that unreflective use of the msm category frustrates HIV prevention efforts. As amfAR expressed in 2006:

> The nature of MSM activity across the [Asian] continent is so diverse that it forces us to rethink the basic strategies of fighting AIDS … The most prominent feature of MSM identities in Asia is their diversity. MSM identities include transgender individuals, feminine-acting MSM, their masculine-acting partners, gay-identified men, and men who have situational sex with each other. All of this diversity is in theory covered by the term MSM, which focuses on behaviour rather than identity, but unfortunately in some locations even this broad term has become associated with single groups – often those that are most visible (e.g., feminine acting MSM) or most politically active (e.g., gay-identified MSM). Within these broad categories of MSM there is still more diversity. In each country, MSM have their own set of behaviours and interactions with other MSM groups. (amfAR, 2006, p. 1)

Complementing amfAR's *MSM Initiative*, the Global Fund committed an additional $349 million from 2002 to 2010, or about 10% of total funding for HIV prevention, to addressing HIV prevention in most-at-risk populations, including msm, sex workers, and injection drug users (Avdeeva, Lazarus, Aziz, & Atun, 2011).[7] In contrast to most other donors and organisations working in HIV/AIDS, the Global Fund incorporates msm in their programmes on gender. At a meeting in November 2007, the Global Fund's Board explicitly recognised the importance of addressing gender issues in the fight against AIDS, Tuberculosis, and Malaria, placing a 'particular focus on the vulnerabilities of women and girls and sexual minorities' (Global Fund, 2007). At the same meeting, the Board authorised the Global Fund Secretariat to develop a strategy to ensure gender equitable responses to AIDS, TB, and malaria, to open three new staff positions including a senior-level 'Champion for Gender Equality', and to provide technical guidance and encourage grant applicants to submit proposals addressing the vulnerabilities of women, girls, and sexual minorities. Within a year, the Global Fund developed a parallel strategy on Sexual Orientation and Gender Identity (SOGI) and appointed new SOGI staff to increase the ability of msm, transgender people, and female, male, and transgender sex workers to access and benefit from Global Fund grants (Global Fund, 2009). The Global Fund's unique attention to 'sexual minorities' within gender frame brings greater visibility to linkages between gender inequality and sexual inequality, as well as issues of social and economic inclusion of msm, discrimination in healthcare settings, and the needs of lesbian women and transgender people in addition to msm.

A third major player in the development and diffusion of msm in HIV programmes and policy is the US PEPFAR. Despite its conservative and ideologically driven beginnings, in the late 2000s PEPFAR has attempted to reinvent itself as a 'data-driven' funder by incorporating attention to HIV among msm. In contrast to the original bill authorising PEPFAR (US Congress, 2003), the 2008 reauthorisation of PEPFAR (US Congress, 2008) was redrafted to include msm as a specific target population on grounds that new evidence on HIV among msm in some PEPFAR countries showed disproportionate rates of infection and were likely high elsewhere. Under this second PEPFAR bill, the US Congress explicitly authorised the use of funds to '(i) gather epidemiological and social science data on HIV; and (ii) evaluate the effectiveness of prevention efforts among men who have sex with men, with due consideration to stigma and risks associated with disclosure' (§ 301/C/3/F) and support partner countries by providing 'assistance for appropriate HIV/AIDS education programmes and training targeted to prevent the transmission of HIV among men who have sex with men' (§ 301/C/1/K).[8] Three years later, PEPFAR administrators developed technical guidance to inform countries about the epidemiology of HIV transmission among msm and the types of prevention programmes that PEPFAR funding would support for msm (PEPFAR, 2011). Through these changes in legislation and the dissemination of technical guidance documents on msm, PEPFAR has diverged from its previous model of earmarked allocations for ideologically determined programmes to a model that, at least for the sake of appearances, espouses research data and epidemiological trends.[9] A key issue identified in PEPFAR reporting reflects the aggregation problems associated with the msm category writ large. As amfAR's review of PEPFAR programmes targeting msm concludes, 'In national statistics and some country-level PEPFAR data, MSM are often subsumed under the general category of "most-at-risk populations", making it difficult to determine which services are targeting MSM specifically' (amfAR, 2011, p. 2).

Discussion

Over the last two decades, msm have been incorporated into global and national responses to AIDS in ways that were unthinkable at the beginning of the epidemic. This paper examines the inclusion of gay and other men who have sex with men in that response with attention to how categories – homosexual, gay, bisexual, and more recently msm and sexual minorities – structure understandings of and responses to the epidemic. From this, I demonstrate that a key element in seeing HIV among msm in developing countries is first seeing msm at all. It is decidedly not 'homosexual', 'gay', or 'behaviourally bisexual' men that have been made visible in global and national AIDS policies and prevention programmes, but rather a general – and ever expanding (Boellstorff, 2011) – category of 'men who have sex with men', within which there is wide variation in identity, behaviour, and social and economic circumstance. 'Making up' msm, to use Hacking's (1990) phrase, was an early necessary condition for constructing notions of risk and disease that were sufficiently broad to accommodate the diverse needs of global policy-makers, international and local activists, governments, and scientists.[10] Although GPA did not mount a successful policy response to HIV among gay and bisexual men despite growing evidence of the importance of HIV among populations of msm, conversations begun at GPA around variation in sexual identity and behaviour laid the groundwork for UNAIDS to take a stronger policy response in the late 1990s. Ultimately, new measures of accountability ratified by states in the 2001 *Declaration of Commitment on HIV/AIDS* provided a window of opportunity to include msm in national AIDS programmes.

Yet, widespread use of the msm category has not been without its critics and challenges, especially as various international and national actors have attempted to implement global policy recommendations. Understandings of who constitutes msm and what should be done to prevent HIV infection vary considerably within and across actors and contexts. When employed as a broad, inclusive category in HIV research and surveillance, the msm category also imposes serious challenges to collecting and using data to inform prevention activities by obscuring the ways that identity, communities, and institutions shape sexual behaviour and exposure to HIV. As early as 1992, GPA recognised the inadequacy of aggregating same-sex sexual behaviours under the umbrella of msm and the complications that this category posed for recognising and acting on HIV infections among behaviourally bisexual men. Moreover, the myopic focus on behaviour runs into substantial difficulty when organisations attempt to plan and implement prevention programmes that are responsive to diverse identities and interests (Khan, 1997). Thus, as Boellstorff writes, while 'it is neither possible nor desirable to put the msm genie back into the bottle of epidemiological categorization' (2011, p. 290), the way forward requires greater attention to how different understandings of msm have shaped our knowledge and response to HIV among diverse groups of msm over time.

Disclosure statement

No potential conflict of interest was reported by the author.

Notes

1. Throughout, I reflect the language that is used in a particular historical moment or by a given actor. In my own discussion and analysis, I have used msm in lowercase following Epprecht (2008) in order to describe elements of this mutable and contested category rather than the uppercase 'msm' which further reifies the category as stable and cohesive.
2. Word choice is deliberate here on the part of stakeholders who make a distinction between 'bisexual' – often used unreflexively to convey sexual preference, identity, or practice – and bisexual behaviour, which was deemed most important to HIV/AIDS transmission.
3. However, GPA continued to reiterate the need for more research throughout the 1990s. For example, the 1994–1995 Annual Report, which summarises all activities conducted by GPA from 1987 to 1995, identifies as one of 10 'Intervention Research Priorities for the 1990s' the need to "determine the most feasible, relevant and effective interventions targeting homosexual and bisexual behaviours amongst various groups and situations of men who have sex with men in developing countries, including interventions with emphasis on: (a) reaching those persons practicing bisexual and/or homosexual behaviours who do and do not identify themselves as such; (b) situations with large numbers of male or transgender prostitutes; and (c) different forms of situational homosexuality (e.g. the military, migrant labour communities, prisons)." (GPA, 1997, p. 16) Yet, in contrast to detailed summaries of almost a decade of prevention activities targeting women, youth, and even drug injectors, the 74 page report does not include any additional discussion of the agency's activities targeting gay, bisexual, or other msm.
4. Because the composition of countries submitting reports varies each report year and missing data decreases with each subsequent report year, the percentage of countries at each level of prioritization should be read as demonstrating a general trend toward stronger prioritization rather than absolute gains or losses over time.
5. Buckley's (2008) report on estimating HIV prevalence in the Southern Caucasus provides an intriguing and commendable exception in this area.
6. Prior to amfAR's *MSM Initiative*, private foundations like the Ford Foundation and the Bill and Melinda Gates Foundation, and other development organizations such as Family Health International and Population Services International used their general mandates to improve health and prevent HIV to make several individual awards to local and national HIV and LGBT organizations working with gay men and other msm.
7. 2002 is used as it is the start date for the Global Fund; however, nearly all of the Global Fund's funding for msm is stacked towards the last few years of this time series.

8. Unfortunately, PEPFAR does not report specifically on program expenditures targeting msm, and tracking the flow of resources from US agencies is extremely difficult due to the number of sub-contracts to other international, national, and government organisations. Still, evaluations of PEPFAR note progress in targeting msm through PEPFAR-funded and community-led activities in some countries, for example in China, Côte d'Ivoire, Ukraine, and Vietnam (see amfAR's (2011) evaluation of PEPFAR). In Asia, PEPFAR also supports the Purple Sky Network, a transnational advocacy organisation which works to reduce HIV among msm by strengthening msm community groups, improving clinical services, and engaging with governments to establish a supportive environment for HIV prevention.
9. amfAR and others continue to criticize PEPFAR for its neglect of msm and a lack of transparency in where funds go once they get in-country (amfAR, 2011).
10. See also Martucci (2010) on how the ambiguity of the msm category has structured US blood screening policy.

ORCID

Tara McKay http://orcid.org/0000-0001-5076-6483

References

Aggleton, P., & Parker, R. (2015). Moving beyond biomedicalization in the HIV response: Implications for community involvement and community leadership among men who have sex with men and transgender people. *American Journal of Public Health, 105*(8), 1552–1558. doi:10.2105/AJPH.2015.302614

amfAR. (2006). *An interview with Shivananda Khan –Standing up for MSM in South Asia*. Bangkok: TREAT Asia.

amfAR. (2011). *MSM and the global HIV/AIDS epidemic: Assessing PEPFAR and looking forward*. Washington, DC: American Foundation for AIDS Research.

Avdeeva, O., Lazarus, J., Aziz, M. A., & Atun, R. (2011). The Global Fund's resource allocation decisions for HIV Programmes: Addressing those in need. *Journal of the International AIDS Society, 14*, 51–61. doi:10.1186/1758-2652-14-51

Baral, S., Trapence, G., Motimedi, F., Umar, E., Iipinge, S., & Dausab, F. (2009). HIV prevalence, risks for HIV infection, and human rights among men who have sex with men (MSM) in Malawi, Namibia, and Botswana. *PLoS ONE, 4*(3), e4997. doi:10.1371/journal.pone.0004997

Biehl, J. (2007). *Will to live: AIDS therapies and the politics of survival*. Princeton, NJ: Princeton University Press.

Biruk, C. (2012). Seeing like a research project: Producing 'high-quality data' in AIDS research in Malawi. *Medical Anthropology, 31*(4), 347–366. doi:10.1080/01459740.2011.631960

Boellstorff, T. (2011). But do not identify as gay: A propleptic geneology of the MSM category. *Cultural Anthropology, 26*(2), 287–312. doi:10.1111/j.1548-1360.2011.01100.x

Boulton, M., & Weatherburn, P. (1990). *Literature review on bisexuality and HIV transmission: Report commissioned by the social and behavioural research unit, global programme on AIDS, world health organization*. Geneva: World Health Organization.

Buckley, C. (2008). *Myths, meanings, and measurement: Estimating HIV prevalence in the Southern Caucasus*. Seattle, WA: National Council for Eurasian and East European Research.

Carballo, M. (1990). WHO global programme on AIDS: Social and behavioural research. *Disasters, 14*(3), 276–281. doi:10.1111/j.1467-7717.1990.tb01072.x

Carballo, M., Cleland, J., Carael, M., & Albrecht, G. (1989). A cross national study of patterns of sexual behaviour. *Journal of Sex Research, 26*(3), 287–299. doi:10.1080/00224498909551516

Center for Global Development. (2009). *Report of the UNAIDS leadership transition working group*. Washington, DC: Center for Global Development.

Chin, J., & Mann, J. M. (1988). The global patterns and prevalence of AIDS and HIV infection. *AIDS, 2*(suppl. 1), s247–s252.

Chin, J., Sato, P. A., & Mann, J. M. (1990). Projections of HIV infection and AIDS cases to the year 2000. *Bulletin of the World Health Organization, 68*(1), 1–11.

Cleland, J. G., & Ferry, B. (1995). *Sexual behavior and AIDS in the developing world.* Bristol, PA: Taylor & Francis.

Coxon, A. P. (1993, June). *Results of WHO/GPA 7-nation homosexual response studies.* Paper Presented at the International AIDS Conference, Berlin, Germany.

Coxon, A. P., & Carballo, M. (1989). Research on AIDS: Behavioral perspectives. *AIDS, 3*, 191–198.

Coxon, A. P., Davies, P. M., Hunt, A. J., Weatherburn, P., McManus, T. J., & Rees, C. (1990). The structure of sexual behavior. *Journal of Sex Research, 29*(1), 61–83.

CPA. (1986). *Global WHO strategy for the prevention and control of acquired immunodeficiency syndrome.* Geneva: World Health Organization.

Dowsett, G. (1989 May). *'You'll never forget the feeling of safe sex!' AIDS prevention strategies for gay and bisexual men in Sydney, Australia.* Paper presented at the WHO/GPA Workshop on AIDS Health Promotion Activities Directed Towards Gay and Bisexual Men, Geneva, Switzerland.

ECOSOC. (1995). *Report of the committee of co-sponsoring organizations of the joint and co-sponsored United Nations Programme on HIV/AIDS (E/1995/71).* Geneva: United Nations.

Epprecht, M. (2008). *Heterosexual Africa? the history of an idea from the age of exploration to the age of AIDS.* Athens, OH: Ohio University Press.

Esacove, A. (2010). Love matches: Heteronormativity, modernity, and AIDS prevention in Malawi. *Gender & Society, 24*(1), 83–109. doi:10.1177/0891243209354754

Finnemore, M. (1999). The politics, power and pathologies of international organizations. *International Organization,* 699–732. doi:10.1162/002081899551048

Gibbons, A. (1990, June 15). New head for the WHO global program on AIDS. *Science, 248*(4961), 1306–1307.

Global Fund. (2007). *Sixteenth board meeting, 12–13 November.* Kunming, China: The Global Fund to Fight AIDS, Tuberculosis and Malaria.

Global Fund. (2009). *The global fund strategy in relation to sexual orientation and gender identity.* Geneva: The Global Fund to Fight HIV/AIDS, Tuberculosis and Malaria.

Godlee, F. (1994). The World Health Organization. The regions – too much power, too little effect. *British Medical Journal, 309*, 1566–1570.

Government of Bangladesh. (2012). *Country progress report: Bangladesh.* Dhaka: Ministry of Health and Family Welfare.

Government of Malawi. (2012). *2012 Global AIDS response progress report: Malawi country report for 2010 and 2011.* Lilongwe: Government of Malawi.

Government of Malawi. (2015). *Malawi AIDS response progress report 2015.* Lilongwe: Government of Malawi.

Government of Romania. (2010). *UNGASS country progress report: Reporting period January 2008–December 2009.* Bucharest: Government of Romania.

Government of Romania. (2012). *Country progress report on AIDS: Reporting period January 2010 – December 2011.* Bucharest: Government of Romania.

Government of Tuvalu. (2012). *Global AIDS response progress reporting: Country progress report, January 2010–December 2011.* Funafuti: Tuvalu National Aids Committee.

GPA. (1988a). *London declaration on AIDS prevention.* Geneva: World Health Organization.

GPA. (1988b). *Progress report number 4.* Geneva: World Health Organization.

GPA. (1992a). *1991 Progress report.* Geneva: World Health Organization.

GPA. (1992b). *Informal consultation of interventions to prevent HIV transmission among behaviorally bisexual men.* Geneva: World Health Organization.

GPA. (1997). *Global programme on AIDS 1987–1995. Final report with emphasis on 1994–1995 Biennium.* Geneva: World Health Organization.

Hacking, I. (1990). *The taming of chance.* Cambridge: Cambridge University Press.

Hafner-Burton, E. M., & Tsutsui, K. (2005). Human rights in a globalizing world: The paradox of empty promises. *American Journal of Sociology, 110*(5), 1373–1411. doi:10.1086/428442

Islamic Republic of Afghanistan. (2012). *Country progress report 2012.* Kabul: Ministry of Public Health.

Khan, S. (1997). *Sex, secrecy, and shamefulness: Developing a sexual health response to the needs of males who have sex with males in Dhaka, Bangladesh*. London: Naz Foundation International.

Khan, S. (2009). *Final report: Rapid assessment of male vulnerabilities to HIV and sexual exploitation in Afghanistan*. London: Naz Foundation International.

Mann, J. M. (1988). *The global picture of AIDS: An address presented 12 June 1988 at the IV International Conference on AIDS. Stockholm, Sweden*. Geneva: World Health Organization.

Mann, J., & Kay, K. (1991). Confronting the pandemic: The World Health Organization's global programme on AIDS, 1986–1989. *AIDS, 5*(suppl. 2), s221–s229.

Mann, J., Chin, J., Piot, P., & Quinn, T. (1988). The international epidemiology of AIDS. *Scientific American, 259*(4), 82–89.

Martucci, J. (2010). Negotiating exclusion: MSM, identity, and blood policy in the age of AIDS. *Social Studies of Science, 40*(2), 215–241. doi:10.1177/0306312709346579

NSO. (2011). *Malawi Demographic and Health Survey 2010*. Zomba: Author.

Orkin, A. (1990). Sixth International AIDS conference featured some notable absentees. *Canadian Medical Asociation Journal, 143*(5), 407–410.

Parker, R. G., & Carballo, M. (1990). Qualitative research on homosexual and bisexual behavior relevant to HIV/AIDS. *Journal of Sex Research, 27*(4), 497–525. doi:10.1080/00224499009551578

Parker, R. G., Guimarães, C. D., & Struchiner, J. D. (1989, May). *The impact of AIDS health promotion for gay and bisexual men in Rio de Janeiro, Brazil*. Paper presented at the WHO/GPA Workshop on AIDS Health Promotion Activities Directed Towards Gay and Bisexual Men, Geneva, Switzerland.

Parker, R. G., Herdt, G., & Carballo, M. (1991). Sexual culture, HIV transmission, and AIDS research. *Journal of Sex Research, 28*(1), 77–98. doi:10.1080/00224499109551596

Parker, R., Khan, S., & Aggleton, P. (1998). Conspicuous by their absence? men who have sex with men (MSM) in developing countries: Implications for HIV prevention. *Critical Public Health, 8*(4), 329–346. doi:10.1080/09581599808402919

PCB. (2005). *Report of the NGO representative*. Geneva: UNAIDS.

PEPFAR. (2011). *Technical guidance on combination HIV prevention for men who have sex with men*. Washington, DC: Author.

Shiffman, J. (2006). Donor funding priorities for communicable disease control in the developing world. *Health Policy and Planning, 21*(6), 411–420. doi:10.1093/heapol/czl028

Treichler, P. (1999). *How to have theory in an epidemic: Cultural chronicles of AIDS*. Durham, NC: Duke University Press.

UN. (2001a). *Resolution adopted by the General Assembly: S-26/2. Declaration of commitment on HIV/AIDS: 'Global Crisis – Global Action'*. New York, NY: Author.

UN. (2001b). *United Nations system strategic plan for HIV/AIDS for 2001–2005*. Geneva: Author.

UNAIDS. (1998). *AIDS and men who have sex with men: UNAIDS point of view*. Geneva: Author.

UNAIDS. (1999). *The UNAIDS report*. Geneva: Author.

UNAIDS. (2000). *AIDS and men who have sex with men: UNAIDS technical update*. Geneva: Author.

UNAIDS. (2001a). *Global crisis –Global action: Reversing the HIV/AIDS epidemic: Critical issues*. Geneva: Author.

UNAIDS. (2001b). *The global strategy framework on HIV/AIDS*. Geneva: Author.

UNAIDS. (2003). *AIDS epidemic update: December 2003*. Geneva: Joint United Nations Programme on HIV/AIDS and the World Health Organization.

US Congress. (2003). *United States leadership against HIV/AIDS, tuberculosis, and malaria act of 2003*. Washington, DC: One Hundreth Eigth Congress of The United States of America.

US Congress. (2008). *Tom Lantos and Henry J. Hyde United States global leadership against HIV/AIDS, tuberculosis, and malaria reauthorization act of 2008*. Washington, DC: One Hundreth Tenth Congress of The United States of America.

Watkins, S. C., Swidler, A., & Hannan, T. (2012). Outsourcing social transformation: Development NGOs as organizations. *Annual Review of Sociology, 38*, 285–315. doi:10.1146/annurev-soc-071881-145516

WHO. (1992). *The global AIDS strategy*. Geneva: Author.

WHO. (2002). *Follow up on the United Nations general assembly special session on HIV/AIDS: Work of WHO*. Geneva: Department of HIV/AIDS.

Wirtz, A. L., Jumbe, V., Trapence, G., Kamba, D., Uman, E., Ketende, S., ... Baral, S. D. (2013). HIV among men who have sex with men in Malawi: Elucidating HIV prevalence and correlates of infection to inform HIV prevention. *Journal of the International AIDS Society, 16*(4 Suppl. 3), 1–11. doi:10.7448/IAS.16.4.18742

Young, R. M., & Meyer, I. H. (2005). The trouble with 'MSM' and 'WSW': Erasure of the sexual minority person in public health discourse. *American Journal of Public Health, 95*(7), 1144–1149. doi:10.2105/AJPH.2004.046714

From MSM to heteroflexibilities: Non-exclusive straight male identities and their implications for HIV prevention and health promotion

Héctor Carrillo and Amanda Hoffman

ABSTRACT
This article examines the logics of self-identification among men who have same-sex desires and behaviours and consider themselves to be straight. We draw from interviews conducted in the USA with 100 straight-identified men who have same-sex desires and 40 partners of such men. Our data allow us to reject two misconceptions. One is the idea that these men are actually gay or bisexual but refuse to accept those identities. We argue instead that these men see themselves as straight and therefore it is important to understand what specifically they mean by that. The second misconception links straight-identified men who have same-sex desires and behaviours to the racialised discourse of the so-called down low (or 'DL') in the USA. While the DL typically is depicted as involving African American and Latino men, most of our participants are White. Moving beyond these misconceptions, we propose that health educators must acknowledge flexibilities in the definition of heterosexuality and use an expanded definition as a starting point to envision, together with these men, how to more effectively engage them in HIV prevention and health promotion.

Introduction: MSM, heteroflexibilities, and the down low

When epidemiologists in the USA studying HIV/AIDS coined the behavioural category MSM (men who have sex with men) more than two decades ago, one of their primary goals was to better count non-gay-identified MSM within HIV statistics and epidemiological research. As Young and Meyer (2005) have noted:

> [B]y using identity-free terms, epidemiologists sought to avoid complex social and cultural connotations that, according to a strict biomedical view, have little to do with epidemiological investigation of diseases. Accordingly, *MSM* was introduced to reflect the idea that behaviors, not identities, place individuals at risk for HIV infection. (p. 1144)

The limitation of identity-based categories was also perceived by HIV prevention researchers and educators, who realised that straight-identified MSM were not being appropriately reached by HIV prevention messages targeting either gay men or the so-called general population (Boellstorff, 2011). Straight-identified MSM engaged in sex with men furtively and were perceived as being in denial about their bisexual or gay orientation, making them 'hard to reach' with HIV prevention messages (Pathela et al., 2006). The label MSM thus was believed to hold 'the promise of sidestepping identity' (Boellstorff, 2011, p. 293). Focusing on sexual behaviour rather than identity might facilitate reaching these men, which seemed crucial to reduce the potential for a so-called bisexual bridge that could lead to a more generalised HIV epidemic among heterosexual people in the USA – particularly heterosexual women (Malebranche, 2008; Phillips, 2005; Shearer, Khosropour, Stephenson, & Sullivan, 2012; Siegel, Schrimshaw, Lekas, & Parsons, 2008). This concern centred more recently on the growing HIV/AIDS epidemic among African American men and women (Malebranche, 2008; Phillips, 2005).

In practice, the use of the behavioural category MSM did not fulfil its promise, in part because the label did not resonate with those whom it intended to reach (Muñoz-Laboy, 2004; Young & Meyer, 2005), and also because it became a global quasi-identity label increasingly recognised as a euphemism that is safer than the label 'gay' (Boellstorff, 2011). The use of MSM as a euphemism for gay, however, had the effect of excluding the very men that the label and its associated behavioural category originally were meant to include.

Given this failure of the MSM category to incorporate non-exclusively straight men, in this article we explore an alternative. In place of a sole focus on sexual behaviour, we propose that public health efforts must acknowledge and seek to understand the sexual desires and identities of those men, avoiding in the process the tendency to simply see them as anomalous because of their lack of concordance with strict definitions of heterosexuality, bisexuality, and homosexuality. We do just that by closely examining the logics of self-identification among a subset of these men, as well as the implications of such identification for future HIV prevention and health promotion work.

We draw from interviews conducted with 100 non-exclusively straight men in the USA (supplemented by interviews with 40 female and male partners of such men). We begin by examining how these men make their sexual behaviours consistent with a straight identity, and also explore nuanced secondary patterns of self-identification that emerge in our data. Then we discuss in more detail how the meanings they attach to their behaviours inform their interpretations of same-sex desires and their constructions of sexual identities as straight. By this route we reject the presumption that such men necessarily and in all cases should be seen as 'really' gay or bisexual but refusing to acknowledge it. Throughout our analysis, we respond to a growing perceived need to 'move beyond MSM' (Muñoz-Laboy, 2004, p. 59; Young & Meyer, 2005) in search of more nuanced understandings of these men's sexualities and better ways of addressing their HIV/AIDS and other sexual health needs.

The patterns that emerge in our data are generally connected to the notion of 'heteroflexibility', a term that refers to the incorporation of same-sex desires and practices into the definition of heterosexuality. Such incorporation in effect turns heterosexuality into an elastic category, which in turn makes room for the idea that straight-identified individuals may recognise some interest in being sexually involved with both women and men without perceiving a need to give up their identity as straight or heterosexual as a consequence. We must clarify that, although some people use the term 'heteroflexible' as a descriptor of identity (among other labels, including 'mostly straight' and 'bicurious'; see Ambrose, 2009–2010; Cohen & Savin-Williams, 2010; Essig, 2000; Savin-Williams

& Vrangalova, 2013; Thompson & Morgan, 2008; Vrangalova & Savin-Williams, 2012), we propose that 'heteroflexibility' – or the plural 'heteroflexibilities' – can also serve as a general conceptual framework for studying a range of sexual identities that depart from, but are closely aligned with, heterosexuality.

In the article we also briefly attend to yet another complication that emerged in the USA as attempts progressed to understand the sexuality of non-gay or non-bisexually identified MSM. Those sexualities became heavily racialised as they increasingly became associated with the so-called down low (or 'DL') among African Americans and Latinos (Ford, Whetten, Hall, Kaufman, & Thrasher, 2007; Goldbaum, Perdue, & Higgins, 1996; González, 2007; Malebranche, 2008; Phillips, 2005). The perception that non-gay-identified MSM (particularly men of colour who are on the DL) are secretive and deceitful about their same-sex behaviours, and put their female partners at high risk for HIV infection, became central to popular explanations about growing HIV transmission in African American and Latino/a communities (Dodge, Jeffries IV, & Sandfort, 2008; Goldbaum et al., 1996; González, 2007; Kalichman, Roffinan, Picciano, & Bolan, 1998; Malebranche, 2008; Pathela et al., 2006; Phillips, 2005; Shearer et al., 2012; Siegel et al., 2008; Stokes, McKirnan, Doll, & Burzette, 1996). Some of the extant research, however, has also noted that the levels of disclosure of same-sex behaviours and protection against HIV infection among 'men on the down low' are possibly more varied than is commonly assumed (Dodge et al., 2008; Malebranche, 2008).

Some scholars have challenged the assumption that the DL applies only to African American and Latino men, indicating that White straight-identified men also engage in the kinds of secrecy and other management strategies that are commonly associated with the DL (see, for instance, Ford et al., 2007; Goldbaum et al., 1996; Siegel et al., 2008; Ward, 2008). In fact, in our own study most of the straight-identified participants are White, and our findings add to critiques of how the stereotypical understanding of the DL draws on racialised perceptions of sexual cultures – by which we mean 'the systems of meaning, of knowledge, beliefs and practices, that structure sexuality in different social contexts' (Parker, Herdt, & Carballo, 1991, p.79) – that depict communities of colour as 'pre-modern'.

Finally, we explore how HIV/AIDS prevention programmes could best address the specific needs of non-exclusively straight men. We argue that health educators should seek to better understand heterosexual flexibility rather than merely sidestepping them in favour of a focus purely on sexual behaviour. In addition, we argue for the need to avoid imposing normative expectations about sexual orientation. We emphasise the importance of reconsidering expectations about consistency between sexual identity and behaviour (according to conventional definitions of sexual orientation categories), as well as reconsidering whether disclosure and 'coming out' are required for effective HIV prevention.

Methods

We conducted our study in two phases. During the first phase, we recruited and interviewed 100 straight-identified US men in the 'Men4Men (relationships)' and 'Men4Men (casual encounters)' sections of Craigslist.org, a popular online personals website where people seek friendships, relationships, or sex. These men were physically located across the USA. Our criteria for inclusion were: (1) self-identification as straight, (2) having experienced same-sex desires after the age of 13, and (3) being 18 or older. All interviews were conducted by three female interviewers, primarily using an online chat function. Before the interview, participants were asked to provide informed consent and also filled out a short demographic survey.

Online interviews lasted between 2 and 3.5 hours (sometimes including pauses during which participants attended to other personal matters). This method proved helpful because it is convenient to participants, it provides a sense of anonymity and possibly enhances participation, it allows participants to read their responses before submitting them (possibly promoting reflexivity), it provides an instant transcript and, importantly, it lines up nicely with the techniques and strategies used by these straight-identified participants to pursue and manage their same-sex desires and behaviours online. Minor disadvantages are the potential for distraction and the absence of non-verbal cues, but we compensated by asking for clarification when the meaning or intention of any given answer was not immediately clear.[1] We protected our participants' confidentiality by creating a chat room that did not require them to use their personal email addresses, as well as unique screen names and passwords that we changed immediately after the interview ended.

During interviews, we asked participants about their sexual identities; sex lives, partners, and relationships; sexual desires, practices, and fantasies; and how they manage their same-sex desires. (Twenty four men also participated in a follow-up interview, during which we asked them further details about their sexual lives and experiences.)

Most straight-identified men in our study described themselves as White ($N = 78$), with the remaining 22 being Latino ($N = 11$), African American ($N = 5$), Native American ($N = 3$), Asian American ($N = 2$), and Middle Eastern/White ($N = 1$). Most were in a relationship ($N = 59$), including 38 who were married to a woman. Finally, their ages ranged from 18 to 72 and were well distributed within that span.

During a second phase, we recruited and interviewed 40 partners of non-exclusively straight MSM (not partnered to the men in phase one of our study), including 19 gay men and 21 women. We used the same procedures and recruited participants primarily from Craigslist and through Facebook ads. For the purposes of this article, however, we focus almost exclusively on the interviews with straight-identified men and only draw a few selected quotations from our interviews with gay male and female partners.

All interview transcripts were coded and organised with the aid of Atlas.ti, a software package for qualitative analysis. We carried out the following analytical tasks: We read our interviews and created approximately 20 codes for each set of interviews. Three coders independently coded a sample of transcripts, achieving an average rate of 82% intercoder reliability, which was calculated based on the number of times that all coders assigned the same codes to specific text passages (Miles & Huberman, 1994). We then coded all interviews and conducted thematic searches to identify patterns in the data. We also considered disconfirming cases and re-contextualised selected passages in relation to the individual cases from which they were drawn. In the sections that follow we present our findings regarding the diversity of identities among the straight MSM in our study, the logics that inform such self-identification, and the implications of their identities and sexualities for HIV prevention and public health work. We primarily draw from our interviews with straight-identified men but also include some perspectives provided by partners of such men.

Straight MSM

Among the 100 men who self-identified as straight during recruitment, half ($N = 50$) confirmed during interviews that the labels 'straight' or 'heterosexual' fully describe them. The remaining half additionally described themselves using secondary labels that denoted more nuanced interpretations of their heterosexuality. Twenty-three had adopted labels that denote heteroflexibility, or a sense that they are straight but their sexualities depart somewhat from exclusive heterosexuality, and 27 reported that in private they might call themselves bisexual. Men in this latter group, however, typically said they would never publicly adopt a bisexual identity, choosing instead to maintain a public identity as straight.

These men's primary identification as straight reflects several intertwined issues. First, these men live in a society where, in spite of the many achievements of the gay movement, being straight (and a straight man in particular) is still widely considered a better option than being anything else (Dean, 2014). As Devon (39, White), one of our participants, put it, 'society teaches people to be straight'. Thus, boys and young men are assumed to be heterosexually oriented unless they give signs that they are not (often based on perceptions of conventional or even hegemonic masculinities, Connell & Messerschmidt, 2005), and they are also expected to grow up to become heterosexual men leading 'normal' straight lives. 'Who wouldn't prefer a hetero lifestyle?' said Frank (24, White). 'It is what is expected of us by the society at large'.

Second, because of the strong social value placed on heterosexuality, any man who can legitimately claim being sexually and romantically interested in women is assumed to qualify as straight. For example, Chayton (25, Native American) said, 'I tell people I am straight, and I've never been asked to define my sexuality, today is the first [time]'. Chayton's comment reflects 'heteronormativity' – a term defined by Dean (2014, p. 26) as 'the privileging of heterosexuality as normal, natural, and right over homosexuality' – and the accompanying sense that heterosexual people have no sexual identity or any need for one (Watney, 2000 [1993]). Heteronormativity may thus explain why non-exclusively straight men emphasise their attraction to women and consider that their same-sex attraction is of a lesser importance, a result that allows them to remain firmly on the heterosexual side of an imagined spectrum of sexual orientation.

The same logic helps explain why such men might prefer to understand heterosexuality as flexible rather than adopt a public identity as bisexual. They thus adopt descriptors such as 'heteroflexible' (Miles, 30, White; and Corey, 24, White), 'mostly heterosexual' (Sterling, 34, White), 'bi-curious, but mostly straight' (Sean, 30, White), 'straight with bi tendencies' (Travis, 20, White), 'straight with a pinch of bi' (Peter, 40, White), and 'straight with a little weirdness from time to time' (Lawrence, 57, White). These men rationalise that heterosexuality is an elastic category and come to see their own sexuality as one among many ways in which heterosexuality could be expressed. This view is consistent with what Dean (2011, 2014) calls 'queer heterosexualities', some forms of which allow exploration of same-sex sexualities.

Finally, as we noted before, some men recognise that they themselves could be called 'bisexual' given their sexual behaviours. However, they learn to keep this awareness private and separate it from their public persona. As Simon (27, White) put it,

> I think everybody is a little bi. Isn't that what this research is about? ... I think I'm probably bi but what I present to the world is a heterosexual man. Internally I'm bi, but that's not something most people know. I'm not ashamed, but the majority of people are ignorant and closeminded.

As Simon implies, these men's reluctance to adopt a public bisexual identity stems from awareness that bisexuality is socially stigmatised, and the expectations that such stigma would be damaging in their personal lives.

Careful management of the disclosure of same-sex desires is thus seen as warranted, as in the case of Dustin (28, White), who indicated that he is 'not openly bisexual to society except in sexual situations', further clarifying that he is openly bisexual 'only with men behind closed doors'. In such a space, some of these men trust that they can acknowledge being bisexual without fearing that the gay world would reject them, even if some gay men might view them as closeted gay men.

The construction of heterosexuality as an elastic category

As suggested by the previous section, to maintain their identities as straight these men must become convinced that they are significantly different from strictly bisexual or gay men. They achieve this by relying on a number of indicators that tell them that their choice of identity terms is justified despite their sexual interest in men. We now turn to examining more deeply some of those indicators and the sexual meaning around which straight MSM construct their identities. In particular, we focus on four of the patterns that emerged in our data. First we analyse their assessments of their relative sexual and romantic attraction toward women and men. Second, we discuss the meanings that they assign to specific sexual practices. Third, we examine their desire to escape the constraints of masculinity and pursue the excitement of transgressive sexual adventure. Finally, we explore a sense among some of these men that they first explored same-sex sexualities out of a wish to please female partners.

Attracted to women, not to men

The straight men in our study consistently emphasised that they are primarily attracted to women, which is a cornerstone of their ability to identify as straight. In Scott's (22, White) words, 'I guess I would say I'm on the part of the scale that is mostly women with a little bit of cock thrown in for excitement every now and then'. Feeling threatened by the interviewer's question about his self-identification, he retorted: 'I feel like you are implying that acts of homosexuality automatically make you bi and I would reject that notion'.

These men's opinions are bifurcated, however, in terms of their sexual attraction to men. Some do acknowledge that they have some level of attraction to men (although they often are also quick to clarify that their attraction toward women is much greater), while others deny having any attraction to men.

As an example of the first group, Sean (34, White), who thought of himself as 'bi-curious but also straight', spoke about his attractions to women and men in the following terms:

> If I'm out in a social situation, I'm almost 100% looking at women, and not at men ... Bisexual is closer to 50/50 in terms of attraction to both sexes ... Bi-curious, to me, tends to be more attracted to the opposite sex and more likely not openly identifying as interested in homosexual sex.

For Sean, his attraction toward women was permanent, as opposed to men 'who are on their way to being openly bisexual or even openly gay or exclusively homosexual'. He did pay attention to men's 'dress, size, [and] weight' and recognised that he found some men attractive, 'but not the same attraction that I have toward women'. He clarified that he can look at a woman 'and think "I would do her", and men don't do that [for me] ... they have to work on me ... show me that they are interested, and that there is a part of them that I can be attracted to'.

Men in the second group, however, unambiguously stated that they have no attraction toward men. Rodolfo (22, Latino) said: 'I never feel attracted to men physically, never have I looked at a guy and say, "wow, good looking guy"'. In a similar vein, Charlie (32, White) indicated:

> Women are hot ... I can see a beautiful woman walk down the street and I instantly can become hard and get horny. I don't think I've ever seen a guy walking by and got a boner. Also, I would not want to kiss or make out with them or love them. They would be more like a sexual experience.

As Charlie's comment also implies, these men commonly perceive that their lack of attraction to men is confirmed by the fact that they could never imagine developing romantic feelings toward another man (on this, see also Reback & Larkins, 2010). Ajay (22, Asian American) said: 'I can't see myself with a guy in anything more than sex ... With a girl I can see myself [spending] the rest of my life'. And Reggie (28, African American) emphasised his romantic interest in women and discounted any interest in being affectionate with a man. 'I would kiss a woman. ANYWHERE. I can barely hug a man', he said.

In the absence of any romantic desire toward men, non-exclusively straight men assess that their interest in men is thus purely sexual. As Rodolfo (22, Latino) put it, 'it is more about the sex part'. Others went even further. Freddie (25, Latino) firmly stated, 'I don't enjoy men. I use them; I guess you would say ... I only really like women'. Freddie's comment strongly indicates sexual objectification, which some of the non-exclusively straight men in our study took to yet another level. They claimed that they are not aroused by male bodies, but they do feel strongly interested in, and attracted by, a man's penis as a sexual object. For instance, Ajay (22, Asian American) expressed that 'every time I did anything with a guy it mostly depended on their cocks. I didn't really care what they looked like'. Other men argued that penises are merely a better alternative to a dildo. Josh (21, White) indicated that a penis 'is much hotter than a toy made out of some material made to look or slightly feel like the male penis', and Sam (42, White) characterised his male sexual partners as being 'only living and breathing dildos'.

In summary, these non-exclusively straight men rationalise that they have a primary attraction to women, and many feel that they are not attracted to men. They find confirmation of the latter in their sense of a lack of romantic interest in men and the fact that male bodies do not arouse them. They thus interpret their interest in men as purely sexual, or believe that their interest in men is limited to penises as a source of sexual pleasure. They also sometimes solve potential tensions inherent in the notion of desiring sex with men while not being attracted to them by emphasising their simultaneous interest in women and penises. Finally, some even seek other creative ways of solving this tension by fantasising about or seeking sex with pre-op trans women who, as Josh put it, have 'the features of a girl's body ... and the most "exciting" part of a guy'.

The management and meanings of sex with men

In the same manner in which some of the non-exclusively straight men in our study played down their sexual attraction to men, some also believed that sex with men is not comparable in any way to having sex with women in terms of pleasure, meaning, or significance. For instance, Scott (22, White) said the following:

> I told you, I'm very attracted to women, almost exclusively ... in my encounters with men by the time they're over I'm ready to get out of there and [I] lose all interest, which is certainly not the case with women.

Shaun (30, White) said that he felt 'intrigued' and 'curious' when a specific man proposed to give him oral sex. They first chatted online and by phone, and then they met in person at a bar. Shaun described these interactions as consistently 'flirty'. At the bar they first talked 'like guys' about things like 'sports, cars, [and] drinking', but the other man eventually made a sexual advance. They went to the man's house, where this man gave Shaun oral sex. Shaun merely 'played with [the man's] cock a little through his jeans'. 'I came and that was about it', said Shaun, adding that after finishing he felt 'odd ... it wasn't the same afterglow that I would have with a woman ... the feel good feeling after sex'. Shaun recognised that this male partner made him 'cum harder', and yet 'afterward it was odd shifting back to guy talk'. Shaun had sex again with this man, and this time they went farther: they kissed, the man rimmed him, and Shaun also performed oral sex. However, when the man made a move toward anal intercourse, Shaun stopped him. 'He situated me to put his cock into my ass, and I couldn't do it', says Shaun, 'and [instead he] stroked me until I came'.

Gay male partners of straight men who participated in our study felt that straight partners who are reluctant to be anally penetrated see that practice as the point of no return. For instance, Graham (27, White) explained:

> Some guys want to try everything, but I'd say 95% of the guys I've been with I knew identified as straight absolutely refuse receiving anal sex. I'm just speculating here, but I think that's the line between gay behaviour and straight behaviour for them.

Similarly, Stewart (46, White), talked about a male partner who:

> ... enjoyed mutual masturbation, and he enjoyed receiving blow-jobs. He was also capable of (I think the word is frottage?) rubbing our naked bodies together to get off. But he had no interest in anal sex, which I enjoy being on the receiving end of ... He always just said that that didn't interest him at all. But I honestly think it was that he considered [it] to be 'too' gay for him.

In these interpretations, sex is conflated with anal intercourse (Boellstorff, 2011), and being anally penetrated with gayness. These interpretations are also reminiscent of findings about male homosexualities in the global South or among men of colour in Western societies, including, for instance, among Latin American men or Latino men in the USA (among many examples, see Carrillo, 2002; González, 2007; Muñoz-Laboy, 2004; Parker, 1999).

On the other hand, our findings in terms of sexual behaviour do not fully support the conclusion that straight-identified men perceive being anally penetrated as a strict point of no return. Although more reported engaging in oral sex with male partners (59 receiving, 53 giving) than in anal intercourse (34 receptive, 20 insertive), these latter figures are not trivial. For instance, Miles (30, White) was one of the men who described enjoying 'anal play ... both giving and receiving, toys and also participating in anal sex'. Other men, however, stressed that they had only been anally penetrated by women using a dildo (a practice known as 'pegging', see Burke, 2014), although some also added that had fantasised about being anally penetrated by a man. That was the case for Matt (41, White), whose wife first penetrated him with a dildo and who continued using dildos on himself after they divorced. '[Dildos] felt good, I enjoyed them. I imagined that must be similar to what it really feels like [being penetrated by a man]'. In his interview, Matt also described elaborate fantasies about being penetrated by a man, after which he felt compelled to state 'Wow, I am a pervert!!!!!' These findings may reflect shifting senses of masculinity (Anderson, 2012; Connell & Messerschmidt, 2005; Dean, 2014), and possibly even shifts in attitudes about anal pleasure among heterosexually identified men (Burke, 2014). This is a topic that we believe merits further investigation.

The constraints of conventional masculinity

These men's fantasies also reflect a desire for having a space in which they can seek relief from the pressures of being a man – at least in terms of conventional or hegemonic masculinities (Connell & Messerschmidt, 2005). Matt himself discussed this issue in the following terms: 'I am an alpha male in a male dominated profession ... I am aggressive, a decision maker. Masculine means the ability to do guy stuff and be strong ... fix things, be brave, provide', and Russell (54, White) put it in even more poignant terms:

> For most of my sex life I'm in control of things. I'm not a boss at work anymore but I've been in situations where I've managed a hundred people at a time. I take care of my family. I take care of my kids. I'm a good father. I'm a good husband in providing material things for my wife ... I'm in charge in a lot of places ... There's times when I don't want to be in charge and I want someone to be in charge of me ... that's what brings me over [to] the bisexuals ... it's kind of submitting to another guy or being used by another guy.

Men such as Matt and Russell assume that having sex with men can provide them a respite from the burdens of hegemonic forms of masculinity, particularly since such sex happens in a space that that they feel is kept apart from everyday lives in which they feel they are expected to perform prescribed roles as heterosexual men. Those expectations, they perceive, include being dominant, and commanding others as part of their conventional roles as bosses, husbands, and fathers.

However, these participants feel that finding a space of respite from the burdens of masculinity requires secrecy, and, moreover, they view such secrecy as exciting and erotic. As

Gerard (57, White) put it, none of his friends nor his girlfriend, 'know that I sometimes like to stroke with a guy. I think that's part of the attraction … that it's a secret', and Josh (21, White) found that 'the thought of having sex with a guy is a big turn on, maybe 'cause it's so taboo'. These men's eroticisation of the secrecy surrounding their sexual interactions with men stands in contrast to the greater comfort with publicly engaging in homoerotic intimacy that Anderson (2012) detected among young, straight-identified male athletes.

Pleasing women

Finally, some of the straight-identified men in our study claimed that they began to engage in sex with men only after steady female partners asked them to help diversify and spice up their sexual lives as a couple by involving other sexual partners. Clark (54, White) was one of those men. Responding to a question about how he began to pursue sex with men, Clark pointed out that his girlfriend wanted him to do so, 'I didn't. [The] more I thought about it, the more aroused I became, eventually tried it'. His girlfriend, he said, 'thought it would be hot to see me with a guy'. Similarly, for Peter (40, White) his same-sex sexual explorations were prompted by a series of events that he described as a kind of slippery slope. His female partner wanted them to participate in threesomes involving a second man. 'After the third or fourth time, the guy went down on me. A couple of times after that, he asked me to do the same for him, and she encouraged it'.

Some of the female partners of non-exclusively straight men partially confirmed this idea. Silvie (31, White) described threesomes involving her male partner and another man, during which, for her, 'the most arousing part … was being the centre of attention'. She appreciated her male partner's flexibility to engage in sex with a man and openly stated that she found 'the fantasy of straight identified men (or hetero-flexible?) being sexual together arousing. Maybe it's because it's a taboo, or just the reverse of the common lesbian fantasy/porn that so many men seem to find attractive'. Josephine (37, Asian American) expressed having similar fantasies. She said that 'man-on-man action is just plain hot' and appreciated being with a male partner who is as open as she is. And Shawna (31, African American) kept in her 'fantasy list for us to have a threesome with a man that is penetrating my husband'. In more conventional couples, however, non-exclusively straight men usually did not share with their female partners any information about their same-sex desires and explorations, deciding instead to pursue them secretly on the side.

Discussion

Our findings further problematise the usefulness of the category MSM in HIV/AIDS prevention work as a catch-all behavioural category meant to address the public health needs of any and all men who engage in same-sex behaviours. As Boellstorff (2011) has noted, the category MSM has been radically transformed from its original formulation as purely behavioural, and has come to ambiguously serve as: (1) a signifier for men who do not identify as gay 'because they will use other terms' (p. 295); (2) a signifier for men who '"do not identify" at all in terms of sexual practice' (p. 295), which implies that 'such men have no sexual identity whatsoever' (Watney, 2000 [1993], p.76; quoted in Boellstorff,

2011, p. 295), and (3) a euphemism for gay men, particularly in the global South, leaving the actual term 'gay' as a referent for Western, White men.

The men in our study do have a clear sense of their sexual identity. Simply put, they are straight. But in constructing their primary identities as straight, and then supplementing them with secondary descriptors that denote a sense of heteroflexibility, they reconceptualise the category of heterosexuality to allow it to encompass same-sex desires and behaviours. This does not necessarily mean, however, that they incorporate their same-sex desires seamlessly into their straight identities. On the one hand, as part of their identities they seem eager to challenge social prescriptions about what being a straight man – and a masculine straight man, for that matter – means. But on the other hand, they also seem to fear the social consequences – in terms of their images as men, and as masculine straight men – of publicly revealing their same-sex behaviours or publicly adopting identities that do not have the word 'straight' in them.

These various issues can easily get lost if we solely focus on behaviour, or if we presume that all 'MSM' fit a single mould for the purposes of HIV prevention and sexual health programmes. Losing sight of such issues can also make it difficult to deeply consider them in designing HIV/AIDS prevention efforts – including behavioural, structural, and biomedical approaches – that could be more responsive to the needs of non-exclusively straight men. We thus view the idea of sidestepping identity (as Boellstorff, 2011 put it) that is implied by the behavioural category MSM as ill-conceived. Instead, similarly to Young and Meyer (2005), we propose that giving a deeper consideration to the links between sexual identity, attraction (desire), and behaviour is necessary – that a focus on identity can illuminate the multiple meanings that sexual behaviours may acquire within specific interpretations of identity, which seems crucial for understanding how preventive measures can be incorporated into people's sexual lives. We concur with other scholars who have argued that sexual health programmes must embrace the challenge of understanding the social, cultural, and historical aspects of sexualities and working with them (see, for instance, Brown & Maycock, 2005; Dodge et al., 2008; Ford et al., 2007; González, 2007; Kippax & Race, 2003; Malebranche, 2008; Muñoz-Laboy, 2004; Phillips, 2005).

Moreover, the presence among US White men of the various interpretations and management strategies that we detected further destabilises pervasive assumptions about the DL (as well as about the sexualities of MSM who live in the Global South). First, they challenge the perception that the DL exclusively characterises so-called men of colour – the illusion that there is not also such a thing as a 'White Down Low' (Ford et al., 2007). This view that has been paradoxically maintained in spite of the significant number of prominent US straight white men, including religious figures and politicians, who have been found to be living 'on the Down Low' in recent years (Phillips, 2005; Ward, 2015).

Second, our data also destabilise racial stereotypes that tend to split MSM into those who identify as gay (defined as White or Western) and those who do not identify as gay (defined as non-White or non-Western), creating what Boellstorff (2011) called a 'teleological hierarchy privileging Western, middle-class, white gay men' (p. 293). As Cantú (2009) has observed, this perception is sustained by 'cultural deficit models' – by the notion that the sexual cultures of non-White groups or non-Western societies are culturally deficient and, in effect, pre-modern. Such a perception not only reproduces colonial interpretations of the sexualities of 'the other', but may also easily lead to the conclusion that, as a prerequisite for effective implementation of HIV prevention, all MSM must first become educated about, and adopt, 'modern' categories of sexual identity (Saleh & Operario, 2009). And linked to this notion are normative expectations about 'coming out' and disclosure, which are commonly seen as a central tenet of a global gay model, as prerequisites for HIV risk reduction (Decena, 2008; Malebranche, 2008). Our findings challenge these presumptions, including the notion that straight identities among MSM are not also a White phenomenon, especially since we did not detect particular differences by race (a topic that we believe needs further investigation).

Overall, based on our findings, we believe that it may be productive for educators concerned with HIV/AIDS and other health issues to fully acknowledge the elastic definitions of heterosexuality that straight-identified men such as those in our study have reflectively created. They can then take those identities – and not just same-sex behaviours – as a starting point to envision, together with these men, how to effectively engage them in health promotion. Those efforts might in fact involve addressing the pernicious effects of heteronormative expectations that prevail within these men's social worlds – especially those that result in the secrecy that often surrounds their same-sex desires, which signals both a socially produced sense of shame and unequal power dynamics in the relationships some of these men have with women – but without assuming that their lack of a public self-identification as bisexual or gay is the core problem to be overcome. In addition, we would call attention to the fact that heteroflexibilities is a term in the plural. This means that strategies that address heterosexuality as an elastic category of sexual orientation will likely vary according to the specific logics of interpretation used by men in particular groups and settings. Although we have challenged reified conceptions of racial difference, it is certainly possible that programmes for heteroflexible men might appropriately be tailored to racial, cultural, as well as sexual identity.

Note

1. Similar advantages and disadvantages have been noted in an evaluation of online interviewing conducted by Hinchcliffe and Gavin (2009).

Acknowledgements

Our thanks go to Christine Wood and Pavithra Prasad, who conducted and coded interviews. We are grateful to Steven Epstein for commenting on drafts of this article, and to the journal's reviewers for their insightful comments.

Disclosure statement

No potential conflict of interest was reported by the authors.

Funding

This work was supported by the American Institute of Bisexuality and the Sexualities Project at Northwestern (SPAN).

References

Ambrose, E. (2009–2010). Heteroflexibility: Bending the existing label triangle. *Journal of Student Affairs, XVIII*, 69–75. Retrieved from http://www.sahe.colostate.edu/Data/Sites/1/documents/journal/2009_Journal_of_Student_Affairs.pdf#page=71

Anderson, E. (2012). Shifting masculinities in Anglo-American countries. *Masculinity and Social Change, 1*(1), 40–60. doi:10.4471/MCS.2012.03

Boellstorff, T. (2011). But don't identify as gay: A proleptic geneology of the MSM category. *Cultural Anthropology, 26*(2), 287–312. doi:10.1111/j.1548-1360.2011.01100.x

Brown, G., & Maycock, B. (2005). Different spaces, same faces: Perth gay men's experiences of sexuality, risk and HIV. *Culture, Health and Sexuality, 7*(1), 59–72. doi:10.1080/13691050412331271425

Burke, K. (2014). What makes a man: Gender and sexual boundaries on evangelical Christian sexuality websites. *Sexualities, 17*(1/2), 3–22. doi:10.1177/1363460713511101

Cantú Jr., L. (2009). *The sexuality of migration: Border crossings and Mexican immigrant men*. New York: New York University Press.

Carrillo, H. (2002). *The night is young: Sexuality in Mexico in the time of AIDS*. Chicago: University of Chicago Press.

Cohen, K. M., & Savin-Williams, R. C. (2010). *Can men have sex with men and still call themselves straight?* Retrieved from http://www.alternet.org/story/148876/can_men_have_sex_with_men_and_still_call_themselves_straight

Connell, R. W., & Messerschmidt, J. W. (2005). Hegemonic masculinity: Rethinking the concept. *Gender & Society, 19*(6), 829–859. doi:10.1177/0891243205278639

Dean, J. J. (2011). The cultural construction of heterosexual identities. *Sociology Compass, 5*(8), 679–687. doi:10.1111/j.1751-9020.2011.00395.x

Dean, J. J. (2014). *Straights: Heterosexuality in post-closeted culture*. New York: New York University Press.

Decena, C. U. (2008). Profiles, compulsory disclosure and ethical sexual citizenship in the contemporary USA. *Sexualities, 11*(4), 397–413. doi:10.1177/1363460708091741

Dodge, B., Jeffries IV, W. L., & Sandfort, T. G. M. (2008). Beyond the down low: Sexual risk, protection, and disclosure among at-risk black men who have sex with both men and women (MSMW). *Archives of Sexual Behavior, 37*, 683–696. doi:10.1007/s10508-008-9356-7

Essig, L. (2000). *Heteroflexibility: The latest semantic ploy to keep sexual options open really pisses me off*. Retrieved from http://www.salon.com/2000/11/15/heteroflexibility/

Ford, C. L., Whetten, K. D., Hall, S. A., Kaufman, J. S., & Thrasher, A. D. (2007). Black sexuality, social construction, and research targeting "the down low" ("the DL"). *Annals of Epidemiology, 17*, 209–216. doi:10.1016/j.annepidem.2006.09.006

Goldbaum, G., Perdue, T., & Higgins, D. (1996). Non-gay-identifying men who have sex with men: Formative research results from Seattle, Washington. *Public Health Reports, 111*(Suppl. 1), 36–40. Retrieved from: http://www.ncbi.nlm.nih.gov/pmc/articles/PMC1382041/pdf/pubhealthrep00044-0038.pdf

González, M. A. (2007). Latinos on da down low: The limitations of sexual identity in public health. *Latino Studies, 5*, 25–52. doi:10.1057/palgrave.lst.8600238

Hinchcliffe, V., & Gavin, H. (2009). Social and virtual networks: Evaluating synchronous online interviewing using instant messenger. *The Qualitative Report, 14*(2), 318–340. Retrieved from http://www.nova.edu/ssss/QR/QR14-2/hinchcliffe.pdf

Kalichman, S. C., Roffinan, R. A., Picciano, J. F., & Bolan, M. (1998). Risk for HIV infection among bisexual men seeking HIV-prevention services and risks posed to their female partners. *Health Psychology, 17*(4), 320–327. doi:10.1037/0278-6133.17.4.320

Kippax, S., & Race, K. (2003). Sustaining safe practice: Twenty years on. *Social Science & Medicine, 57*, 1–12. doi:10.1016/S0277-9536(02)00303-9

Malebranche, D. (2008). Bisexually active black men in the United States and HIV: Acknowledging more than the "down low". *Archives of Sexual Behavior, 37*, 810–816. doi:10.1007/s10508-008-9364-7

Miles, M. B., & Huberman, A. M. (1994). *Qualitative data analysis: An expanded sourcebook.* Thousand Oaks, CA: Sage.

Muñoz-Laboy, M. (2004). Beyond 'MSM': Sexual desire among bisexually-active Latino men in New York City. *Sexualities, 7,* 55–80. doi:10.1177/1363460704040142

Parker, R. G. (1999). *Beneath the equator: Cultures of desire, male homosexuality, and emerging gay communities in Brazil.* New York: Routledge.

Parker, R. G., Herdt, G., & Carballo, M. (1991). Sexual culture, HIV transmission, and AIDS research. *The Journal of Sex Research, 28*(1), 77–98. doi:10.1080/00224499109551596

Pathela, P., Hajat, A., Schillinger, J., Blank, S., Sell, R., & Mostashari, F. (2006). Discordance between sexual behavior and self-reported sexual identity: A population-based survey of New York City men. *Annals of Internal Medicine, 45*(416–425). doi:10.7326/0003-4819-145-6-200609190-00005

Phillips, L. (2005). Deconstructing "down low" discourse: The politics of sexuality, gender, race, AIDS, and anxiety. *Journal of African American Studies, 9*(2), 3–15. Retrieved from http://www.jstor.org/stable/41819081

Reback, C. J., & Larkins, S. (2010). Maintaining a heterosexual identity: Sexual meanings among a sample of heterosexually identified men who have sex with men. *Archives of Sexual Behavior, 39,* 766–773. doi:10.1007/s10508-008-9437-7

Saleh, L. D., & Operario, D. (2009). Moving beyond 'the down low': A critical analysis of terminology guiding HIV prevention efforts for African American men who have secretive sex with men. *Social Science and Medicine, 68,* 390–395. doi:10.1016/j.socscimed.2008.09.052

Savin-Williams, R. C., & Vrangalova, Z. (2013). Mostly heterosexual as a distinct sexual orientation group: A systematic review of the empirical evidence. *Developmental Review, 33,* 58–88. doi:10.1016/j.dr.2013.01.001

Shearer, K., Khosropour, C., Stephenson, R., & Sullivan, P. S. (2012). Do bisexual men tell their female partners about having male partners? Results from a national online HIV prevention survey in the United States. *International Journal of Sexual Health, 24*(195–204). doi:10.1080/19317611.2012.686965

Siegel, K., Schrimshaw, E. W., Lekas, H.-M., & Parsons, J. T. (2008). Sexual behaviors of non-gay identified non-disclosing men who have sex with men and women. *Archives of Sexual Behavior, 37*(720–735). doi:10.1007/s10508-008-9357-6

Stokes, J. P., McKirnan, D. J., Doll, L., & Burzette, R. G. (1996). Female partners of bisexual men. *Psychology of Women Quarterly, 20*(2), 267–284. doi:10.1111/j.1471-6402.1996.tb00470.x

Thompson, E. M., & Morgan, E. M. (2008). 'Mostly straight' young women: Variations in sexual behavior and identity development. *Developmental Psychology, 44*(1), 15–21. doi:10.1037/0012-1649.44.1.15

Vrangalova, Z., & Savin-Williams, R. C. (2012). Mostly heterosexual and mostly gay/lesbian: Evidence for new sexual orientation identities. *Archives of Sexual Behavior, 41,* 85–101. doi:10.1007/s10508-012-9921-y

Ward, J. (2008). Dude-sex: White masculinities and 'authentic' heterosexuality among dudes who have sex with dudes. *Sexualities, 11*(4), 414–434. doi:10.1177/1363460708091742

Ward, J. (2015). *Not gay: Sex between straight white men.* New York: New York University Press.

Watney, S. (2000 [1993]). Emergent sexual identities and HIV/AIDS. In S. Watney (Ed.), *Imagine hope: AIDS and gay identity* (pp. 63–80). London: Routledge.

Young, R. M., & Meyer, I. H. (2005). The trouble with 'MSM' and 'WSW': Erasure of the sexual-minority person in public health discourse. *American Journal of Public Health, 95*(7), 1144–1149. doi:10. 2105/AJPH.2004.046714

What is in a label? Multiple meanings of 'MSM' among same-gender-loving Black men in Mississippi

Nhan Truong, Amaya Perez-Brumer, Melissa Burton, June Gipson and DeMarc Hickson

ABSTRACT

Men who have sex with men (MSM) and other same-gender-loving (SGL) men continue to be disproportionately affected by HIV and AIDS, particularly among the Black population. Innovative strategies are needed to support the health of this community; however, public health efforts primarily approach MSM as a monolithic population erasing the diverse identities, practices, and sexualities within and beyond this category. To better understand diversity within MSM in a geographic region with the largest proportion of Black Americans in the U.S.A. and among the most heavily affected by the epidemic, the Deep South, we conducted four focus groups ($n = 29$) with Black men who reported having sex with other men residing in Jackson, Mississippi. Results suggest multiple overlapping usages of MSM as identity and behaviour, reflecting internalisation of behavioural categories and co-creation of identities unique to the Black community. These narratives contribute to the literature by documenting the evolving understandings of the category 'MSM' among Black men to reflect intersections between race, socioeconomic status, sexual behaviour, sexuality, subjectivities, and social context. Findings suggest the current monolithic approach to treating MSM may limit public health efforts in developing effective HIV prevention and promotion programmes targeting SGL Black men in the Deep South.

Introduction

In the U.S.A., men who have sex with men (MSM) have been disproportionately affected by HIV since the start of the epidemic, and Black MSM (BMSM) are the most affected compared to other racial/ethnic MSM groups (Center for Disease Control and Prevention [CDC], 2012). The current status of the epidemic, however, cannot be understood solely in terms of racial and gender difference, but rather geographic concentrations highlight that the largest burden of HIV is in the Southern United States (Nunn et al., 2014; Oster et al., 2011). For example, Mississippi ranks 2nd in states with the greatest proportion of Black residents and among the top 10 states in HIV infection rates (Mississippi State Department of Health, 2010). In 2010, close to 80% of all new cases of HIV were among Black Americans in the state (Mississippi State Department of Health, 2010), and new infections increased by 38% from 2004–2005 to 2006–2007 among young BMSM in the Jackson, Mississippi metropolitan area (CDC, 2009). However, the previously understood risk factors and demographic characteristics do not explain existing disparities among BMSM (Millett, Flores, Peterson, & Bakeman, 2007; Millett et al., 2012). As such, there is an urgent need to assess socio-cultural factors and local realities to better understand key determinants influencing the high HIV rate and maintenance of HIV prevalence among the BMSM community.

To understand risk and vulnerability to HIV for Black men, an acknowledgement of the intersections between race, class, gender, sexuality, and power are necessary to inform their lived reality. A keen starting point is with the category BMSM. Scholars critiquing the term 'MSM' highlight that such a broad term erases diverse identities and decontextualises same-gender sexual behaviour, and the repercussions for culturally relevant prevention and promotion efforts (Boellstorff, 2011; Young & Meyer, 2005). Similarly, Petchesky (2009) critiques the term 'sexual minority' for codifying potentially problematic assumptions about what is 'normal'. These limitations may be particularly salient for Black men and their vulnerability to HIV. As a push beyond MSM, or BMSM, the present paper uses local terms derived from the community, alongside the term same-gender-loving (SGL) in efforts to minimise minoritising discourse that reinforce the hierarchical division between majority ('normal') and minority ('abnormal') groups (Parks, 2001; Petchesky, 2009; Young & Meyer, 2005). Adopting an intersectionality perspective furthers attention to category construction by highlighting the complex interactions between race, gender, class, and sexual identities (Bowleg, 2012; Dworkin, 2005). Intersectionality theory posits that identification with more than one social group is qualitatively unique and intersectional, not additive, and that intersecting identities at the micro-level of individual experience reflect interlocking systems of inequality at the macro-level. Thus, membership of different identity groups can lead to differing behavioural health consequences (Bowleg, 2008; Crenshaw, 1995).

Recent discussions of SGL Black men on the down-low (DL) have problematised the use of DL in relation to Black sexuality suggesting that the term furthers the narrative that Black men are dangerous, sexual predators who have double lives, secretly having sex with other men, while placing their girlfriends or wives at risk for HIV (Ward, 2008; Watkins-Hayes, 2014). Stigma attached to DL may stem from the co-opting of DL by public health in relation to HIV infection and the pressures to adhere to traditional expectations of Black masculinity (Fields et al., 2015; McCune, 2014). In extension, the false notion that DL is unique to SGL Black men and does not occur in other races, including White men reinforces these stereotypes that serve to further stigmatise DL SGL Black men (Robinson & Vidal-Ortiz, 2013; Ward, 2008).

Socially constructed identities and subjectivities within the MSM category among Black men can also be viewed as sexual identities and practices that ebb and flow over time, situational contexts, and within power relations. With regard to HIV vulnerability among young urban SGL Black men, expectations of hypermasculine and anti-feminine behaviour, and failure to meet cultural standards of masculinity influenced feelings of social isolation, low self-esteem, and low awareness of HIV prevention messages (Fields et al., 2015). In extension, some scholars have sought to provide analytic groups to enhance HIV prevention efforts among SGL Black men, suggesting typologies of HIV testing patterns, characterised by sexual identity and behaviour (Hussen et al., 2013). Particularly relevant to SGL Black men, Weber's (2001) research showed that viewing an individual's lived experiences at the intersections of race, class, gender and sexuality reveals influential relationships of hierarchy and interlocking systems of inequality. Interrelations between variation in identities at the micro-social psychological level and the broader society's multiple interlocking race, gender, class, and sexual orientation systems of oppression may further reveal group differences in HIV vulnerability within the SGL Black male community (Collins, 1991).

Given the HIV and AIDS burden among SGL Black men and specifically SGL Black men in the Deep South, there is a need to better understand the multiple intersecting identities and practices within the Black 'MSM' category. Knowledge of diverse and intersecting identities, subjectivities and labelling practices can better inform public health research, HIV/AIDS services and intervention development. Accordingly, this paper explores the diversity of sexual identities and subjectivities within the MSM category and how realities of race, sexuality, and power contribute to HIV sexual risk behaviours for SGL Black men in the Deep South. The aims of the study were to explore: (1) how SGL Black men in Jackson, Mississippi socially construct and define identities and labels within the broad category of MSM and (2) how these identities and labels relate to HIV sexual risk and testing behaviours among this population.

Methods

Participants and procedure

Between July 2014 and August 2014, 29 SGL Black men participated in 4 focus group sessions in Jackson, Mississippi. All participants were part of a larger multisite study, the CDC-funded *Minority HIV/AIDS Research Initiative (MARI)* that examined interpersonal, intrapersonal, and environmental factors associated with HIV and Sexually Transmitted Infections (STIs) among SGL Black men in the Southeastern United States. Full study details are reported elsewhere (Hickson et al., 2015). In brief, eligibility was restricted to participants who self-identified as African American, assigned male sex at birth, identified as a cisgender man, 18 years old or older, reported having had sex with a man in the past six months, and lived in Jackson.

Recruiters contacted active MARI participants who expressed interest in future studies via telephone or text message. All men who indicated interest were scheduled to a session. All sessions were hosted after hours in a private space at a community-based Lesbian, Gay, Bisexual, and Transgender (LGBT) health clinic. Prior to study commencement, participants provided informed consent. Prior to group-based discussion, participants completed a demographic survey. Focus group sessions lasted between 60 and 90 minutes and covered four domains: types of identities and labels within the SGL Black male community in Jackson, Mississippi; dynamics of interaction between identity groups; condom negotiation among identity groups during anal intercourse; and HIV testing behaviours among identity groups. All participants were provided a $35 gift card, condoms and water-based lubricant. The Mississippi State Department of Health, Tougaloo College, and Sterling Institutional Review Boards approved all study procedures.

Analytic approach and data analysis

Focus groups were employed to identify identities within the Jackson SGL Black community, and to illuminate social norms and patterns regarding identities, and HIV sexual risk behaviours within this community (Allen, 2005; Hussen et al., 2013). This allowed exploration of subjectivities, revealing how SGL Black men manage their own sexual, gendered, racial, and class memberships through discussions about identities and labels within the 'MSM' category and HIV risk.

Focus groups were audio recorded and transcribed verbatim. Analysis was guided by intersectionality theory (Crenshaw, 1995), and study aims. The analytic framing revolved around social category memberships and power relations between groups and social roles in relation to the identities and labels within the MSM category. Qualitative data were analysed for saturation of focus group patterns and themes by two independent coders, trained in qualitative data analysis (Stewart, Shamdasani, & Rook, 2007; Weiss, 1995). Coders analysed the data through: (a) highlighting excerpts from transcripts, (b) developing codes based on excerpts, (c) linking codes to excerpts, and (d) developing and linking memos to coded excerpts. Coders then reviewed each others' codes and coded excerpts. Themes that emerged from the coded excerpts within and across focus group transcripts were identified. All analyses were conducted using an online qualitative research software program, Dedoose (Version 5.2.0) (http://www.dedoose.com).

Results

Among the 29 participants, ages ranged between 19 and 42 years ($M = 24.8$, $SD = 5.52$). The majority grew up in Mississippi (79%) and 79% reported their sexual orientation as gay or homosexual, while 17% self-identified as bisexual and 3% as other. Across focus groups 37 identities and labels associated with the MSM category were identified (see Table 1). When asked about a distinction, if any, between behaviour and identity, participants generally felt that behaviour and identity frequently overlapped. For instance, performing a sexual role, such as a top, bottom, and versatile, was considered sexual behaviour. Nonetheless, for some, sexual behaviours were interwoven with their sexuality, as well as, a key aspect of their sexual identities. When asked about whether there were differences between labels and identities, participants felt that labels were generally identities imposed upon them by others, from within and outside their community, and the majority were described as being negative (e.g. floor punk and punk). Few identities emerged that were considered positive, including beat girl and professional.

Sexual and social desirability hierarchy

Participants described a hierarchy of sexual and social desirability among sub-labels within the MSM category. The most sexually desirable strata encompassed labels characterised by masculine appearance, mannerisms, and/or talk (e.g. DL, trade, jock), and the most socially desirable strata were labels with high socioeconomic status (e.g. professional). Conversely, the lower strata were typically described as gender bending or feminine characteristics (e.g. floor punk, punk, sissy, trans), lower socioeconomic status

Table 1. Illustrative Quotes from Focus Group Narratives of Terms Associated with 'MSM' among same-gender-loving Black men in Jackson, Mississippi.

Identity/Label	Illustrative Quotes
Top/Bottom	"A top penetrates. A bottom takes it." [FG2]
Fudge packer	"… a behavior of sex … pack fudge … So the top in which penetrates the bottom when you're pounding him." [FG4]
Verse-top	"… boys are very funny because we may top you and bottom for somebody else." [FG4]
Verse-bottom	"Ain't no more straight tops and straight bottoms." [FG4]
Power-bottom	"a person that can take the whole Interstate 55 up their anus. That means they don't have a hole. They done lost the grip." [FG1]
DL	"And DL, or down low is from my understanding a man who's more conservative, really conscious about … how people are perceiving him and he doesn't want to be perceived as a part of the homosexual community." [FG2]
Trade	"… dudes who are usually willing to do sexual things very discreetly for a trade off of something, whether it be money, a place to stay, you know, support in some type of way." [FG2]
Homo thug	"So, homothug would be part of this DL/Trade, ultra masculine group." [FG3]
Jock	"… the ones that go to the gym all the time, and those people they're very desirable." [FG1]
Professional	"Pretty much everyone that's career oriented." [FG1]
Floor punk/Floor sissy	"… the gay people that sleep on the floor of somebody else's house. It's the closest thing to homeless. Like, they'll circulate from friend to friend." [FG1]
Club head	"You know the people that you see in the club every time you go." [FG1]
Masc	"Masc is masculine." [FG2] "More aggressive … Controlling … You can't be dating anyone else, but they can be messing with God knows who else." [FG 3]
Femme	"Femme [means] … really gay." [FG2]
Daddies/Sugar daddies	"Older men who wanna take care of younger guys … some people are smart enough not to allow the daddies to control their acts, but then some people need the money … like the floor punks." [FG1]
Punk	"I think as it relates to Jackson, punk kind of takes every idea of stereotypical of a homosexual in the South or a Black homosexual and puts it under one label … Lazy … very promiscuous, very feminine, bummish, doesn't work really. At the club every weekend." [FG2]
Sissy	"… more sort of a conservative, but flamboyant guy." [FG4]
Beat girl	"… they work/walk the beat … So beat girls and street walkers can kinda go together." [FG1] "They're the pretty girls … guys that will come to the club in makeup but will wear regular guy clothing. And it's no hair or anything; it's just a pretty face. It's masculine dress." [FG1]
Bitch	"A label or a taunt even. Same way another female will call another female a bitch and mean it in a bad way." [FG4]
Drag queen	"Female impersonation … some people just do it for the clubs as a career and some do it in real life." [FG1]
Butch queen	"They are like feminine guys, but they're more masculine. They wear the beard … the regular male hair like a fro or bald head but they have on like full make-up." [F G1]
Stunt queen	"It comes from stunt which is slang for trying to be more than what you are … someone who tries to identify something to which they really don't ascribe." [FG1]
Church queen	"When they are at church most of them will not say they are gay or anything, but they are the most flamboyant human beings in the church. Their identity is tied to their religious affiliation … They don't express their sexuality even though everyone in church knows (through) their actions and gestures … Like the tambourine player, how they stereotype that to be like the only gay male in church." [FG1]
Fag/Flaming faggot	"Words from transvestite to flaming faggot those ain't no positive words at all you gone get to fighting if you say that." [FG4]
Homo	"The abbreviation of homosexual is offensive." [FG2]
J-setter	"It's a group of male dancers … within the MSM community. It's a certain style of dance that is made popular by Jackson State j-setters … a group of girls, who perform certain distinctive moves that are indicative of that group." [FG1]
Fish	"… someone who's extremely feminine probably to the point where they could probably fool you into thinking they are a real woman, but not necessarily a transgender." [FG2]
House boy	"… they are guys that have sex just to stay at somebody's house and clean up and have sex with them just to stay there." [F G1]
Porn star	"They make gay porn … and they do it for the money." [FG1]
Street walker	"… a prostitute … that dress-up as a woman in drag … " [FG1]
Powder head	"Cocaine … They come together and do the same kind of drugs and they party a different kind of way but in the same venue as others." [FG1]

(Continued)

Table 1. Continued.

Identity/Label	Illustrative Quotes
Pill popper	"[Guys who are also high on] … codeine, xanax, umm yeah molly. Codeine, molly, crazy stuff. And anti depressants." [FG1]
Thirsty/THOT	" … THOT, and thirsty are terms that just very openly sexual individuals who have no boundaries. THOT … An acronym for 'That Hoe Over There' … individuals that basically anything goes." [FG4]
Trannies	" … they classify themselves as trannies you know like Carmen Carrera, got up, she don't like to be labeled as a trannie, but technically she is because she's transgendered. But trannies just a short term word for it … but to her its offensive." [FG4]
Trans	" … trans, transgendered, transgendered men are a part of the MSM lifestyle because technically they have not had a gender reassignment are still men sleeping with men, other enhancements to live their life as a female." [FG4]
Transvestite	" … some people consider transvestites as those who haven't gone through the surgery but they're still going around as a female. But they're still men." [FG2]

FG is an abbreviation for Focus Group

(e.g. floor punk, punk, street walker, porn star), and drug use (e.g. powder head, pill popper) (see Figure 1). Across narratives, the intersection of social membership categories (e.g. race, gender, class, sexual behaviour) and the power relations between groups were reflected in the hierarchical construction of identities and labels. Labels used within this community were reported as having unique social meanings tied to recognition and respect both within and beyond their immediate community. One participant discussed the intersection between gender, power, and desirability:

> Sometimes we just label each other in order to climb the hierarchy … and then on top of that when you get to the outside world, the world is like (also) labeling (us) … and most times the labels are negative. Like if I'm considered a queen, then I'm disrespected by a top because the top feels like this is a guy that thinks that he is a woman, but that queen might not think he is a woman. He's just feminine, and so the top sees him (the queen) as, you know, nothing, or he (the top) is more powerful in a sense. (FG1)

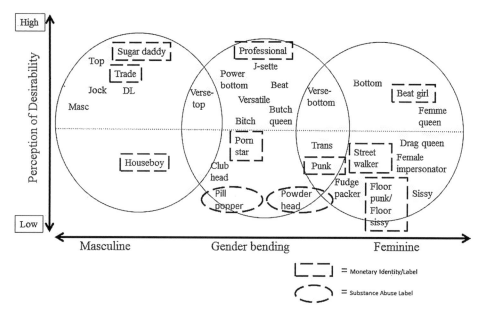

Figure 1. Conceptual Mapping of Identities and Labels Associated with Understandings of MSM in Jackson, Mississippi.

The above quote highlights the underlying topography of power differentials based on gender that parallel existing social inequities. For example, 'sometimes we just label each other in order to climb the hierarchy' suggests intention and that labels are not given passively. Linking to the intersection between gender and power, the section, 'He's just feminine, and so the top sees him (the queen) as, you know, nothing, or he (the top) is more powerful in a sense' speaks to the ways in which the already existing ordering of masculinity at the societal level is presented in a different form, where dominant (masculine top) and subordinate (feminine queen) positions are viewed at the intersection of gender and sexual role positions. As such, the majority of participants highlighted that masculine identities were perceived as more sexually desired than feminine identities because they were more controlling, dominant and aggressive.

Perceptions of desirability were particularly relevant to discussions regarding HIV prevention efforts. When discussing narratives of sexual intimacy and condom negotiation, participants reported more masculine associated labels as having the 'upper hand' in facilitating the occurrence of the sexual event and negotiating HIV prevention (e.g. condom use). Nonetheless, participants also stated that sex 'just happens' and that factors beyond perceived masculinity impact condom use. For example, when discussing sex between two bottoms, participants combined labels such as 'professional-bottom' or 'j-setter-bottom' to further delineate economic standing (FG4). Overlapping labels allowed participants to express their intersecting economic status and sexual role position identities and labels, which additionally were described as influencing a partner's ability to negotiate condom use or non-use.

The descriptions of power dynamics within this perceived hierarchy were also linked to class characteristics. Labels associated with more economic stability were also described as more sought after as a sexual partner and labels associated with economic disparities were intertwined with perceptions of HIV risk. When asked what other factors influence condom use, participants discussed drug use and engagement in a sexual economy, such as, exchanging of sex for money and basic necessities (e.g. food and shelter). The use of sex to obtain money, drugs, etc. was perceived as socially undesirable and in extension sexually undesirable. As described by participants, sexual commodification is prevalent in the lower stratum of the social and sexual hierarchy. Sub-labels used to describe these practices, and in extension identities, included powder heads, pill poppers, beat girls, street walkers, houseboys, floor punks, and porn stars. The accumulation of multiple undesirable characteristics can be additionally evidenced through the intersection of race and sexual identities with (low) economic stability and (high) drug use statuses. Across discussions, economically marginalised SGL Black male subgroups were perceived to be at higher risk for HIV infection and less likely to be able to negotiate condom use during a sexual encounter. For instance, when participants were asked which groups needed the most immediate public health interventions, they identified street walkers and substance abusers (powder heads and pill poppers):

> I would say the ones who like y'all said earlier that situational sex, those who use sex in exchange for some other service. Those are the ones who probably engage in more impulsive behaviors I would assume, or the ones with impaired judgment ... Those that need something. (FG1)

Gendered sexual scripts and hypermasculinity

Several participants mentioned an expectation for gay coupling to mimic heterosexual norms: composed of a masculine-top/feminine-bottom dyad. Descriptions also detailed expectations regarding appropriate ways to have sex and to display masculine behaviour. These gendered sexual scripts highlighted masculine/feminine power dynamics but additionally intersected with culture, race and class. For example, the interrelationships between gender role expectations and Black sexuality, homophobia, living a double life, engaging in unprotected anal intercourse, and not getting tested were reflected in the following quotes from participants across three focus groups:

> … Historically, African American men are seen as hypermasculine and that's a culture that's been bred to be African American masculine men, you have to be hypermasculine … (FG1)

> … I feel like when homosexuals were like shunned by like society, that forced them into the shadows and into the dark doors, and the undercovers, you know, sneaky, you gotta be in, you gotta be out. So, the whole preparation and the whole thinking about oh we need to be using protection, it kind of goes out of the window if y'all meeting up outta nowhere and randomly doing it because you don't want everybody to know. (FG2)

> … one of the reasons why they're [referring to DL and trade] so afraid to come in [to a clinic] because they don't want to know because if it is that they have something, the girl's gonna be wanting to know who you've been messing with, and then that's when problems arise. (FG3)

Focus group participants also described bottoms as more promiscuous, a perception also noted to be prevalent in the SGL Black male community. Combined with the sexually desired and highly sought after masculine tops, bottoms become at high risk for HIV infection:

> But I know for the bottoms, they're typically more promiscuous. And so if I'm the bottom and I'm chasing after you and my top doesn't want to use a condom, I want to have sex with my top so we're not going to use a condom because I still want to have sex. (FG2)

Narratives of hypermasculinity specific to the Black community emerged as a hegemonic masculinity script facilitating the strict policing of feminine behaviours, mannerisms, and talk that occurs both outside and within the SGL Black male Jackson community:

> To be African American men, you have to be hypermasculine which means you can't be anything remotely gay. If you took a risk, you're seen as feminine. If you talk a certain accent, if you don't talk Black and you don't talk country, if you talk with a certain professional air [of confidence] then they [define] you as feminine. If you wear pants that are at your waist, you're seen as feminine. So being hypermasculine is what's desired and that's very relative and very specific, I think to Black MSMs. (FG1)

Discussions of hypermasculinity and gendered expectations were linked to expected sexual roles. Participants frequently noted that the association with hypermasculinity and role was often a stereotype that did not accurately represent intimate encounters. Participants stated that though stereotypes helped structure the hierarchy of sexual desirability, the reality of sexual role practices that occurred during sex were flexible. Beyond the bedroom, these stereotypes influence access to HIV prevention services for DLs. For example, when asked about which SGL male subgroups would be least likely to access medical care, participants stated:

> Trade ... DL. Because ain't that how women get STDs, because of DL? You know they don't get checked out ... They don't want to be seen there .....they not going to go to any clinic until it's an extreme, and then they going to the hospital. And the reason I say that is because (DL and), trade feel as if they're exempt ... because like I said, those that are sleeping with men and women think that they're exempt from anything happening to them. (FG4)

Across focus groups, participants perceived that DLs were least likely to get tested for HIV and some participants additionally noted that unprotected anal intercourse legitimised DL masculinity. Participants also discussed parallels between DLs and trades getting tested for HIV and heterosexual men getting tested for prostate cancer – noting that they think that they are 'too real of a man' and 'stubborn' to seek a health professional. Black men are supposed to 'be strong all the time' (FG2). Moreover, when asked why trades and DLs are less likely to use condoms during sex, focus group participants stated:

> And if you're tryna imitate what an everyday man is as a trade or a DL, you're probably like it's ok not to have sex with a condom because my cousins do it or my uncles do it and everybody else, all the dudes I know do it. That's what I'm tryna be like. (FG2)

Paradox of 'DL'

As highlighted in Theme 2, the term DL is not only a term but also a label, which embodies gendered sexual scripts, hypermasculinity, and practices beyond intercourse. However, DL also emerged as a label of particular prominence when discussing what MSM means and how it influences sex and sexual identities. Participants described a tension between the sexual desirability of DLs and HIV infection and transmission associated with DL and trades in the broader society. Participants describe how DLs are portrayed as the infectors or carriers of HIV due to the secrecy of having unprotected sex with other men and also women, infecting their female partners with HIV. For example, participants described how the majority of Black women who have HIV and STIs were infected by DL SGL Black men:

> ... 85% of women get HIV/AIDS from men that are, have HIV, that [are] DL, trade guys ... because openly, women are not supposedly going to sleep with a openly gay man. (FG4)

This quote shows that the perception of secrecy is a central characteristic of DLs and places them at 'fault' for HIV transmission. However, viewing the experiences of DLs at the intersection of (Black) race, (masculine) gender, and (same-sex attraction) sexuality within larger social structural forces (e.g. homophobia) indicates that both the perception of secrecy and HIV transmission attached to their DL identity feed into each other and serve to simultaneous eroticise and stigmatise DLs. Participants also highlighted that having sex with a DL is particularly erotic because in many cases risky/illicit sex is a secret and intimacy is heightened due to the sharing of an illicit event:

> DL is ... very much something that a lot of people look for. Not because it's forbidden. It's kinda like that secrecy. (FG2)

The emphasis of secrecy, seen above as erotic, was also described as needing to be maintained. The pressure to maintain secrecy of who is DL can pose physical danger for those involved in the community. One participant discussed how a DL can act violently towards another SGL Black man who has knowledge of his same-sex sexual interest:

> Now DL is a guy who's down-low and he don't identify as gay but he still mess with men and if you tell somebody he'll shoot you in the face (laughter). (FG1)

This juxtaposing between the erotic and the violent was further compounded by the laughter that was present during the conversation. Although the participant laughed following his comment of being shot in the face by a DL, it triggered a conversation among the focus group participants about DLs' engagement in interpersonal violence to maintain secrecy.

The duality of DL, embodying both negative and positive aspects, is reflected in the narratives of men speaking about DLs. This complexity highlights that secrecy occurs at multiple levels; within the community and in the context within which SGL Black men are nested. Jointly, perception of HIV transmission and secrecy both serve to maintain non-disclosure of same-sex sexual behaviours to sexual partners among DLs, increasing likelihood of DLs' engaging in unprotected intercourse and therefore risk for HIV infection.

Resistance narratives

Counter narratives against the prevailing gender stereotypes were described as influencing sexual roles and sexual identities. These counter narratives described the liminal periods and spaces when condom negotiations between more masculine-aligned labels versus feminine-aligned labels (e.g. tops and bottoms) shift in power, and where gendered sexual scripts are turned on their head. Power dynamics regarding condom use and safer sex practices can shift, dissolve, and/or be reconstructed. As noted by one participant, 'strong' bottoms have the 'self-control' to refuse engaging in anal sex without a condom:

> If you are a strong bottom ... when it comes to, 'Hey babe I don't want to use a condom', then you know you have some bottoms that are like, 'Whoa, then we're not having sex' and no matter how much they kiss on you and try to put hickies on your neck and all of that, you have to have that kind of self control to where you're like, 'Well we're not having sex without condoms'. (FG2)

Similarly, other focus group participants echoed the notion that feminine stereotyped sexual practices, such as being bottom, can be powerful and dominate condom negotiation. One participant explained how some DL tops want to go 'raw', with him but will 'get their heads beaten' by someone like him, a dominant bottom (FG3).

Finally, focus group participants discussed fluidity of sexual identities and sexualities, as being mutable and contextual. Role switching was described as common, irrelevant as self-identification as a top or bottom, and can occur in the context of relationships. Participants described how they would change their motives for the man that they care for and love:

> I've seen tops become bottoms ... Let's say I'm in a relationship. I'm a top, you're a bottom. But if we get in a relationship where we really care for each other, we love each other, we want to switch it. If you really love (him), you will do that for that person. (FG3)

Moreover, participants commonly described mobility within strata of the social and sexual desirability hierarchy within SGL Black male sub-labels as associated with economic fluctuations:

> But it does happen, like throughout a lifetime, maybe I'm a floor punk at 21, but I don't want to be a floor punk all my life ... So I try to man up or maybe something else at 28 or 31, you know ... They can get up and go get a job ... (FG2)

The shift from (younger) floor punk to (older) professional over the participant's life course reflected the intersection of age and class identities and movement through other social structures. The shift to occupying a higher position in the desirability hierarchy indicated agency, a reclaiming of subjectivity, and exploration of alternative possibilities.

Discussion

Our results suggest that the contemporary epistemological configurations of sexual identities, behaviours, and meanings impacting the lives and well-being of SGL Black men are not readily captured by the category 'MSM'. The diversity of labels and identities highlight a fundamental tension between the needs of the diverse SGL Black male community and the existing provision of HIV and AIDS-related interventions and services. Importantly, discussions around SGL Black male subgroups and HIV risk reflect how these individuals manage their racial, gendered, sexual, and class subjectivities. In this context, the use of labels and identities were a process, constantly being reconfigured across social contexts and stages in life, which included identification and dis-identification, and tensions between agency and social structure.

According to these narratives, the prominent social, political, and cultural factors that structured HIV vulnerability were gender, economic disparities, and substance use and abuse. These factors were reflected in descriptions of sub-labels within the term MSM and their ordering in a sexual and social desirability hierarchy. Privileged statuses, meaning those associated with positive attributes and/or power, included labels associated with masculine gender and higher socioeconomic class characteristics. Conversely, non-privileged statuses represented in sub-labels were associated with feminine gender, lower socioeconomic status, and perception of substance use or abuse. Men's intersectional positions were woven into narratives of how these identities can be lived, and how these intersecting identities influenced social and biomedical prevention efforts. For instance, the heterosexual male role (e.g. DL and trade) were described as avoiding HIV care and having limited engagement with HIV prevention strategies, as were those individuals who displayed more feminine characteristics (e.g. floor punk, punk, trans, sissies). Other labels that were perceived as most 'risky' or vulnerable to HIV infection and transmission were those that intersected with other social categories, such as low socioeconomic status (e.g. floor punk, street walker, porn star), and drug use (e.g. powder head and pill popper).

When discussing more masculine SGL Black male sub-labels, such as DLs and trades, participants noted the challenges with masculine/feminine identities and labels and their prescribed behaviours, the stigma attached to the DL identity and the pressure to maintain the Black heterosexual male role. These findings echo previous literature noting that the construction of the DL top as a reservoir of infection and as a bridge between the Black SGL male and heterosexual communities creates moral and cultural panic in both communities (McCune, 2014). Moreover the stigma of having same-sex relationships might be increased among masculine SGL Black men in the Deep South as these individuals are situated in communities that often stigmatise homosexuality, while, simultaneously expected to adhere to cultural norms which fuel notions of Black hypermasculinity and anti-feminine appearance and mannerisms (Fields et al., 2015). Participants described acting masculine as both a gender performance and a form of role flexing, paralleling other literature suggesting that these traits may be adaptive strategies to avoid suspicions from friends, family, and others in the heterosexual community (Balaji et al., 2012; Butler, 1999). Jointly, being subjected to the stigma attached to DL and gender role strain both serve to negatively affect HIV testing behaviours and condom use during anal intercourse. Emergent themes also highlighted the incongruence of masculine/feminine identities and expected sexual behaviours; for instance, a jock who may prefer to be a bottom. These findings indicate a need for HIV prevention strategies that seek to actively dispel gender stereotypes and expectations by promoting an awareness of multiple sexual identities, eroticism, and pleasure as factors influencing sexual behaviours.

Focus group discussions described the DL paradox as the simultaneous stigmatisation of DLs from society and the Black community, and eroticisation of the secrecy of DL sexual behaviour within the SGL Black community. McCune (2014) discussed the DL paradox around a common descriptor pervasive within the media, 'the Down-Low Brotha', whereby DLs are blamed by society and the Black community for Black women's increase in HIV infection rates, which create a moral panic around the Black family. However, McCune's work disregards psychological processes at play within the SGL Black community. Understandings of this paradox can best be captured through an intersectional lens that involve both social structural forces (e.g. homophobia and hypermasculinity) and internalised pathways (eroticisation of DL). The application of an intersectional analysis exposed the nuance of multiple identities, labels, and subjectivities and the interactions with social structural forces at the community and societal level that influence behaviours and understandings of self.

Echoing Mocombe's (2008) notion of practical consciousness, focus group participants described how feminine bottoms and floor punks chose alternative practices and life choices upon reflecting on behaviours prescribed to their non-privileged identities, thereby showing the ways in which SGL Black men resist stereotypes. These examples of resistance underscores that terms cannot be presumed or taken for granted since such identities and labels (and the meanings associated with them) are the product of the field of power where the boundaries are constantly being contested. Furthermore, the fluidity of identities and their subjective meanings in the focus groups' narrative accounts suggest that these identities are constantly being re-configured over time and across social contexts (Wetherell, 2008). As an example of these nuanced identity terms, in some of the focus group narratives, feminine bottoms emerged as an identity that can assert power over condom negotiation when engaging in anal intercourse with masculine tops, and role switching can occur in intimate relationships and across time with varying partners. Here, shared narratives of agency in the face of stereotypes regarding HIV infection in their community revealed that negotiations over safer sex are contextual and situational (He & Ross, 2012; Weis & Fine, 2004). Participants also discussed how SGL Black men in the lower strata of the social and sexual hierarchy (e.g. floor punks) can shift towards becoming members of the higher strata (e.g. professionals) over their life course. This suggests that HIV prevention interventions need to not only adapt to diversity and overlap in identities and labels, but also to ongoing processes of change.

These findings are particularly relevant for informing the implementation and acceptability of HIV prevention strategies among SGL Black men. Despite advances in biomedical technology, behavioural and community-based approaches continue to be a crucial component to HIV prevention acceptability and sustainability (Aggleton & Parker, 2015). As evidenced in this study, the diverse sexual identities within 'MSM' among SGL Black men in the Deep South and their associated meanings in relation to HIV and AIDS are locally and culturally distinct from other MSM communities within the U.S.A. and worldwide (Meyer, Costenbader, Zule, Otiashvili, & Kirtadze, 2010). Importantly, understanding how SGL Black men in the Deep South experience these unique local identities at the intersection of race, class, gender, and sexuality in relation to social structural forces (stigma, discrimination, poverty, low education) is crucial to understanding differential HIV patterning and effective ways to ameliorate the burden of HIV among those most impacted.

There are important limitations to consider when interpreting the impacts of this study. Nuanced identity terms, such as local identities that reflect the diverse practices, sexualities, and subjectivities in these men's everyday lived experiences cannot be captured within labels. Furthermore, the terms, definitions, and/or labels presented here are not static and are amenable to change. The space where the focus groups sessions were held, a clinic that focused on providing health services to the LGBT community, may have influenced the narratives and discussions evoked during the focus groups. In efforts to minimise the potential for social desirability bias, all focus group discussions were held after hours and no clinic staff were present when participants arrived or at any point during study procedures. Despite this potential bias, the clinic provided a comfortable and non-threatening space that was conducive to productive discussions on sensitive topics. We did not explore environment and place as a potential factor to capture HIV risk levels among MSM identities in various situations. For scholars interested in this research, pile sorting and ethnography may be valuable methods to explore how sexual identities within 'MSM' interact with public/private locations where sex occur (e.g. clubs, cars, parks, rest stops, public restrooms, prisons, homes) to produce differential HIV sexual risk behaviours. As an exploratory qualitative study, the results from this study pertained only to those individuals directly engaged in our study and their reflections of the communities within which they live which is Jackson, Mississippi.

Nonetheless, this study furthers existing public health literature by highlighting and describing the diverse range of sexual identities and subjectivities within 'MSM' in a SGL Black male community located in a region of the U.S.A. disproportionately burdened by HIV and AIDS. The use of intersectionality theory to frame how the experiences of SGL Black men intersect with race, gender, and class to pattern differences between sexual identities within 'MSM' to produce differential HIV vulnerability may be key to future HIV and AIDS research, services and interventions targeting SGL Black men in the Deep South. These results seek to focus attention on the need to further investigate the multiple identities, labels, and subjectivities circulating within and around the term MSM among Black men to make visible the factors that directly and indirectly fuel HIV vulnerability.

Acknowledgements

The authors give thanks to all study participants for their time and effort. We thank Dr Leandro Mena for the informal conversations that helped the initial development of the study. We also thank Nikendrick Sturdevant, Gerald Gibson, and Reginald Stevenson for the recruitment of focus group participants. Finally, we would like to acknowledge Dr Simon Obendorf for his theoretical insights on power relations between gender and sexuality in SGL populations.

Funding

This work was funded by APA's (American Psychological Association) ProDIGs (Promoting Psychological Research and Training on Health Disparities Issues at Ethnic Minority Serving Institutions) (PI: Truong) and SPSSI's (Society for the Psychological Study of Social Issues) Grant-In-Aid (PI: Truong). Support was also provided by Eunice Kennedy Shriver National Institute of Child Health & Human Development [T32 HD049339] (PI: Nathanson) and National Institutes of Mental Health [R25 MH083620] (PI: Flanigan). This study was also funded in part by Centers for Disease Control and Prevention [U01 PS003315-04] (PI: Hickson).

Disclosure statement

No potential conflict of interest was reported by the authors.

References

Aggleton, P., & Parker, R. (2015). Moving beyond biomedicalization in the HIV response: Implications for community involvement and community leadership among men who have sex with men and transgender people. *American Journal of Public Health*, 105(8), 1552–1558. doi:10.2105/AJPH.2015.302614

Allen, L. (2005). Managing masculinity: Young men's identity work in focus groups. *Qualitative Research*, 5(1), 35–57. doi:10.1177/1468794105048650

Balaji, A. B., Oster, A. M., Viall, A. H., Heffelfinger, J. D., Mena, L. A., & Toledo, C. A. (2012). Role flexing: How community, religion, and family shape the experiences of young Black men who have sex with men. *AIDS Patient Care and STDs*, 26, 730–737. doi:10.1089/apc.2012.0177

Boellstorff, T. (2011). But do not identify as gay: A proleptic genealogy of the MSM category. *Cultural Anthropology*, 26, 287–312. doi:10.1111/j.1548-1360.2011.01100.x

Bowleg, L. (2008). When Black + Lesbian + Woman ≠ Black Lesbian Woman: The methodological challenges of qualitative and quantitative intersectionality research. *Sex Roles*, 59, 312–325. doi:10.1007/s11199-008-9400-z

Bowleg, L. (2012). The problem with the phrase women and minorities: Intersectionality – An important theoretical framework for public health. *American Journal of Public Health*, 102, 1267–1273. doi:10.2105/AJPH.2012.300750

Butler, J. (1999). Bodily inscriptions, performative subversions. In J. Price & M. Shildrick (Eds.), *Feminist theory and the body: A reader* (pp. 416–422). New York: Routledge.

Center for Disease Control and Prevention. (2009). HIV infection among young black men who have sex with men – Jackson, Mississippi, 2006–2008. *Morbidity and Mortality Weekly Report*, 58, 77–81. Retrieved from http://www.cdc.gov/mmwr/preview/mmwrhtml/mm5804a2.htm

Centers for Disease Control and Prevention. (2012). Estimated HIV incidence among adults and adolescents in the United States, 2007–2010. *HIV Surveillance Supplemental Report 2012*, 17(4), 1–26. Retrieved from http://www.cdc.gov/hiv/pdf/statistics_hssr_vol_17_no_4.pdf

Collins, P. H. (1991). *Black feminist thought: Knowledge, consciousness, and the politics of empowerment*. New York: Routledge.

Crenshaw, K. (1995). Mapping the margins: Intersectionality, identity politics, and violence against women of color. In K. Crenshaw, N. Gotanda, G. Peller, & K. Thomas (Eds.), *Critical race theory: The key writings that formed the movement* (pp. 357–383). New York: The New Press.

Dworkin, S. L. (2005). Who is epidemiologically fathomable in the HIV/AIDS epidemic? Gender, sexuality, and intersectionality in public health. *Culture, Health & Sexuality, 7*, 615–623. doi:10.1080/13691050500100385

Fields, E. L., Bogart, L. M., Smith, K. C., Malebranche, D. J., Ellen, J., & Schuster, M. A. (2015). "I always felt I had to prove my manhood": Homosexuality, masculinity, gender role strain, and HIV risk among young black men who have sex with men. *American Journal of Public Health, 105*, 122–131. doi:10.2105/AJPH.2013.301866

He, M. F., & Ross, S. (2012). Narrative of curriculum in the South: Lives in-between contested race, gender, class, and power. *Journal of Curriculum Theorizing (Online), 28*(3), 1–9. Retrieved from http://journal.jctonline.org/index.php/jct/article/download/378/pdf

Hickson, D. A., Truong, N., Smith-Bankhead, N., Sturdevant, N., Stanton, J., Gipson, J., … Mena, L. (2015). *Socio-ecological study of sexual behaviors and HIV/STI among African American men who have sex with men in the Southeastern United States (U.S.): Rationale, design and methods. PLoS ONE, 10*(12), e0143823. doi:10.1371/journal.pone.0143823

Hussen, S. A., Stephenson, R., del Rio, C., Wilton, L., Wallace, J., & Wheeler, D. (2013). HIV testing patterns among Black men who have sex with men: A qualitative typology. *PLoS ONE, 8*(9), 1–9. doi:10.1371/journal.pone.0075382

McCune Jr., J. Q. (2014). *Sexual discretion: Black masculinity and the politics of passing.* Chicago, IL: University of Chicago Press.

Meyer, W., Costenbader, E. C., Zule, W. A., Otiashvili, D., & Kirtadze, I. (2010). 'We are ordinary men': MSM identity categories in Tbilisi, Georgia. *Culture, Health & Sexuality, 12*, 955–971. doi:10.1080/13691058.2010.516370

Millett, G. A., Flores, S. A., Peterson, J. L., & Bakeman, R. (2007). Explaining disparities in HIV infection among black and white men who have sex with men: A meta-analysis of HIV risk behaviors. *AIDS, 21*, 2083–2091. doi:10.1097/QAD.0b013e3282e9a64b

Millett, G. A., Peterson, J. L., Flores, S. A., Flores, S. A., Hart, T. A., Jeffries, W. L.4th, … Remis, R. S. (2012). Comparisons of disparities and risks of HIV infection in black and other men who have sex with men in Canada, UK, and USA: A meta-analysis. *The Lancet, 380*, 341–348. doi:10.1016/S0140-6736(12)60899-X

Mississippi State Department of Health. (2010). *State of Mississippi 2010 STD/HIV epidemiologic profile.* Retrieved from http://msdh.ms.gov/msdhsite/_static/resources/3591.pdf

Mocombe, P. C. (2008). *The soul-less souls of Black folk: A sociological reconsideration of Black consciousness as Du Boisian double consciousness.* Lanham, MD: University Press of America.

Nunn, A., Yolken, A., Cutler, B., Trooskin, S., Wilson, P., Little, S., & Mayer, K. (2014). Geography should not be destiny: Focusing HIV/AIDS implementation research and programs on microepidemics in US neighborhoods. *American Journal of Public Health, 104*, 775–780. doi:10.2105/AJPH.2013.301864

Oster, A. M., Pieniazek, D., Zhang, X., Switzer, W. M., Ziebell, R. A., Mena, L. A., … Heffelfinger, J. D. (2011). Demographic but not geographic insularity in HIV transmission among young black MSM. *AIDS, 25*, 2157–2165. doi:10.1097/QAD.0b013e32834bfde9

Parks, C. W. (2001). African-American same-gender-loving youths and families in urban schools. *Journal of Gay and Lesbian Social Services, 13*, 41–56. doi:10.1300/J041v13n03_03

Petchesky, R. P. (2009). The language of "sexual minorities" and the politics of identity: A position paper. *Reproductive Health Matters, 17*, 105–110. doi:10.1016/S0968-8080(09)33431-X

Robinson, A. R., & Vidal-Ortiz, S. (2013). Displacing the dominant "down low" discourse: Deviance, same-sex desire, and Craigslist.org. *Deviant Behavior, 34*(3), 224–241. doi:10.1080/01639625.2012.726174

Stewart, D. W., Shamdasani, P. N., & Rook, D. W. (2007). *Focus groups: Theory and practice.* Thousand Oaks, CA: Sage.

Ward, J. (2008). Dude-sex: White masculinities and 'authentic' heterosexuality among dudes who have sex with dudes. *Sexualities, 11*, 414–434. doi:10.1177/1363460708091742

Watkins-Hayes, C. (2014). Intersectionality and the sociology of HIV/AIDS: Past, present, and future research directions. *Annual Review of Sociology, 40*, 431–457. doi:10.1146/annurev-soc-071312-145621

Weber, L. (2001). *Understanding race, class, gender, and sexuality: A conceptual framework.* New York, NY: McGraw-Hill.

Weis, L., & Fine, M. (2004). *Working method: Research and social justice.* New York, NY: Routledge.

Weiss, R. S. (1995). *Learning from strangers: The art and method of qualitative interview studies.* New York, NY: The Free Press.

Wetherell, M. (2008). Subjectivity or psycho-discursive practices? Investigating complex intersectional identities. *Subjectivity, 22,* 73–81. doi:10.1057/sub.2008.7

Young, R., & Meyer, I. H. (2005). The trouble with "MSM" and "WSW": Erasure of the sexual-minority person in public health discourse. *American Journal of Public Health, 95,* 1144–1149. doi:10.2105/AJPH.2004.046714

Switching on After Nine: Black gay-identified men's perceptions of sexual identities and partnerships in South African towns

Joanne E. Mantell, Jack Ume Tocco, Thomas Osmand, Theo Sandfort and Tim Lane

ABSTRACT
There is considerable diversity, fluidity and complexity in the expressions of sexuality and gender among men who have sex with men (MSM). Some non-gay identified MSM are known colloquially by gay-identified men in Mpumalanga, Province, South Africa, as 'After-Nines' because they do not identify as gay and present as straight during the day but also have sex with other men at night. Based on, key informant interviews and focus group discussions in two districts in Mpumalanga, we explored Black gay-identified men's perceptions of and relationships with After-Nine men, focusing on sexual and gender identities and their social consequences. Gay-identified men expressed ambivalence about their After-Nine partners, desiring them for their masculinity, yet often feeling dissatisfied and exploited in their relationships with them. The exchange of sex for commodities, especially alcohol, was common. Gay men's characterisation of After-Nines as men who ignore them during the day but have sex with them at night highlights the diversity of how same-sex practicing men perceive themselves and their sexual partners. Sexual health promotion programmes targeting 'MSM' must understand this diversity to effectively support the community in developing strategies for reaching and engaging different groups of gay and non-gay identified men.

Introduction

Queer sexual identities in South Africa are inextricable from the shifting politics of race, class and gender that have characterised the country's complex history. During Apartheid, sexual intercourse between men was punishable by up to seven years in prison. Yet, homosexuality flourished in the single-gender institutions instituted by the Apartheid government, including mining hostels, prisons and single-sex schools (Aldrich, 2003; Cameron & Gevisser, 1995; Epprecht, 2008). Until the late 1980s, gay organisations were often divided along racial lines and by the larger political question of Apartheid. For men who are not from the European-descended minority population, a specifically 'gay' subjectivity did not emerge in South Africa until the 1980s and was spawned largely by exposure to media from outside the country (Donham, 1998; McLean & Ngcobo, 1994). For these men, the emergence of a specifically 'gay' subjectivity occurred in the context of more racially inclusive anti-Apartheid activism that was also inclusive of lesbian and gay civil and human rights (Donham, 1998), and was primarily expressed in urban settings.

Post-Apartheid political and social transformations created space for public discourse about queer sexualities in South Africa in the 1990s. The synergistic forces of globalisation, urbanisation, news and entertainment media, the solidarities of the anti-Apartheid movement, and subsequently of the AIDS epidemic fostered a blossoming of queer organising and sexual identities unique on the African continent. The country's 1996 constitution became the first in the world to explicitly protect the rights of sexual minorities (Altman, 2001), outlawing discrimination on the grounds of race, gender and sexual orientation. In 2006, South Africa became the fifth country in the world to legalise same-sex marriages.

Though impressive, these legal achievements have not yielded widespread public acceptance of homosexuality (Roberts & Reddy, 2008). In 2013, only 32% of South Africans said that society should accept homosexuality (Pew Research Center, 2013). Perhaps unsurprisingly in light of South Africa's heterogeneity, post-Apartheid legal achievements have neither resulted in a unified national gay community, nor in a unified way of understanding sexual and gender variance. Some South Africans with same-sex attractions openly self-identify as 'gay', but many others do not. Reasons for this dis-identification include homophobia, stigma and discrimination, marginalisation (Sandfort, Parker, Gyamerah, Lane, & Reddy, 2012), and the perceived inapplicability or limitations of the label.

Like 'gay', 'homosexual' and 'bisexual', the all-encompassing referent label 'men who have sex with men' (MSM), widely used for HIV/AIDS surveillance, funding streams, and programming, may not convey the diversity, nuances and fluidity of same-sex desires, behaviours, identities and gender expressions. This may render the experiences of some men as invisible (Cáceres, Aggleton, & Galea, 2008; Sharma et al., 2008; Young & Meyer, 2005) and mask potentially important differences in behaviours. Moreover, the 'MSM' label in public health discourse may establish the link between HIV/AIDS and homosexuality at the expense of embracing broader sexual well-being and health needs. Finally, 'MSM' may obscure locally popular characterisations of same-sex desires and practices, the nuances of which are critical to effective health programming (Reddy, 2006).

In this paper, we explore the diversity of sexual and gender identities and labels from the perspective of Black self-identified gay men ('gay men') in Mpumalanga, South Africa. We focus specifically on gay men's relationships with a group of non-gay identified, stereotypically straight-acting men whom they refer to as 'After-Nines' – so called because they present publicly as 'straight' men, generally express antipathy towards gay men in public during the day, but make themselves available to gay men for clandestine sexual encounters at night ('after nine o'clock').

Methods

Participants and procedures

The data analysed here were collected during targeted ethnography (Wainberg et al., 2007) undertaken to adapt Mpowerment, a community-level HIV prevention intervention for young gay and bisexual men of proven efficacy in the USA (Kegeles, Hays, & Coates, 1996) to the South African context (known presently as Project *Boithato*). Between March and September 2011, field workers conducted 150 hours of structured observations in 'MSM-friendly' venues, eight focus group discussions (FGDs) with three to eight MSM per group ($N = 52$) and 41 in-depth semi-structured key informant interviews (KIIs) in two district municipalities in Mpumalanga Province, South Africa – Gert Sibande and Ehlanzeni. Like other Black South African communities, these municipalities were structurally disadvantaged by Apartheid, and continue to experience significant economic, social and health disparities as compared to the minority White population in the region. Data in this paper are based on the FGDs and KIIs.

We used purposive sampling via snowball techniques through social networks to recruit local 'experts' on the MSM community, including informal MSM community leaders, proprietors of formal or informal MSM-friendly venues and health professionals. All FGD participants and 29 of the 41 key informants reported having partners that included other men and were between the ages of 18 and 49. The study protocol was approved by the Committee on Human Research at the University of California San Francisco and the University of the Witwatersrand Human Research Ethics Committee (Medical).

The FGDs and KIIs lasted each approximately two hours, and were conducted either in English, *isiZulu* (Gert Sibande) or *SiSwati* (Ehlanzeni) by ethnographers. The ethnographers were four social science researchers between 23 and 27 years of age who were trained at the University of the Witwatersrand. One was a gay-identified man, one a straight-identified man, and two were straight-identified women. They worked in teams of two on FGDs (one facilitating whilst the other took notes) and individually for KIIs. The ethnographers were all at least trilingual, and when needed, could switch between languages during interviews. All FGDs and KIIs were digitally recorded and transcribed verbatim; *isiZulu* and *SiSwati* narratives were translated into English.

Prior to data collection, the ethnographers were trained in qualitative research methodology, research ethics, community entry and MSM sensitisation, data management and on standardised interview and group facilitator guides. Familiar with South African urban gay culture, all ethnographers immersed themselves in Mpumalanga's rural and gay subcultures during a six-month period of community entry prior to formal ethnographic fieldwork. The KII guide was developed to cover topics related to growing up as a MSM in South Africa, MSM community formation, sex and relationships in the lives of MSM, HIV/AIDS, how MSM communicate with each other, and ways and strategies to mobilise the MSM community. The FGD guide used a community participatory mapping approach, asking the participants to help the research team understand how the MSM community and membership is defined, structured, and networked, including identifying venues and events where MSM socialise and find sexual partners. Finally, the FGD participants were prompted to discuss challenges living as MSM in the general community.

Analysis

Initially, we used a thematic analysis approach to the data. Ethnographers and study investigators read a subset of transcripts together (three FGDs, six KIIs) to develop topical codes related to the main study questions about community structure, social life, sexuality and relationships, and health. Grounded theory was used to identify and code emergent themes (Glaser & Strauss, 1967). Coding consensus and refinement of the codebook were achieved through team meetings between the ethnographers and investigators. We used Atlas.ti software to code and manage the data. In this paper, the analysis is based on the topical codes of 'sexual identity', 'sexual partnerships' and 'intimacy' from the FGD and KII data. Two of the authors read the coding reports and developed additional thematic categories within these topical codes.

Results

Two key themes emerged in gay men's narratives with regard to sexual and gender categories and how they are situated in sexual relationships: (1) diversity within gay communities and (2) relationships between gay men and a subset of non-gay identified male sexual partners whom gay men referred to as After-Nine men. We did not discern differences between geographic communities or data collection method, and have thus aggregated results.

Sexual and gender diversity within gay communities

When speaking to self-identified gay men, the ethnographers asked them to define who they considered to be part of the gay community. Participants characterised the community broadly, illustrating the heterogeneity of categories of sexual identity and gender expression. Groups gay men considered part of the larger gay community included gays, transgenders, drag queens, bisexuals and lesbians. Many also included 'After-Nines' and other non-gay identified MSM who had 'not yet accepted that they are gay'.

> We don't say wena [you] belong to another kraal, or you belong to another community .... you can be whatever. You belong in the family. You are gay.

> To me, whether you are bisexual or 'After-Nine', you still fall under the category of homosexual because if you were straight you would not be sleeping with men.

Being 'gay' was described in a number of different ways: as an inner feeling unrelated to physical appearances ('you can look straight ... .It's basically a feeling, it is something that is internal'); as a gender dysphoria ('a boy trapped in a girl's body') and as a sexual desire unrelated to feminine gender presentation ('you are a man that is interested in another man. So I must keep it like that, dress like a man, walk like a man, do things like a man because I know my identity'). Being the receptive partner in anal sex was often associated with being gay, and vice versa.

> My ex did not want to be called gay. To him, being gay meant that you were a bottom. If you are not a bottom, then you are not gay. This doesn't mean that he is hiding what he is doing. In actual fact, he didn't have a problem with what he was doing, but the name 'gay' didn't sit well with him, because to him, once you use the term 'gay', this means you are sissy-like. He believed you can't be a man and be gay.

Some gay-identified participants expressed tolerance of and preference for unique and fluctuating gender expressions among gay men.

> We are in between the male and the female; we have best of both worlds.
>
> Men must understand that once you are gay it's obvious that you will be forward and you will be sissy-like. Sometimes we also want to be treated like ladies. In my relationships I demand to be treated like a lady. I tell the guy I'm seeing, 'You are the man, treat me like a lady.'

Whether 'gay' explicitly signified femininity and obligated one to behave in a stereotypically feminine way was a point of contention. For those who self-identified as 'gay', the meaning of the term was open to interpretation. The distinction between 'gay' and 'transgender' was not absolute, nor was 'transgender' a commonly claimed identity. More common were references to being a 'drag queen', feeling 'trapped' in men's bodies or being 'gay women'.

> There was not even one gay man wearing pants, and he [a gay man dressed in drag] said [to me], 'No, when you are in [a gay club] and you are gay, you have to drag'. And I said, 'No, that's not it. Who told you that?' And he said, 'We were told by the elders such and so and so.'

> Personally, I feel like a woman, but I don't go around telling people I'm a woman trapped in a man's body. By doing that I would be fighting with my creator. He knew that he was creating a gay man. Now why must I fight that. I tell them that I'm not a girl, I'm a woman, a gay woman.

Where some gay men celebrated femininity, others sought to conceal appearances of homosexuality by refraining from what were perceived as overtly gay behaviours and rejecting stereotypically feminine gender expression – at least in public social spaces. Dressing and behaving in conventionally masculine ways were strategies to avoid stigmatisation. Some participants voiced concerns towards gay men who openly embrace a stereotypically feminine expression of their 'gayness' and believed that this should only be expressed in the presence of gay friends.

> People know I am gay, but I do not just share that with everyone so that they don't disrespect me and call me 'girlfriend' or 'girl'. Being gay does not mean I am a girl; I am a boy.

> You don't have to show everyone that you are gay. But you can only do that when you are around your friends. Then you can reveal your true gay self. We as gay people like to perform and act gay in public and we should only do that amongst family and friends.

> You will never see me wearing a skirt or a dress. I would be forgetting who I am if I did that. Who I am is a man; the inner me is a woman. … There is a time for mini-skirts and there is a time for everything else.… You can wear a mini-skirt at a party, but not at a funeral.

Gay men who described themselves as feminine voiced desires for relationships with 'real men', and expressed little desire for sexual relationships with other gay men who, like them, were perceived to display more female expressions of gender. Moreover, such gay-identified men felt strongly that gay-identified men expressing more fluidity with their gender presentation was undesirable.

> I do not want to be with a girl; I want to be with a real man. So now all of a sudden when [he] turns on me and starts acting feminine, it turns me off and I end up leaving him because he is not what I was looking for.

Participants also described some gay men as 'straight-looking gay guys', or 'straight gays', meaning men who consider themselves gay but look and act in a stereotypically masculine or straight manner. As such, they were seen as objects of sexual desire. 'Straight gays' were described as only having other men as their sexual partners. Nevertheless, some participants characterised them as being in denial about being gay. 'These are men who will act like he is straight, but when you pass by him, he will be busy pinching you to get your attention'. But more frequently, men in this category were described as sexually desirable.

> You see those gay men understand gays and the way that gay people behave. For example, my husband is a gay man, he is masculine and I am feminine.

> Some guys, they don't want drag queens; they are looking for those straight-looking gays because they don't want to be seen around gay people. When walking with a straight-looking gay guy, they don't feel embarrassed.

'After-Nine' men were distinguished from 'straight gays' and described by gay men in various ways: 'dating women', 'being with a woman and a man', and 'hiding their sexuality under the table' to avoid disclosure of their sexual proclivities. 'There are people who define themselves as straight but they do sleep with gay men, but at the same time, they do not consider themselves as part of us.' These descriptions conveyed that After-Nine men were stereotypically masculine, behaviourally bisexual, and generally the insertive partner during anal sex. However, After-Nine men's masculinity was not always a guarantee that they assumed the 'top' role in their sexual encounters with gay men.

> There are those [After-Nines] who say that they are straight, but they are also bottoms in bed. So when you are out with him, you need to treat him like a boyfriend and you need to act like a lady because you are gay – but it is a different story when you have sex.

One gay man characterised After-Nine men as not yet accepting they are 'gay' or being uncertain about their same-sex desires.

> They can't find a key. Or, they have it, but they are just struggling to open the door and pave their way.

Some gay men did not consider After-Nine men to be part of local gay communities because After-Nine men did not overtly experience anti-gay stigma and discrimination, and even were seen to perpetuate it. However, some gay men still supported including After-Nines as part of the gay community.

> I think that as a gay community we can still do more because even though they are After-Nines, they still need our support because one day their secret will be out in the open and it will be difficult for them.

Gay men's relationships with After-Nine sexual partners

Despite the fact that many gay men expressed desire to have After-Nine men as sexual partners, many expressed frustration and dissatisfaction with these relationships. They were disappointed by and resented After-Nine men's abrupt switch from pursuing gay men as sexual partners in the evening to avoiding them the next day. Some gay men said, 'During the day, they [After-Nine men] act like they hate gay people'.

> You will greet them and they will not respond. They will just walk past you in a passage. All they know is just how to strut, 'left, right, left, right', as if there is no one there.

> I think during the day, they do not want to be seen talking to gay men and most of them are very homophobic and do not want to want to be associated with gay men. Because to them this would mean that they are not manly enough. But when no one is watching, they become very friendly toward gay people.
>
> Then at night, he is the first one to come to you and say 'Baby I love you, I am bisexual.' Then I say, 'But wasn't it you that was swearing at me saying I am gay? You now sleep with gays?'

Some gay men expressed being hurt by After-Nine men's inconsistent behaviour towards them.

> … when After-Nines see a gay man who is out of the closet, they are not happy about that because they are still in the closet. Their time to be out is only at night or whenever they have that opportunity … .Sometimes … I will be at a party and sleep with [an] After-Nine. After that night, that particular After-Nine will do all that he can to sabotage and hurt me.

Gay men expect that their After-Nine partners have girlfriends, wives, and other female sexual partners. Not all were upset about this.

> In life I cannot choose for a person. I can't tell them that they shouldn't be with a woman, but be with me only. As long as he satisfies me, then it's fine, because he deserves a vaginal [vagina] and an anal [anus]. As long as he is able to satisfy me and keep me happy on my side, just as he has to satisfy his girlfriend as well.

Some gay men expressed desires for public validation of their relationships with After-Nine men. However, they knew that this public validation was reserved for After-Nine men's female partners.

Others, however, expressed a desire for public validation of the relationship with the After-Nine man that was reserved for his female partners.

> … As an After-Nine, you come to me. You keep telling me that you love me, but during the day, you are with your wife. I can't be seen anywhere with you. You know that I am like ecstasy, I'm addictive. You keep on taking me when nobody is looking at you, but on the other hand, I want to be seen out with you.

Sex, gender, power and exchange

Gay men's relationships with After-Nine men are characterised by exchanges of sex for goods. Gay men buy alcohol for their After-Nine partners in exchange for sex; other items of exchange included food and mobile phone airtime. A less common description of the transactional nature of these relationships was aligned with expected gender roles, manifest by After-Nines providing for more feminine gay men.

> They can say they bought us. He'll be buying you drinks and everything you ask for. He'll buy and you know that at the end of the night, you are going to be going home with him to sleep with him.

It was far more common for gay men to describe providing the material benefits in exchange for sex with After-Nine men.

> After-Nines just think that all you need to do to get a gay guy is tell him you love him and he will just melt and end up buying you beers and sleeping with you.

These types of transactional relationships were frequently based on the reality or perception that gay men were financially well-off and had disposable income. Although the exchange of cash for sex between men was uncommon, some gay men referred to them as 'rent boys'.

> It's about power and money because people think that gays have money. So After-Nines use gay people to buy them drinks and food.

> They sell their bodies. Even though we do not give them hard cash, the fact [is] that you buy them alcohol and then [he is] going to come home with me and eat my food and sleep in my blankets.

> … you will find someone who will say, 'Buy me a beer. I want to go with you'. So in a way I would say, according to my understanding, that man is selling sex–not monetary, but alcohol-wise.

Gay men's narratives about these exchanges frequently conveyed the sense that After-Nine men were opportunistic, and left their gay partners disappointed with the terms of the exchange.

> For straight guys, they only want to ejaculate. That's all. And you can't have sex with them the whole night because after they ejaculate they are done with you.

> You pick this person up at [a tavern], you take him home, you sleep with him and as soon as he has reached climax, he says he needs to be somewhere. He has done what he was there for.

One participant articulated the entanglement of material, sexual and emotional affect that many gay men experienced in their relationships with After-Nine men.

> … The relationship between MSM that do not identify themselves as gay and gay men causes tension because you're telling yourself that you are in a relationship with this person. But in actual fact, this person has other agendas. It could be money or just to have fun and drink alcohol, and the sex is not good. … the one that you find at a tavern, for example, you have basically bought him with alcohol and once you get to your place to have sex, he is only concerned about getting it over and done with. At 11 PM when he is done having sex with you, he'll put on his clothes and leave. It's not true love.

Unrequited desire for intimacy

Emotionally unfulfilling relationships with After-Nine sexual partners were a source of dissatisfaction for gay men. Sexual encounters were frequently described as one-night stands, devoid of commitment or emotional intimacy, and solely centred on achieving sexual pleasure. A common theme in gay men's descriptions of relationships with After-Nine men, whether they were transactional and fleeting, or established over time, was a well-articulated sense of disappointment that they could not achieve any intimacy with After-Nine partners. 'One-night stands' were particularly non-reciprocal and had the potential for physical altercations if gay men pursued them further.

Gay men perceived they had no control over the behaviour of their After-Nine partners in public settings.

> It's not nice because sometimes you could be really in love with that person but you are not able to prove how much you love him. The only relations that the two of you will have is meeting up at clubs that weekend maybe on a Friday then the next day he'll disappear. He's basically playing with your heart. But he'll still say that you are his boyfriend amongst your friends.

One participant admonished gay men generally for falling for straight men when the outcome of these relationships was almost never satisfying.

> Some of us, actually most of us, tend to fall in love with straight people. Where are you going to find love from a straight person? ... At least if you are looking for someone that is straight-looking, that is okay – as long as they are gay. But you cannot try and find love from someone who is completely straight. It won't happen; he will never even introduce you as his partner to his family.

The hidden nature of After-Nine men's relationships with gay men was a source of frustration for most and emotionally traumatic for some.

> Just imagine waiting on the rain. You are basically waiting, waiting for the day that he will come out and be comfortable to be with you. Whereas, on the other hand, you want him badly. Can you imagine how much it hurts? We get hurt; it's a fact. That's why I think there are high cases of suicide amongst gays because you are basically waiting on this one person.

There was also tacit acceptance of the lack of commitment by After-Nine men.

> Sometimes you go into this knowing that it is a no-strings attached relationship, so it doesn't matter if they do not talk to you the next day.

Discussion

Our study provides insight into how Black gay South African men living outside of that country's major metropolitan areas articulate their sense of a community defined by a shared sexuality, and how gay men make sense of their own sexual expression and those of their sexual partners, specifically men that are labelled as 'After-Nines'. Participants' narratives suggest that they understand that the social and sexual dynamics that exist among various groups within the 'gay community' in Mpumalanga are complex and often marked by tension, particularly with the non-gay identified group of After-Nine men. The data presented here support Young and Meyer's (2005) caution against using MSM interchangeably with gay identity in public health discourse. However, the data also show that the meaning of gay identity is itself contested by gay men in these communities, who frequently articulated an inclusive community identity that incorporates non-gay identified men as sexual partners.

Participants primarily characterised gender expression among MSM as a masculine–feminine binary. This gender binary has been reported in other studies of gay and other MSM in South Africa (Lane, Mogale, Struthers, McIntyre, & Kegeles, 2008; McLean & Ngcobo, 1994; Rabie & Lesch, 2009; Reid, 2005; Sandfort et al., 2012). Gay men associated their own and others' gay identity less commonly with masculine gender conformity than with feminine gender non-conformity. They perceived After-Nine non-gay identified men as well as straight, non-gay identified MSM, who were the objects of their desire, as masculine gendered. Fluidity in gender expression was described, with participants characterising themselves in terms of being both feminine and masculine. Some categorised After-Nine men as 'straight', while others considered them bisexual, or secretly gay. They distinguished After-Nine men from straight gay men in that the former also had sex with women. The inversion of gender roles that gay men described in their relationships with After-Nine sexual partners in Mpumalanga, whereby a more feminine partner attracts and attempts to hold the attention of a more masculine partner by giving material goods, is comparable to the dynamics in gender-stratified homosexual relationships reported elsewhere in South Africa (Masvawure, Sandfort, Reddy, Collier, & Lane, 2015) and in other countries, for example, in Cote d'Ivoire (Brooks & Bocahut, 1998) and Brazil (Kulick, 1998).

Although some participants enjoyed exploring aspects of their feminine feelings, they recognised the need to present publically in a more masculine manner, with a preference for reserving overt female gender expression for private contexts and specifically gay spaces. These gay men consciously embodied a more masculine style as a way to conceal homosexuality, foster public acceptance and command respect. Whereas gay identity in South Africa has traditionally been associated with feminine gender presentation (Rabie & Lesch, 2009; Reid, 2005), there is some evidence for the emergence of a new form of identity and desire that is not based exclusively on a binary gender system. Participants' mapping of the diversity of identities revealed that sexuality and gender were not necessarily discrete categories, as Valentine (2007) theorised in his ethnography of the emerging transgender category in New York City. Gay men had a broad conception of anyone not strictly heterosexual and not strictly cisgender as part of the 'gay' community, including individuals who in a western context would likely be identified as 'transgender'.

The exchange of commodities such as sex, alcohol and money between gay and After-Nine men who meet in 'gay-friendly' bars and taverns in the towns and townships of Mpumalanga was assumed to be a basic feature in their relationships. Power inequities in these relationships were manifest in two ways. The perception that gay men were relatively affluent gave them advantage for attracting sexual partners, including After-Nine men. Gay men were expected to buy alcoholic drinks, cell phone airtime, and other material goods in exchange for sex and companionship with After-Nine men. At the same time, After-Nine men held power over gay men as objects of their sexual desire. This suggests that within the gay community, normative masculinity is another sought-after commodity, one that all straight-identified MSM possess and that After-Nine men use to their advantage in their interactions with gay men.

Power and exploitation in relationships between gay men and their After-Nine partners can be understood through the lens of a social exchange framework (Emerson, 1976) which considers attributes of the relationship between actors as key, rather than attributes of individual actors. Relations are viewed as a process of reinforcing rewards (financial gains and attention) and minimising costs (exploitation and lack of intimacy). This bi-directional exchange of power allowed for sexual transactions as a social exchange. Gay men desired and longed to be desired by After-Nine men, and believed that After-Nine men sought to reap material benefits from them. However, our data indicate that gay men experienced the transaction as asymmetrical. Despite being perceived as having money to spend, and despite deploying resources in a transactional sexual context, they experienced themselves as nonetheless disadvantaged in getting what many desired from After-Nine men beyond a simple fuck: a relationship that included emotional intimacy and love.

The problematic nature of these relationships for gay men in Mpumalanga must also be seen in the context of the narrow pool of openly gay men in our study communities. The secrecy imposed by After-Nine men was attributed to the closeted nature of their sexuality, which, in turn, was related to homophobia. This social distance between gay and 'straight' men was also reported in Lorway's (2006) study in Namibia, with the latter group only socialising and having sex with gay men they met at clubs at night. This covert sexual dynamic also bears similarities to that of 'down-low' men in the US context (Bond et al., 2009; Sandfort & Dodge, 2008).

Our study has several limitations. First, our ethnographic sample was composed largely of self-identified gay men recruited through snowball sampling, most of whom embraced binary sexual and gender identities of gay and non-gay identified men, including After-Nine men. Second, the data do not include the perspectives of non-gay identified men. We acknowledge that understanding how After-Nine men perceive their own sexual and gender identities and their relationships with gay men and other sexual partners is important to fully understanding relationship and sexual dynamics, and their impact on HIV risk-reduction and health-promoting behaviours. Notwithstanding these limitations, the study contributes to the fields of sexuality studies and public health by describing the diversity of homosexual identities and sexualities in the narratives of Black gay men in rural South African townships that, in public health discourse, are generally subsumed under the 'MSM' category.

Fish (2008) points to the need to consider intersectionality theory (Crenshaw, 1991) and the interconnectedness of the multiple identities of gender, race and class associated with oppression and social inequality among LGBT communities. This is especially salient in South Africa, where such intersections have been the sites of considerable contestation and change in recent decades.

As we continue to consider the utility and limitations of the MSM category, there is a need to interrogate sexual and gendered discourses, vocabularies and identities. Recognising that sexual minority community identities do not map neatly onto public health categories invented to describe them, there is equally a need to understand that sexual behaviour and HIV risk are not bounded by the sexual identity terms that sexual minority communities may employ to describe themselves. Emic terms like 'After-Nines' cannot be adopted wholesale into prevention programming because who and what behaviours such terms encompass is not static. Moreover, those to whom such labels are applied are likely to reject them as derogatory – particularly if health programmes considered exogenous to the communities from which such categories originate appropriate them.

Conclusion: implications for HIV prevention

Non-gay identified After-Nine men are an integral part of the sexual networks of gay men in Mpumalanga. The social and sexual interactions between gay and non-gay identifying MSM are critical to understanding HIV risk and effective targeting of sexual health-promoting interventions. However, the secretive nature of After-Nine men's sexual relationships with gay men and their antipathy towards overt identification with gay men presents a challenge to community-based HIV prevention approaches to addressing the needs of all MSM in Mpumalanga. Though difficult to identify and recruit because of lack of organised social networks, our findings underscore the need for future research to explore After-

Nine men's perspectives on sexuality, gender, sexuality, and risk to improve HIV programming for men who engage in sex with men. At the same time, sexual risk-reduction interventions with gay men and those who defy strict identity categorisation must assist in building safer-sex self-efficacy to manage challenging circumstances with any sexual partners.

Acknowledgments

We wish to thank the participants in this study for sharing their time and experiences with us. We also thank the two anonymous reviewers who provided helpful comments on earlier versions of this article. The content is solely the responsibility of the authors and does not necessarily represent the official views of NIAID, NIMH, or the NIH.

Disclosure statement

No potential conflict of interest was reported by the authors.

Funding

This research and analysis were supported by grants from the U.S. National Institute of Allergy and Infectious Disease ([grant number R01-AI089292]; Principal Investigator: Tim Lane, Ph.D.); and a centre grant from the U.S. National Institute of Mental Health to the HIV Center for Clinical and Behavioral Studies at NY State Psychiatric Institute and Columbia University ([P30-MH43520]; Principal Investigator: Robert H. Remien, Ph.D.). Dr. Tocco was supported by a training grant from the U.S. National Institute of Mental Health ([T32 MH19139], Behavioral Sciences Research in HIV Infection; Principal Investigator: Theo Sandfort, Ph.D.).

References

Aldrich, R. (2003). *Colonialism and homosexuality*. London: Routledge.
Altman, D. (2001). *Global sex*. Chicago, IL: University of Chicago Press.
Bond, L., Wheeler, D. P., Millett, G. A., LaPollo, A. B., Carson, L. F., & Liau, A. (2009). Black men who have sex with men and the association of down-low identity with HIV risk behavior. *American Journal of Public Health*, 99, S92–S95. doi:10.2105/AJPH.2007.127217
Brooks, P.(Producer), & Bocahut, L. (Director). (1998). *Woubi cherí*. France & Côte d'Ivoire: California Newsreel.
Cáceres, C. F., Aggleton, P., & Galea, J.T. (2008). Sexual diversity, social inclusion and HIV/AIDS. *AIDS*, Suppl 2, S45–S55. doi:10.1097/01.aids.0000327436.36161.80
Cameron, E., & Gevisser, M. (Eds.). (1995). *Defiant desire: Gay and lesbian lives in South Africa*. New York, NY: Routledge.
Crenshaw, K. (1991). Mapping the margins: Intersectionality, identity politics, and violence against women of color. *Stanford Law Review*, 43, 1241–1279. doi:10.2307/1229039
Donham, D. (1998). Freeing South Africa: The "modernization" of male-male sexuality in Soweto. *Cultural Anthropology*, 13, 3–21. doi:10.1525/can.1998.13.1.3
Emerson, R. M. (1976). Social exchange theory. *Annual Review of Sociology*, 2, 335–362. doi:10.1146/annurev.so.02.080176.002003
Epprecht, M. (2008). *Heterosexual Africa? The history of an idea from the age of exploration to the age of AIDS*. Athens: University of Ohio Press.
Fish, J. (2008). Navigating queer street: Researching the intersection of lesbian, gay, bisexual and trans (LGBT) identities in health research. *Sociological Research Online*, 13, 1–12. doi:10.5153/sro.1652

Glaser, B. G., & Strauss, A. L. (1967). *The discovery of grounded theory: Strategies for qualitative research*. Chicago, IL: Aldine.

Kegeles, S. M., Hays, R. B., & Coates, T. J. (1996). The Mpowerment Project: A community-level HIV prevention intervention for young gay men. *American Journal of Public Health*, 86, 1129–1136.

Kulick, D. (1998). *Travesti: Sex, gender, and culture, among Brazilian transgendered prostitutes*. Chicago, IL: University of Chicago Press.

Lane, T., Mogale, T., Struthers, H., McIntyre, J., & Kegeles, S. (2008). "They see you as a different thing": The experiences of men who have sex with men with healthcare workers in South African township communities. *Sexually Transmitted Infections*, 84, 430–433. doi:10.1136/sti.2008.031567

Lorway, R. (2006). Dispelling "heterosexual African AIDS" in Namibia: Same-sex sexuality in the township of Katutura. *Culture, Health & Sexuality*, 8, 435–449. doi:10.1080/13691050600844262

Masvawure, T. B., Sandfort, T. G., Reddy, V., Collier, K. L., & Lane, T. (2015). 'They think that gays have money': Gender identity and transactional sex among Black men who have sex with men in four South African townships. *Culture, Health & Sexuality*, 17(7), 891–905. doi:10.1080/13691058.2015.1007168

McLean, H., & Ngcobo, L. (1994). Abangibhamayo bathi ngimnandi (those who fuck me say I'm tasty): Gay sexuality in reef townships. In M. Gevisser, & E. Cameron (Eds.), *Defiant desire* (pp. 158–185). New York, NY: Routledge.

Pew Research Center. (2013). *The global divide on homosexuality*. Retrieved from http://www.pewglobal.org/files/2014/05/Pew-Global-Attitudes-Homosexuality-Report-REVISED-MAY-27-2014.pdf

Rabie, F., & Lesch, E. (2009). 'I am like a woman': Constructions of sexuality among gay men in a low-income South African community. *Culture Health & Sexuality*, 11, 717–729. doi:10.1080/13691050902890344

Reddy, G. (2006). Geographies of contagion: Hijras, kothis, and the politics of sexual marginality in Hyderabad. *Anthropology & Medicine*, 12, 255–270. doi:10.1080/13648470500291410

Reid, G. (2005). 'A man is a man completely and a wife is a wife completely': Gender classification and performance amongst 'ladies' and 'gents' in Ermelo, Mpumalanga. In G. Reid, & L. Walker (Eds.), *Men behaving differently: South African men since 1994* (pp. 205–227). Cape Town: Double Storey.

Roberts, B., & Reddy, V. (2008). Pride and prejudice: Public attitudes toward homosexuality. *HSRC Review*, 6(4), 9–11. Retrieved from http://www.hsrc.ac.za/uploads/pageContent/1607/Pride%20and%20Prejudice.pdf

Sandfort, T., & Dodge, B. (2008). " … And then there was the down low": Introduction to Black and Latino male bisexualities Archives of Sexual Behavior. *Archives of Sexual Behavior* 37, 675–682. doi:10.1007/s10508-008-9359-4

Sandfort, T. G. M., Parker, R., Gyamerah, A., Lane, T., & Reddy, V. (2012, July). *After-nine, 429, he-she, stabane, and gay, bisexual and other 'men sleeping with men': Diversity in Black South African MSM identities and implications for HIV prevention*. Poster session presented at the International AIDS Conference, Washington, DC.

Sharma, A., Bukusi, E., Gorbach, P., Cohen, C. R., Muga, C., & Holmes, K. K. (2008). Sexual identity and risk of HIV/STI among men who have sex with men in Nairobi. *Sexually Transmitted Diseases*, 35, 352–354. doi:10.1097/OLQ.0b013e31815e6320

Valentine, D. (2007). *Imagining transgender. An ethnography of a category*. Durham, NC: Duke University Press.

Wainberg, M. L., Alfredo González, M., McKinnon, K., Elkington, K. S., Pinto, D., Gruber Mann, C., & Mattos, P. E. (2007, July). Targeted ethnography as a critical step to inform cultural adaptations of HIV prevention interventions for adults with severe mental illness. *Social Science and Medicine*, 65, 296–308. doi:10.1016/j.socscimed.2007.03.020

Young, R. M., & Meyer, I. H. (2005). The trouble with "MSM" and "WSW": Erasure of the sexual-minority person in public health discourse. *American Journal of Public Health*, 95, 1144–1149. doi:10.2105/AJPH.2004.046714

Intersections and evolution of 'Butch-trans' categories in Puerto Rico: Needs and barriers of an invisible population

Alíxida G. Ramos-Pibernus, Sheilla L. Rodríguez-Madera, Mark Padilla, Nelson Varas-Díaz and Ricardo Vargas Molina

ABSTRACT
Public health research among transgender populations globally has primarily focused on HIV/AIDS. However, trans men remain outside of this conceptual framework, with distinct but overlapping social contexts and needs. In Puerto Rico (PR), the trans men population has remained largely hidden within the 'butch' lesbian community. The objective of this article is to document the identity construction of trans men and 'buchas' (local term to refer to butch lesbians) in PR and its relation to their bodily practices and overall health. We conducted an exploratory qualitative study with 29 trans men and *buchas* based on ethnographic observation, focus groups, audio-recorded in-depth interviews, and critical discourse analysis. Findings emphasise two domains to be addressed by health policies and initiatives: (1) bodily representations and gender performance, and (2) the meanings of female biological processes. This small-scale ethnographic study represents an initial step towards understanding the social context of this 'invisible' community and significant implications for their health and well-being. We provide several recommendations to address public health concerns of this understudied, marginalised community.

Global public health research among transgender/transsexual (heretofore referred to as 'trans') populations has almost exclusively focused on HIV/AIDS (Bockting, Huang, Ding, Robinson, & Rosser, 2005; Melendez & Pinto, 2007). Because trans women (people who were assigned a 'male' sex at birth and have a female gender identity and/ or expression) have been described in public health literature as more vulnerable to engaging in risk behaviour for HIV infection, research and funding have focused primarily on addressing this concern (Kosenko, 2011; Wilson, Garofalo, Harris, & Belzer, 2010). In Puerto Rico (PR), most studies on the trans community have similarly focused on the impact of HIV on trans women and factors influencing their vulnerability (Rodríguez-madera, 2009; TRANSforma Project, 2014). The focus on HIV among trans women has come at a cost to trans men, who are often neglected in research on trans communities, partly due to their presumed low prevalence (Rowniak, Chesla, Rose, & Holzemer,

2011), resulting in a lack of research on the social context of health and illness among trans men.

Examining the embodied experiences of gender and sexuality among trans men is critical to understand the health disparities this community faces. The objective of this article is to document identity constructions of trans men and 'buchas' (a local category analogous to masculine-identified butch lesbians) in PR and to critically examine the effects these constructions have in their bodily practices and health. We will explore how these categories are manifested, and identify some health-related needs and vulnerabilities they face.

Cultural context of Puerto Rican trans men and buchas

PR is the smallest of the Greater Antilles in the Caribbean, characterised by strong cultural adherence to traditional gender roles, including *machismo* (a gender ideology that encourages cisgender males to engage in a range of social practices such as dominance over women or sexual prowess) and *marianismo* (a gender identity that encourage cisgender females to be pious, maternal, and faithful) (Burgos & Díaz Pérez, 1986; Saez, Casado, & Wade, 2009; Wood & Price, 1997). One of the consequences of the social value placed on these models is a high degree of intolerance for gender non-normativity (Kulick, 1998; Parker, 1999). Such intolerance results in stigma and discrimination, heightened vulnerability to HIV, lack of social support, reduced access to healthcare services, unemployment, and poverty (Bockting et al., 2005; Padilla et al., 2008).

The *transgender* concept has been often described as a macro-level category (Sevelius, Scheim, & Giambrone, 2010) that encompasses a wide range of gender presentations and identifications that are culturally variable. In PR, the population of trans men has remained largely hidden within the lesbian community, which has itself been described in Latin America as 'invisible' (Padilla, Vásquez del Aguila, & Parker, 2007). Given the lack of information and resources, trans men and *buchas* have found social support in a community that shares some of their struggles, but does not represent their particular realities or needs (Rodríguez-Madera, Ramos-Pibernus, & González-Sepúlveda, 2012). In PR, the term *bucha* derives some of its social meanings from the English term *butch*, which refers to a woman who assumes social roles typically attributed to cisgender males (Torres, 2007)[1].

Locally, trans women have been studied more extensively (Rodríguez-Madera, Ramos-Pibernus, Padilla, & Varas-Díaz, 2016) and there is a gap in knowledge of trans men. It was not until the 1990s that the presence of gender transgressive identities became evident in local vernacular (Aponte-Parés, Arroyo, Crespo-Kebler, La Fountain-Stokes, & Negrón-Muntaner, 2007). Studies regarding the lesbian community have been mainly approached from a feminist perspective and presented in the form of poetry or literature. Configurations of the *bucha* identity in PR have been studied largely from the perspective of migration. Certain strands of Puerto Rican culture undergird intolerance towards diverse sexual orientations and gender identities, resulting in migration of gender non-conforming people to the U.S.A. (La Fountaion-Stokes, 2005). Migrations have played a role in the configuration of non-normative sexual and gender identities, but there is still much descriptive ethnographic research to be done to understand their transformations.

Trans people face major barriers to employment, non-discrimination, public accommodations, and general social acceptance (Bradford, Reisner, Honnold, & Xavier, 2013; Mizok & Mueser, 2014; Rodríguez-madera, 2009, 2012). However, vulnerabilities of trans men have been largely overlooked (Califia, 1997; Cromwell, 1999)[2]. Emphasis on trans women prevents the development of a fuller understanding of needs and appropriate public health initiatives for trans men (Pollock & Eyre, 2011). The lack of attention granted to trans men has contributed to a slower diffusion of *transgender* terminology and self-identification in PR. Prior research on HIV has been shown to shape identification practices of sexual minorities, which social science researchers have described as the medicalisation of sexuality and sexual terminology (Epstein, 1996; Muñoz-Laboy, 2004; Patton, 1990, 1996). Trans men have been largely ignored in HIV/AIDS research and intervention, and this has contributed to their relative invisibility in public discourse and health initiatives.

Border wars: intersections and distinctions between trans and bucha categories

There is an ongoing debate in the scientific literature regarding differences and similarities between trans men and butch lesbians (Halberstam, 1998; Hale, 1998). Halberstam (1998) and Hale (1998) have described the semantic tensions between these gender categories as 'border wars' (Cromwell, 1999). The debate is in part due to the overlap of identity constructions and social characteristics between both. Crawley (2002) states that trans and butch categories are similar in their gender presentation and ambivalence towards the feminine body, but markedly differ in their gender identification. Trans men often self-identify as *men* and butch lesbians as *women* (Cromwell, 1999). Halberstam (1998) stresses that trans men are associated with a desire for 're-embodiment', while butch women are associated with a playful desire for masculinity and gender deviance.

In PR, a distinction between categories is far from clear, with much overlap and inconsistency in self-definitions of gender. These fine-grained distinctions between the Puerto Rican cultural context and those described in other settings are critical in addressing health vulnerabilities and gaps in public health services.

Health-related issues in the trans and butch community in PR

In PR, the absence of social research on trans men and *buchas* health is related to lack of theoretical conceptualisations of health and illness. Health, as a social process with biological implications, has been conceptualised as a system of classification that assigns specific labels to individuals (Turner, 1999, 2001). Sick/healthy, normal/deviant, and male/female are just a few examples of binary pairs used through medical and health discourses to redistribute individual variability into bipolar categories (Lupton, 2003; Peterson & Lupton, 2000). Once individuals fall outside the confines of normative, 'healthy' categories, medical and health discourses have difficulties with categorisation, an essential step in identifying health problems and establishing treatment plans or guidelines (Riggs, 2005). Such categorisation of individuals, and their embodiment of 'disease' or 'deviance', is an integral part of social regulation of marginalised communities and maintenance of bipolar gender categories that these groups challenge through their embodied practices (Nettleton, 2000). Social stigma is a common response from the medical and health establishment when faced with people who transgress such categorisations (Nettleton, 2000). Medical institutions are often sites that exclude or delegitimise trans bodies and identities and their unique clinical needs. Too often, healthcare services and health promotion campaigns contribute to trans invisibility and marginality, with adverse health consequences for them.

A wide range of health conditions associated with stigma and discrimination disproportionately affect trans populations, including substance abuse (Ann Finlinson, Colón, Robles & Soto, 2007), mental health conditions (Blosnich et al., 2013; Bockting, Miner, Swinburne Romine, Hamilton, & Coleman, 2013), and cancer (Brown & Tracy, 2008). Lack of preventive care and the delay of urgently needed care constitute major health risks for trans men and butch lesbians (Grant et al., 2011). This is due in part to fear of being discriminated against, misunderstood, or stigmatised by health professionals. Moreover, because trans men and butch lesbians have remained understudied, there is lack of information regarding incidence of chronic health conditions such as cancer or strategies to address them (Ashbee & Goldberg, 2006). These realities have created a gap between the needs and access to social and health-related services and require competent professionals who understand identity constructions and factors related to health in the community of trans men and *buchas*. PR is perhaps an extreme case of such gaps in services and knowledge.

Methods

We conducted a qualitative exploratory study using different methodological approaches, implemented sequentially in three phases: (1) ethnographic observations, (2) focus groups, and (3) individual semi-structured in-depth interviews. The study protocol was reviewed and approved by the Institutional Review Board of our institution. All participants were recruited by convenience using snowball sampling from key contacts identified through ethnographic observations in social settings frequented by the population, including a popular lesbian nightclub in San Juan, key gathering point for trans men and *buchas*. Total sample consisted of 29 participants who self-identified as *hombres trans* (trans men) or *buchas*. Inclusion criteria were: being at least 21 years of age (legal age of adulthood in PR) and self-identifying as a trans man or *bucha* (see Table 1 for socio-demographic characteristics). Inclusion of both trans men and *buchas* was informed by initial ethnographic observations and key informant interviews that revealed that, in PR, the border between these categories is extremely fluid and permeable. We sought to understand how individuals moved between and among these identities. As it can be seen in Table 1, participants used a wide array of labels to describe their gender categorisation. We discuss subtle distinctions between these terms, but they cannot be presumed to be absolute or stable. Ours is an exploratory study aimed at documenting nuances and describing 'shades of grey' in our sample as a starting point to research on this population.

Ethnographic procedures: We conducted ethnographic observations during three months in bars and pubs located in the metropolitan area of San Juan, frequented by trans men and *buchas*. Observations and informal interactions were critical to examine the social and structural factors underlying daily life and identity constructions and health-related practices in this population. Observation involves a structured manner of immersion in local cultural worlds in order to learn about what people do and what it means to them, while also attending to ways in which contextual factors shape and constrain individual and group practices

Table 1. Socio-demographic characteristics of qualitative interviews.

Variable	Frequency
City of residence	
San Juan	4
Río Piedras	2
Cidra	1
Aguada	1
San Diego, CA	1
Education	
High School	1
Some years of college	4
Bachelor's degree	4
Civil status	
Single	5
Living together	4
Employment	
Yes	6
No	3

Note: $n = 9$.

(Bernard, 1994). During ethnographic outings, led by the first author with participation of co-authors, we engaged in informal interactions with owners, employees of establishments, and members of the community of trans men and *buchas*. To gain access to the community, a trans woman who worked as a consultant in another research project introduced us to key gatekeepers of the lesbian/trans men bar scene where most observations were conducted. Gatekeepers or key informants (bar owners) demonstrated genuine interest in our research. They linked our team to key contacts in the community and collaborated with referral of eligible participants. Through frequent and active participation in social and community activities at this key site, we gained trust with potential participants in focus groups, who became interested in the study and informed their peers. Focus groups and interviews were conducted in Spanish.

Data collection involved writing ethnographic field notes and analytic memos and development of provisional hypotheses based on observations further explored in subsequent fieldwork. Towards the beginning of the ethnographic phase, we developed an ethnographic guide to systematise subsequent observations and reflect on the effects of various social and structural factors on health behaviours and practices. The guide focused on issues regarding gender identity constructions, the meanings of community and social affiliation, and tensions or variations in gender representation and performance.

Focus groups: We carried out two focus groups composed of trans men and *buchas* to gather detailed information about topics that have been less explored or might benefit from collective analysis (Babour, 2010). This strategy allowed our team to evaluate shared views regarding a range of topics related to identity construction and health (Robinson, 1999). We recruited 20 participants. Inclusion criteria were: being at least 21 years of age, self-identifying as a trans man or *bucha*, and providing verbal consent. Given that this was an exploratory study and that our preliminary research suggested no clear distinction between *buchas* and trans men, both were integrated into our focus groups. Nevertheless, we diversify the sample by recruiting 10 participants who identified primarily as 'bucha' and 10 as 'trans men'. We used a focus group guide to lead discussion of relevant topics. The guide included questions on: (1) gender identity, (2) meanings of the words *bucha* and *trans men*, (3) bodily modification practices, (4) experiences of

Table 2. Gender identity and sexual orientation of interviews.

Variable	Frequency
Self-description[a]	
Transgender	1
Genderqueer	1
Transgender man	2
Butch	3
Men	1
Fluid identity	1
Sexual orientation	
Heterosexual	2
Bisexual	2
Homosexual	3
Pansexual	1
Not defined	1

Note: $n = 9$.
[a]The terms under the self-description variable are the ones used by each of the participants to describe themselves in terms of gender identity.

stigma and discrimination, and (5) exploration of health-related needs. Focus groups were conducted in the bar's facilities prior to its opening. Discussions were audio recorded for transcription and analysis.

Individual in-depth interviews: In the final phase, we conducted individual semi-structured in-depth interviews with nine participants (see Table 2) to gather additional narrative on experiences related to their social lives and health vulnerabilities in a one-on-one encounter. We selected participants during fieldwork or by referral. Selection criteria were the same as used for focus groups. We used an in-depth interview guide to provide uniformity and to guide conversations while allowing flexibility based on contents addressed by participants. The guide included questions on: (1) identity perception (2) bodily transformations (3) health issues (4) work-related experiences, (5) experiences in affective relationships, and (6) general experiences with society. We included a demographic data questionnaire with questions addressing economic status, gender identification, area of residence, educational level, and sexual orientation among other variables. Confidential interviews lasting 60–75 minutes were conducted in private locations. We provided a monetary incentive of $25.

Data analysis

Audio files were transcribed verbatim into word-processing files. Data obtained were coded and organised using a codebook (Barry, 1998) developed from a grounded, analytic reading of transcripts to identify a core set of issues and inter-related themes. We coded the data using critical discourse analysis to focus on relations between discourse, power, dominance, social inequality, and the position of the researcher in social relationships. Since, we collected and analysed data in Spanish, we translated relevant narratives to English for publication purposes. We made an effort to capture the exact message and included some words in Spanish that we considered had no equal translation to English.

Results

To facilitate the analysis of narratives, we will begin by presenting an ethnographic field note excerpt in order to illustrate the lack or partial incorporation of the category 'hombre trans' (trans man) in this population. Our analysis focuses on two main domains or processes that reflect the intersection and social context of gender identities and the health of trans men and *buchas*. These were: (1) bodily representations and gender performance, and (2) the meanings of female biological processes. We identified each narrative with the participant's self-identified gender category to illustrate the diversity of concepts used to describe their gender identities.

Ethnographic field note excerpt

The following ethnographic field note describes an interaction between the research team, a key informant of another study that is a trans woman, and two participants. This vignette is helpful in situating our analysis within the categorical ambiguity between trans men and *buchas*. It exemplifies the incomplete or inconsistent integration of *trans* identity in this community:

> We started the night at a local bar frequented by the community of lesbian women. Once we got there we noticed that the topic of conversation we were interested in exploring had already started. Owners of the bar, 'Laura' and 'Milagros' [a couple who identified themselves as 'femmes'], welcomed us and the first thing they told us was that we had arrived at the appropriate moment. They were talking with two costumers, 'Sandro' and 'Leon' [who self-identified as *buchas*], about the roles of lesbian women in their relationships. While they identified as *buchas*, they used masculine pronouns to refer to themselves. Sandro and Leon mentioned that two femmes together was a transgression of what is expected for a lesbian couple. For them it was essential that a couple included a *bucha* or that one of the parties assumed the male role. Laura and Milagros disagreed. Leon – who was more vehement in his opinion that lesbian couples should follow heteronormative gender roles – told us that while two femmes together was acceptable, a couple composed of two *buchas* was not. To sustain his viewpoint, he told us a story about a time another *bucha* asked to go to the bathroom with him and that this had disgusted him.
>
> Teresa [a trans woman and key informant] asked Sandro and Leon if they defined themselves as trans men. The answer was: 'we are *buchas*'. Teresa continued to explain the meaning of the trans concept [according to her] and why she thought that Sandro and Leon were actually trans men. Leon clarified that he was a man. 'Here and wherever I go I am attracted to very feminine women', he explained. Leon provided the following explanation to Teresa of what it meant to him to be a *bucha*. He asked Teresa: 'You are a man, right?' to which Teresa replied 'no', and Leon continued: 'You have a dick down there but you see yourself as a woman … Well for me is the same, but the other way around' …

This fragment of the ethnographic field note illustrates a common mixture of different notions of gender that are highly fluid and with blurred boundaries, a phenomenon regularly documented in our field notes. The concept of *trans men* is not clearly integrated into everyday discourse in the community, leading many participants to identify as *bucha*, but describe themselves as *men*. While *bucha* is generally used to refer to a female-bodied lesbian woman who exhibits a masculine gender performance, we found a regular discursive slippage between this category and a more reified notion of 'being a man'. In the above field note, Sandro denies his identity as a 'trans man' by simply excluding the prefix *trans*, and sees no inconsistency between being a *bucha* and being a *man*. Another participant changed the gender of the word *bucha* to *bucho* (a change in the grammatical gender of the term) in order to better describe what he felt he was; once again, he avoided using the term *trans*. When we asked if he defined himself as trans, he stated that he did not know the definition of the term but added that he was 'a man trapped in a woman's body'.

All participants manifested a desire to modify their bodies to be more aligned with a 'masculine' sense of self, which is often described as definitional of *transgender* identity in the scientific literature. In PR, *bucha* is a broader category that encompasses many of the meanings associated with trans identity in the near absence of a distinct label to refer to *trans men*. While three of our interview participants self-identified as *trans* (one as 'transgender' and the other two as 'trans men'), the majority did not use these labels, and many were unsure of its meaning. Interestingly, the category of *trans woman* is recognised and generally understood, whereas *trans man* is a nascent social category that is rarely used in social practice, perhaps because of the broad sub-cultural definition of *bucha*, which subsumes many characteristics associated with *trans*. While this phenomenon needs further study, we believe that it may have important implications for policies, programmes, and interventions, particularly regarding the prominence of the local category *bucha*.

Bodily representation and gender performance

West and Zimmerman (1987) describe 'doing gender' as the interactional process of performing gender identities that reaffirm culturally defined notions of the masculine–feminine binary, even as they may seek to overcome or resist them. The following quote from one of our participants, self-identified as a *trans man*, illustrates how gender identification was described by many of our participants, incorporating a gender binary through which one's own marginal gender identity was experienced or reworked:

> I'm going to describe what I think I am … I feel that I have a masculine mind inside of a feminine body, with feminine sensitivity and the hardness that is needed in order to survive. Maybe If I was completely feminine, I'd still be living with my mother, hide under her skirt because maybe I would be afraid of life, to confront things, or I would have been able to empathize more with who she was, that is, submissive … [Participant self-identified as trans]

This participant attributed characteristics such as 'weakness' (i.e. lack of 'hardness' and a 'submissive' nature) to a feminine role, while exalting male attributes presumably 'needed in order to survive'. Several participants similarly appropriated bipolar notions of gender into their descriptions of self-identity, as illustrated by several participants who described their gender identities in relation to their role as household provider:

> You start to feel like the strongest person in the relationship because you are the one that has more responsibility. At least in my case, I'm the one with the most responsibility. My house lacks nothing … I dress like this and I'm the strong part of the relationship. [Participant self-identified as *bucha*]

> … you try to assimilate all you can from manhood, at least in my case that's what I do and in my house it's like that, I'm the one that provides and the one that says how things are … [Participant self-identified as trans man]

Bodily presentation as a masculine individual was extremely important for trans men and *buchas*. Our participants shared a wealth of intimate information regarding their bodily practices for physical and gender performance and their techniques for projecting a masculine identity.

> At 23 I started to change completely. I changed the way I dressed, but then I have never gone shopping for male clothing. I cut my hair shorter and started to transition. [Participant self-identified as trans man]

> When I was in high school I stole my cousin's swimsuits ... I stole them and wore them and my mother preferred to buy me some male pants to avoid having to steal from my cousin. [Participant self-identified as *bucha*]

> I hated to dress like a girl ... wearing dresses and high heals .... I was a tomboy teenager. Since I was little I dressed as a boy and I used to buy male clothing ... Nowadays, I buy pants in women's department stores because they fit me, but I prefer to buy in the men's area. I also wear male underwear. [Participant self-identified as a fluid identity]

Several participants described biomedical technologies or procedures for body modification in which they had engaged – such as testosterone supplementation, binding of the breasts, and penile prostheses – to embody a more masculine social role. In many instances, the use of these technologies represented significant challenges for daily life and activities:

> I started to change slowly. I began with a haircut and when I felt comfortable, then I started to change my clothing. I started to look to other [trans] men to see what they were doing and it was basically hormone therapy. Until then I just worked on my body by doing exercises and finally, I began self-administering hormones. [Participant self-identified as trans man]

> I wear a super small sports bra and it takes my breath and life away ... I guess it's better than using bandages because they become loose ... Thus you look at yourself like, 'Wow this shit is a *descojón* [huge mess]!' I used to skate board wearing a bandage and always was very ... It was like ... 'I have to go home now or I have to go to the bathroom to fix it'. It's not easy to put it on. I always have to ask my *jeva* [girlfriend] to help me ... They are tiny and painful. Right now I'm talking to you and I look normal and the damn thing hurts. It always hurts. That feeling is not cool. [Participant self-identified as gender queer]

> I use a prosthesis. I bought it on the Internet. I wear it only when I'm going out ... It depends on the shirt I'm wearing and whether it covers my pants or not. It is for my mental peace because people can be looking at you and notice 'that' ... [Participant self-identified as trans man]

> In my case I wear a small prosthesis, but I have to be very careful when I go to the bathroom because on one occasion it fell out. I was lucky that I could grab it quickly. [Participant self-identified as trans man]

In most cases, participants had gone through long periods struggling alone and in silence to align their bodies with their gender, and lacked safe spaces to obtain accurate information about practices and technologies that might be available to them. These practices are entirely invisible in healthcare settings and public health programmes in PR. The social context of use of biomedical technologies, such as testosterone supplementation, was nearly impossible for our participants to discuss with healthcare providers, which strongly constrained their access to appropriate treatment and public health services.

The meanings of female biological processes

The physical body might be described as a signifier that tells others what to expect in terms of social roles. For who is challenging dominant symbols of gender and sexuality, the body betrays or ruptures gender expectations, and becomes a site for social conflict, stigmatisation, and stress (Meyer, 2003). During puberty, mind–body dissonance becomes more evident, as the symbol of the body more intensely contrasts with an underlying sense of one's gender identity (Morgan & Stevens, 2008). A study conducted by Devor (1997) found that most trans participants mentioned not being able to cope with the physical changes they observed during adolescence. Some participants expressed the same feeling of being betrayed by the body during puberty:

> Before puberty I used to wear a pony tail, and I had really long hair and I put it up in a pony tail and pretended I was a boy. You know what? I used to pray to god, please that tomorrow I wake up as a boy. It's really like depressing, but then I say to myself, 'well maybe I will never get my period, maybe my body has a physical problem and that's why I feel this way', but when I got my period all my hopes went away … [Participant self-identified as trans men]

> For me it was something that I was embarrassed of my own body, I couldn't assimilate, I mean, that my breast began to show, that I was developing a woman's body, I couldn't … Sometimes I would lock myself up in my room and cry and say, 'Why, god, if you know I like women, why this, god?' I said, 'why I was born like this, like a woman, I feel like a man and I'm chained to a woman's body'. [Participant self-identified as *bucha* and man]

An important implication of the rejection that these individuals felt towards female anatomy was their attitude towards gynaecological exams and follow-ups. Trans men and butch lesbians visit the gynaecologist less frequently for pap spears and preventive care, which is potentially linked to higher risks for cervical and uterine cancers (Dutton, Koenig, & Fennie, 2008; Tracy, Schluterman, & Greenberg, 2013). One of the reasons for this is the denial of the female body as an expression of gender ambivalence or dissonance (Van Trotsenburg, 2009).

> I say, 'Why go to the gynaecologist if I'm a man and I have confidence in myself?' I'm a man, you know. My body is a carapace … I don't have to. Why let anybody see my body? [Participant self-identified as *bucha* and man]

Another reason for avoiding gynaecological exams was related to discomfort participants experience with their genitals and the pain that accompanies the examination:

> To have those pap spear exams is for me very stressful … I have had it two times, the first one was uncomfortable, but I dealt with it. It did not hurt. But this time it was horrible, it was very painful. I don't know why it hurt so much and I don't know if it was the tension that I had for trying to avoid it. I want to have a hysterectomy to avoid doing it all because I don't want to go through that again. [Participant self-identified as trans man]

Such experiences of being probed in areas of the body that provoked shame and bodily dissonance contributed to a pervasive sense that healthcare facilities are menacing spaces. The lack of clinics specialising in trans health in PR functioned as a significant barrier to accessing basic preventative care and quality treatment, as participants simply did not see the available clinical services open to non-cisgender individuals.

No, I can't [go to the clinic] because there's a bunch of women waiting at the gynaecologist [office] and I can't like be sitting there waiting to be called. I couldn't ... And finding a gynaecologist that can work with you, because you know it's not the same. People look at you ... Unless I had gone with a family member and pretended that it [the appointment] was for her. But then when they called my name ... So no, I couldn't go. [Participant self-identified as trans men]

Even when participants have strategies such as seeking the company of a family member, they do not feel safe. Most of our participants only sought health care during emergency situations. One of them acknowledged that he did not seek preventive care regularly and attributed it to lack of guidance on that matter:

I had never seen [the gynaecologist] but my insurance was going to expire ... So I went and they discovered that I had something that needed surgery. Now I have to go because of the surgery but I had not gone before ... You're right, we don't go regularly to the gynaecologist ... Nobody talks about it, nobody brings this up anywhere. [Participant self-identify as *bucha*]

Non-cisgender constructions were directly linked to problems accessing health care. Participants faced difficulties in understanding how specific healthcare services intended for cisgender females were still applicable to trans men and *buchas* who had female genitalia but masculine gender identities. Clinics and hospitals became sites for uncomfortable, embarrassing, or oppressive social interactions that functioned to stigmatise, undermine, or delegitimise their expressions of self. Individuals who challenge binary notions of gender might face difficulties in accessing services or even understanding the need to access routine health and prevention services that they do not associate with their own bodies or identities. This makes it very unlikely that public health policies and programmes, particularly those related to reproductive and sexual health, to reach trans men and *buchas*, who would not see themselves as target of programmes designed for cisgender women.

Conclusions and recommendations

This study – the first to our knowledge – focused on trans men and *buchas* in PR – represents an initial step in understanding the social context of this 'invisible' community and implications of their experiences for health and well-being. First, our participants described gender identities in their communities using local *butch-femme* categories, in which the masculine figure – the *bucha* – expressed an embodied notion of masculinity that incorporated a variety of practices and bodily technologies. Some of these practices involved non-clinical use of testosterone for body modification, analogous to informal hormone injections that have been described for trans women (Kulick, 1998; Poteat, German, & Kerrigan, 2013), that may contribute to other health risks, particularly when needles are shared. Others described the use of penile prostheses and chest binding, experiencing discomfort and challenges with these practices. *Bucha* is a broad sub-cultural category that is often associated with bodily dissonance and identifications that are akin to most definitions of *transgender* or *transsexual* in the global scholarly literature. While *trans* terminology exists in PR, *bucha* is a dominant cultural category that is inclusive of those who identify themselves as *men* and engage in body modification practices and technologies.

The appropriation of heteronormative models for organising gender relations and the importance of such models for legitimating masculine identities need to be considered in the development of psychological, clinical, or public health initiatives to reach this community. Clinical and public health services for trans men and *buchas* need to include training for personnel on the meanings of these terms and the bodily ambivalence or dissonance that commonly accompany them. Such training should require adaptation to local context and terminology. Sub-cultural realities of trans men and *buchas* are likely to be misunderstood and stigmatised by healthcare providers. This would contribute to avoidance of health care and underlines the importance of developing interventions aimed at promoting preventive care for this population. Stigma reduction interventions and anti-discrimination policies for trans men and *buchas* should be implemented across the healthcare system, even as more trans-specific services are developed.

Participants told many stories of being highly uncomfortable of having their bodies inspected by medical personnel, particularly during gynaecological exams. Bodily ambivalence or dissonance generated strong resistance to healthcare facilities, described as menacing places or sites where they did not belong. It was difficult for them to understand why healthcare services for cisgender females were necessary for *buchas* and trans men, partly due to a tendency to invoke strong contrasts between cisgender women and *buchas*, creating reified notions of differently gendered bodies. In this context, it may be more difficult for trans men and *buchas* to understand how or whether clinical and public health recommendations for cisgender women are applicable to themselves. Future initiatives oriented towards this community should incorporate sub-cultural knowledge inclusive of trans men and *buchas*, to adapt current interventions and outreach programmes, and to create safe spaces where gender non-conformity is welcomed and explored openly. We believe our findings underscore the urgent need for trans-oriented health care and public health programmes in PR.

Notes

1. *Cisgender* is a term often used in social science literature to denote an individual whose self-identity conforms to the gender that is socially assigned to him/her at birth based on biological sex (genitalia). The term is useful, in that it decentres normative gender constructs that might otherwise be essentialised as 'simply natural' (Koyama, 2002).
2. The literature on trans men has been more extensive in the social sciences than it has in the health sciences. Anthropology, cultural studies, and the humanities have contributed to a growing cross-cultural literature on trans men and butch lesbians in recent years (Cromwell, 1999; Green, 2004; Hansbury, 2005; Hiestand & Levitt, 2004; Newton, 2000; Rubin, 2003; Torres, 2007; Weiss, 2008).

Funding

This research was funded by the National Institute of Drug Abuse [grant number 1R21DA032288], [grant number 1K02DA035122]; the Puerto Rico Psychological Association. This article does not represent the opinion of the National Institutes of Health.

Disclosure statement

No potential conflict of interest was reported by the authors.

References

Ann Finlinson, H., Colon, H. M., Robles, R. R., & Soto, M. (2007). An exploratory study of Puerto Rican MSM drug users: The childhood and early teen years of gay males and transsexual females. *Youth & Society, 39*(3), 362–384. doi:10.1177/0044118X07305998

Aponte-Parés, L., Arroyo, J., Crespo-Kebler, E., La Fountain-Stokes, L., & Negrón-Muntaner, F. (2007). Puerto Rican queer sexualities: Introduction. *Centro Journal, XIX*(1), 4–24.

Ashbee, O., & Goldberg, J. (2006). *Medical issues trans people and cancer* (pp. 1–12). Vancouver.

Babour, R. (2010). Focus groups. In I. Bourgeault, R. Dingwall, & R. de Vries (Eds.), *The Sage handbook of qualitative methods in health research* (pp. 327–352). Thousand Oak, CA: Sage Publications.

Barry, C. (1998). Choosing qualitative data analysis software: Atlas/ti and Nudist Compared. *Sociological Research Online, 3*(3), 1–17. doi:10.5153/sro.178

Bernard, H. R. (1994). *Research methods in anthropology: Qualitative and quantitative approaches*. Thousand Oaks, CA: Sage.

Blosnich, J. R., Brown, G. R., Shipherd, J. C., Kauth, M., Piegari, R. I., & Bossarte, R. M. (2013). Prevalence of gender identity disorder and suicide risk among transgender veterans utilizing veterans health administration care. *American Journal of Public Health, 103*(10), e27–e32. doi:10.2105/AJPH.2013.301507

Bockting, W., Huang, C., Ding, H., Robinson, B. B., & Rosser, S. (2005). Are transgender persons at higher risk for HIV than other sexual minorities? A comparison of HIV prevalence and risks. *International Journal of Transgenderism, 8*(2–3), 123–131. doi:10.1300/J485v08n02

Bockting, W. O., Miner, M. H., Swinburne Romine, R. E., Hamilton, A., & Coleman, E. (2013). Stigma, mental health, and resilience in an online sample of the US transgender population. *American Journal of Public Health, 103*(5), 943–951. doi:10.2105/AJPH.2013.301241

Bradford, J., Reisner, S. L., Honnold, J. A., & Xavier, J. (2013). Experiences of transgender-related discrimination and implications for health: Results from the Virginia transgender health initiative study. *American Journal of Public Health, 103*(10), 1820–1829. doi:10.2105/AJPH.2012.300796

Brown, J. P., & Tracy, J. K. (2008). Lesbians and cancer: An overlooked health disparity. *Cancer Causes and Control, 19*, 1009–1020. doi:10.1007/s10552-008-9176-z

Burgos, N. M., & Díaz Pérez, Y. I. (1986). An exploration of human sexuality in the Puerto Rican culture. *Journal of Social Work & Human Sexuality, 4*(3), 135–150.

Califia, P. (1997). *Sex change: The politics of transgenderism*. San Francisco: Cleis Press.

Crawley, S. (2002). Prioritizing audiences: Exploring the differences between stone butch and transgender selves. *Journal of Lesbian Studies, 6*(2), 11–24. doi:10.1300/J155v06n02_04

Cromwell, J. (1999). *Transmen & FTMs: Identities, bodies, genders & sexualities*. Chicago: University of Illinois Press.

Devor, A. H. (1997). *Female-to-Male transsexuals in society*. Bloomington, IN: Indiana University Press.

Dutton, L., Koenig, K., & Fennie, K. (2008). Gynecologic care of the female-to-male transgender man. *Journal of Midwifery & Women's Health, 53*(4), 331–337. doi:10.1016/j.jmwh.2008.02.003

Epstein, S. (1996). *Impure science: AIDS, activism, and the politics of knowledge*. Berkeley: University of California Press.

Grant, J., Mottet, L., Tanis, J., Harrison, J., Herman, J., & Keisling, M. (2011). *Injustice at every turn: A report of the National Transgender discrimination survey* (pp. 1–288). Washington.

Green, J. (2004). *Becoming a visible man*. Nashville, TN: Vanderbilt University Press.

Halberstam, J. (1998). *Female masculinities*. Durham, NC: Duke University Press.

Hale, C. (1998). Consuming the living dis(re)membering the dead in the Butch/FTM borderlands. *GLQ: A Journal of Lesbian and Gay Studies, 4*(2), 311–348. doi:10.1215/10642684-4-2-311

Hansbury, G. (2005). The middle men: An introduction to the transmasculine identities. *Studies in Gender and Sexuality, 6*(3), 241–264. doi:10.1080/15240650609349276

Hiestand, K. R., & Levitt, H. M. (2004). Butch identity development: The formation of an authentic gender. *Feminism & Psychology, 15*(1), 61–85. doi:10.1177/0959-353505049709

Kosenko, K. A. (2011). Contextual influences on sexual risk-taking in the transgender community. *Journal of Sex Research*, *48*, 285–296. doi:10.1080/00224491003721686

Koyama, E. (2002). Cissexual/cisgender: Decentralizing the dominant group [eminism.org]. Retrieved from http://www.eminism.org/interchange/2002/20020607-wmstl.html

Kulick, D. (1998). *Travestí: Sex, gender and culture among Brazilian transgendered prostitutes*. Chicago, IL: University of Chicago Press.

La Fountaion-Stokes, L. (2005). Cultures of the Puerto Rico queer diaspora. In B. Epps, K. Valens, & B. Johnson González (Eds.), *Passing lines: Sexuality and immigration* (pp. 275–309). Massachusetts: Harvard University.

Lupton, D. (2003). *Medicine as culture: Illness, disease and the body in western societies*. London: Sage.

Melendez, R. M., & Pinto, R. (2007). 'It's really a hard life': Love, gender and HIV risk among male-to-female transgender persons. *Culture, Health & Sexuality*, *9*(3), 233–245. doi:10.1080/13691050601065909

Meyer, I. H. (2003). Prejudice, social stress, and mental health in Lesbian, gay, and bisexual populations: Conceptual issues and research evidence. *Psychological Bulletin*, *129*(5), 674–697. doi:10.1037/0033-2909.129.5.674

Mizok, L., & Mueser, K. (2014). Employment mental health, internalized stigma, and coping with transphobia among transgender individuals. *Psychology of Sexual Orientation and Gender Diversity*, *1*(2), 146–158. doi:10.1037/sgd0000029

Morgan, S. W., & Stevens, P. E. (2008). Transgender identity development as represented by a group of female-to-male transgendered adults. *Issues in Mental Health Nursing*, *29*(6), 585–599. doi:10.1080/01612840802048782

Muñoz-Laboy, M. (2004). Beyond 'MSM': Sexual desire among bisexually-active Latino men in New York City. *Sexualities*, *7*(1), 55–80. doi:10.1177/13634607040142

Nettleton, S. (2000). Governing the risky self: How to become healthy, wealthy and wise. In A. Petersen & R. Bunton (Eds.), *Foucault: Health and medicine* (pp. 207–222). London: Routledge.

Newton, E. (2000). *Margaret Mead made me gay*. Durham, NC: Duke University Press.

Padilla, M., Castellanos, D., Guilamo-Ramos, V., Reyes, A. M., Sánchez Marte, L. E., & Soriano, M. A. (2008). Stigma, social inequality, and HIV risk disclosure among Dominican male sex workers. *Social Science & Medicine*, *67*(3), 380–388. doi:10.1016/j.socscimed.2008.03.014

Padilla, M. B., Vásquez del Aguila, E., & Parker, R. G. (2007). Globalization, structural violence, and LGBT health: A cross-cultural perspective. In I. Meyer & M. E. Northridge (Eds.), *The health of sexual minorities: Public health perspectives on lesbian, gay, bisexual and transgender populations* (pp. 209–241). New York, NY: Springer.

Parker, R. (1999). *Beneath the equator: Cultures of desire, male homosexuality, and emerging gay communities in Brazil*. New York, NY: Routledge.

Patton, C. (1990). *Inventing AIDS* (1st ed.). New York, NY: Routledge.

Patton, C. (1996). *Fatal advice*. Durham, NC: Duke University Press.

Peterson, A., & Lupton, D. (2000). *The new public health: Health and self in the age of risk*. London: Sage.

Pollock, L., & Eyre, S. (2011). Growth into manhood among: Identity development among female-to-male transgender youth. *Culture, Health & Sexuality*, *14*(2), 209–222. doi:10.1080/13691058.2011.636072

Poteat, T., German, D., & Kerrigan, D. (2013). Managing uncertainty: A grounded theory of stigma in transgender health care encounters. *Social Science and Medicine*, *84*, 22–29. doi:10.1016/j.socscimed.2013.02.019

Riggs, D. W. (2005). Locating control: Psychology and the cultural production of the 'healthy subject positions'. *Culture, Health & Sexuality*, *7*(2), 87–100. doi:10.1080/13691050412331291405

Robinson, N. (1999). The use of focus group methodology–with selected examples from sexual health research. *Journal of Advanced Nursing*, *29*(4), 905–913. doi:10.1046/j.1365-2648.1999.00966.x

Rodríguez-Madera, S. (2009). *Género Trans: Transitando por las zonas grises*. San Juan: Terranova.

Rodríguez-Madera, S. (2012). TRANS-acciones de la carne: Criminalización de mujeres trans puertorriqueñas que ejercen el trabajo sexual. In S. Serrano Rivera (Ed.), *Registros criminológicos contemporáneos* (pp. 107–150). San Juan: Situm.

Rodríguez-Madera, S., Ramos-Pibernus, A., González-Sepúlveda, O. (2012). *Identity nooks: Gender construction as a social determinant of health and its effects in the Puertorrican trans population.* Presented at the IV Puerto Rican Conference of Public Health, San Juan: Puerto Rico.

Rodríguez-Madera, S., Ramos-Pibernus, A., Padilla, M., & Varas-Díaz, N. (2016). Radiodrafía de las comunidades Trans en Puerto Rico: Visibilizando femeneidades y masculinidades alternas. In M. Vásquez-Rivera, A. Martínez-Taboas, M. Francia-Martínez & J. Toro-Alfonso (Eds.), *LGBT 101: Una Mirada Introductoria al colectivo* (pp. 290–314). San Juan: Publicaciones Puertorriqueñas.

Rowniak, S., Chesla, C., Rose, C. D., & Holzemer, W. L. (2011). Transmen: The HIV risk of gay identity. *AIDS Education and Prevention*, 23(6), 508–520. doi:10.1521/aeap.2011.23.6.508

Rubin, H. (2003). *Self-made men: Identity and embodiment among transsexual men.* Nashville: Vanderbilt University Press.

Saez, P., Casado, A., & Wade, J. C. (2009). Factors influencing masculinity ideology among Latino Men. *The Journal of Men's Studies*, 17, 116–128. doi:10.3149/jms.1702.116

Sevelius, J., Scheim, A., & Giambrone, B. (2010). *What are transgender men's HIV prevention needs?* San Francisco: University of California San Francisco, Center for AIDS Prevention Studies.

Torres, L. (2007). Boricua lesbians: Sexuality, nationality, and the politics of passing. *Centro Journal*, XIX(1), 230–249.

Tracy, J. K., Schluterman, N. H., & Greenberg, D. R. (2013). Understanding cervical cancer screening among lesbians: A national survey. *BMC Public Health*, 13, 442. doi:10.1186/1471-2458-13-442

TRANSforma Project. (2014). *Report on the study "Injection Practices and HIV Risk Behavior among Transgendered Persons in Puerto Rico"* (1R21DA032288) [Brochure]. University of Puerto Rico & Florida International University.

Turner, B. S. (1999). *The body & society.* London: Sage.

Turner, B. S. (2001). The history of the changing concepts of health and illness: Outline of a general model of illness categories. In G. L. Albrecht, R. Fitzpatrick, & S. C. Scrimshaw (Eds.), *Handbook of social studies in health and medicine* (pp. 9–23). London: Sage.

Van Trotsenburg, M. A. A. (2009). Gynecological aspects of transgender healthcare. *International Journal of Transgenderism*, 11(4), 238–246. doi:10.1080/15532730903439484

Weiss, J. T. (2008). The lesbian community and FTMs: Détente in the Butch/FTM borderlands. *Journal of Lesbian Studies*, 11(3–4), 203–211. doi:10.1300/J155v11n03

West, C., & Zimmerman, D. H. (1987). Doing gender. *Gender & Society*, 1(2), 125–151. doi:10.2307/189945

Wilson, E. C., Garofalo, R., Harris, D. R., & Belzer, M. (2010). Sexual risk taking among transgender male-to-female youths with different partner types. *American Journal of Public Health*, 100(8), 1500–1505. doi:10.2105/AJPH.2009.160051

Wood, M., & Price, P. (1997). Machismo and marianismo: Implications for HIV/AIDS risk reduction and education. *American Journal of Health Studies*, 13(1), 44–52.

'You should build yourself up as a whole product': Transgender female identity in Lima, Peru

Lealah Pollock, Alfonso Silva-Santisteban, Jae Sevelius and Ximena Salazar

ABSTRACT

Transgender women in Lima, Peru have, until recently, been grouped together with gay and bisexual men in the category MSM, or men who have sex with men, with little consideration of their unique situation and needs. Transgender women, self-identified in Peru as *travesti*, are a socially vulnerable population with many unmet health needs, including an HIV prevalence of 30%. Understanding specific transgender identities and their contexts will contribute to the improvement and development of HIV prevention programs. Through qualitative open-ended interviews with trans-identified women in Lima, Peru, this study found that the non-normative *travesti* identity is constructed within a conservative homophobic and heteronormative social context. Participants strive towards appearances and relationships perceived as feminine, seeking out silicone injections and abusive men as social markers of this femininity. Sex work is the primary economic activity available and *travestis* are often alienated from their families and communities. Work is needed to increase self-esteem and decrease violence, stigma, and discrimination. There is a need for multilevel HIV prevention campaigns prioritising *travesti* in Lima, utilising a human rights framework.

Introduction

Worldwide, individuals who are born male and have a feminine gender identity are disproportionately affected by HIV infection (Baral et al., 2013). In Peru, a country with an overall adult HIV prevalence around 0.4%, the HIV prevalence among transgender women in Lima is 30% (Silva Santisteban et al., 2012). Qualitative research with transgender women has suggested that gender identity itself may be an important factor in the context of HIV risk, primarily by increasing engagement in sexually risky behaviours (Bockting, Robinson, & Rosser, 1998; Melendez & Pinto, 2007; Operario, Nemoto, Iwamoto, & Moore, 2011; Reisner et al., 2009; Salazar et al., 2006; Sevelius, 2013; Villayzán, personal communication, (L. Pollock), 2010). Fostering understanding of culturally and geographically distinct transgender identities will help clarify the context of transgender HIV risk.

Travesti *identity*

In Latin America, anthropological and sociological study of transgender populations has primarily focused on individuals identified as *travesti*, biological males who manifest a feminine gender identity and adopt traits socially designated female (Barreda, 1993; Kulick, 1998; Vieria Garcia, 2008). Until recently, all public health research in Peru that included *travestis* lumped them together with gay and bisexual men in the category MSM, or men who have sex with men (Cáceres et al., 2008; Salazar & Villayzán, 2009; Salazar, Villayzán, Silva Santisteban, & Cáceres, 2010). As more is known about the HIV epidemic in Peru and its affected subgroups, an understanding has emerged of a community of female-dressing and female-identified *travestis* or *mujeres trans* (trans women), as distinct from gay or bisexual men (Salazar et al., 2010; Salazar & Villayzán, 2009). However, defining this population has proven problematic, because they are often inadequately captured by epidemiological terminology (Cáceres, 1996).

Travesti identity in Lima exists within a context of *machismo* and gender-based violence. According to a government survey in 2014, 72.4% of women have experienced some sort of violence from a spouse or partner (Instituto Nacional de Estadística e Informática, 2014). Seventy per cent reported experiencing verbal or psychological abuse, 32% reported physical abuse, and 8% reported sexual abuse. Among the women who had experienced verbal or psychological abuse, 65% had a partner who had exerted some sort of control, primarily in the forms of jealousy and insistence on knowing where she was at all times. These subtle forms of violence and control are so common as to be considered 'normal' by many Peruvian women.

While much is known about the Peruvian context of discrimination and marginalisation faced by *travestis*, limited qualitative studies have been conducted focusing on *travesti* identity itself in a Peruvian context. Qualitative research in Peru indicates that *travestis* are faced with a daily situation of violence, stigma, discrimination, and low self-esteem; suffer from a lack of education, employment, and housing opportunities; are frequent victims of interpersonal and police violence; and have high rates of substance use (Salazar, 2005; Salazar et al., 2010). The primary economic options available are hairdressing and sex work, which further increases their social vulnerability (Silva Santisteban et al., 2012). Due primarily to a lack of other job opportunities, many *travestis* participate in sex work at some point in their lives (Salazar et al., 2010).

Travestis in Peru have begun to fight for rights and recognition. To build interventions, mobilise an activist movement, and conduct further investigations, it is important to understand what it means to be *travesti*. This study aims to explore contruction(s) of gender identity and the individual and social contexts of *travestis* in Lima, Peru, to clarify the social context of vulnerability, including vulnerability to HIV, in this underserved, at-risk population. The analysis pays special attention to the way in which *travesti* identity is constructed within the social constraints of normative ideas of masculinity, femininity, and heterosexuality.

Methods

Fifteen in-depth open-ended interviews were completed. Investigators worked with field workers familiar with the population to identify and recruit participants. Field workers were asked to locate participants who identify as *trans* or *travesti*, and/or who have a feminine identity and use full-time female dress. Interviews were conducted in five unique neighbourhoods in the Province of Lima. These neighbourhoods ranged from 'inner-city' to more suburban, and were all low socio-economic class. These neighbourhoods were chosen because they were part of a larger ongoing research project involving community centre building, so the researchers had a pre-existing relationship with some community members. In two of the neighbourhoods, the field worker introduced one of the investigators to an individual identified as a *travesti* leader within that neighbourhood. This individual, in turn, identified and helped to recruit other individuals who would be eligible for and interested in the study. In the three other neighbourhoods, the field workers directly identified potential participants, who were approached for recruitment jointly with one of the investigators. Individuals were eligible for participation if they were born male and present as female at least part of the time, were 18 years of age or older, and were able to understand and give informed consent.

The interviews consisted of a series of open-ended and interactive questions, exploring themes related to gender identity, self-esteem, drug and alcohol use, relationships, condom use, sex work, and body modification. Participants were paid 10 Peruvian Soles (approximately $3.50) for their participation and were provided with snacks. The interviews were conducted by a single cis-female American bilingual researcher, lasted between one and two hours, and were recorded and transcribed in Spanish, then translated to English. The interviews were translated by a native Peruvian. The interviewer spot-checked the translations, giving suggestions as the translations were being completed, and double-checked the transparency (i.e. the quality of sounding like a native speaker) and fidelity of the final quotes.

After the initial analysis was complete, two focus groups were held with individuals who had not previously been interviewed for validation of major results. Participants in focus groups had to be at least 18 years of age and identify as *gay, homosexual, mujer trans, transformista,* or *travesti*. One focus group consisted of four participants and another of eight. These focus groups were held in two neighbourhoods different from the initial five, although similar in socio-economic terms. Field notes were taken at both focus groups. The authors chose to start with in-depth interviews to gain insight into individual perspectives on sensitive subject matter and followed up with focus groups to validate the generalisability of our findings.

Human subjects approval was obtained from both the ethics committee at the Universidad Peruana Cayetano Heredia in Lima, Peru, and the Committee on Human Research at University of California, San Francisco.

Analysis

The interviews were analysed by three investigators in both English and Spanish through a process of thematic coding based on template analysis (Crabtree & Miller, 1999). One investigator conducted all of the interviews and initially read all of the transcripts, focusing on particular paragraphs of interest for close analysis to create a coding scheme. Both these emergent codes and other codes used in the authors' previous work and thought to be of potential interest in this study composed the code book, which was modified throughout the analysis, adding new codes that emerged. Using the initial code book, the investigators each coded the same three transcripts. Perceived limitations and needed clarifications were discussed among the coders to generate definitions of each of the codes, which were then employed moving forward. Each coder coded his or her own batch of three to four transcripts, and the primary author reviewed all coded transcripts for consistency of code definition. Once all of the transcripts were coded, important themes were disaggregated and analysed in depth. The qualitative program ATLAS.ti was used to organise the coded text and share the developing analysis among investigators.

Results

The study participants had a median age of 29 (range 18–41). Four worked primarily in hairdressing or cosmetology, one had her own salon where she did hairdressing and sex work, three reported primarily working in sex work, two worked in party planning, one worked in a store, one was maintained by her partner and occasionally worked as an assistant in a salon, and three had no regular employment. Nine lived with immediate family, three lived alone, and three lived in rented rooms in a building with other *travestis*. While not asked explicitly, two reported being HIV positive (Table 1). Each participant was asked what term they use to describe their own identity. These self-identified terms will be used along with the participant's age to identify the source of each quotation in this paper.

Terminology

When asked what words they use to describe themselves and their gender identity or sexuality, the majority of the participants use the term *travesti*, while the rest use variously *trans*, *trans* or *travesti*, *transformista*, and *homosexual*. When asked to further clarify the distinction between these terms, participants indicate that all biological MSM fall under an umbrella category of being *homosexual*, while dress and appearance distinguish an individual as *gay, transformista, or travesti*. Someone who is *gay* has a male appearance and identity, although he may have some feminine traits or occasionally dress in women's

Table 1. Participant characteristics.

	Age	Gender identity	Employment	Living situation	Hormones?	Silicones?	Notes
1	28	*Travesti*	Sex work	Family	No	No	
2	40	*Travesti*	Hairdresser	Family	No	No	
3	40	*Trans*	Hairdresser	Family	No	Yes	
4	18	*Trans*	Salesperson	Alone	Yes	No	
5	41	*Homosexual*	Hairdresser	Family	No	No	
6	24	*Travesti*	Supported by partner, sometimes hairdressing	Rented room	Yes	Yes	
7	37	*Travesti*	Sex work	Rented room	Yes	Yes	HIV+
8	24	*Travesti*	Sex work	Rented room	No	Yes	
9	28	*Transformista*	Party planner	Family	Yes	Yes	
10	29	*Transformista*	Party planner	Family	No	No	
11	25	*Trans*	Cosmetolgist	Family	Yes	Yes	
12	40	*Trans*	Hairdresser and sex work	Alone	No	Yes	
13	29	*Trans*	Odd jobs	Family	Yes	Yes	HIV+
14	35	*Trans*	Unemployed	Alone	Yes	No	
15	28	*Travesti*	Unemployed	Family	No	Yes	

clothes. *Travestis* utilise female dress full time and *transformistas* go back and forth between masculine and feminine appearances.

> *Gays*, now this is generalizing, are the *homosexuals* that appear masculine ... and *travestis* are those that dress like a woman. (*travesti*, 40)

Thus, identity is defined first by sexual behaviour (a *homosexual* has sex with men) and second by outward appearance and dress. To dress full time as a woman reflects a desire to be perceived and accepted as a woman in all aspects of life. On the other hand, *transformistas* often maintain a masculine appearance during the day, in front of their families or for work, and then lead a social life in feminine dress.

> *Transformista* is because, say, during the day I lead a life dressed as a man, but I mostly dress like a woman for the parties, maybe to take a stroll, to go out, that's when I'll dress like a woman, I transform. It's not that I'm dressed like a woman all day long. (*transformista*, 28)

These distinctions set up a continuum of *homosexual* identities, with subtle interplays among appearance, sexual behaviour, and self-perceptions that are not captured by the epidemiologic term 'MSM" or the more colloquial 'gay' or 'transvestite'. It should also be noted that none of these terms incorporate the *macho* men who often have sex with *gays, transformistas, and travestis*, but do not consider themselves *homosexual*.

As we will see, the degree of feminine appearance achieved through body modification and dress affects how a *travesti* individual is received by neighbours and potential sexual partners and feeds back into self-perception and validation as female. Unfortunately, presenting full time as a woman often also has profound negative effects on family relationships and job prospects. Within a binary system of gender, in a *machista*[1] society, there is an advantage to maintaining some fluidity between the two worlds.

While the term *travesti* is universally understood and employed, *trans*, which has come to serve as the Spanish-language umbrella term in the political discourse, is not. Of those who primarily identified themselves as *trans*, most formed part of the same community centre, and another was the youngest participant at 18 years old and was active in a different research-supported community centre. One participant, an identified community leader, describes the recent emergence of the term *trans* as follows:

> They used to be called *travestis*, even now, some of them don't identify themselves as *trans*, and they are still called *travestis* .... The *trans* thing comes from 3 or 4 years ago I believe. Before it was *travesti* and it sounded a little offensive to me. (*trans*, 25)

A group of participants employs some use of the term *trans*, primarily in reference to the *trans* population or the *trans* community, although they do not identify themselves as *trans*.

Becoming travesti

Many of the participants' discussions reflect a deeply embedded belief that the sex into which one is born 'should' be congruous with one of two possible gender categories (man or woman) and all sexual desire 'should' be directed across the invisible aisle. Most participants felt that they could never fully locate themselves in one category, so can never fully *be* women. Rather, they can strive towards feminine appearances and relationships: 'I wanted to appear, not to be a woman, because woman is one thing only, I only wanted to physically look like a woman' (*travesti*, 24).

Most participants recalled having traditionally feminine childhood traits: wanting to dress in women's clothing and makeup, having feminine tendencies or behaviours, or only wanting to play with or be friends with girls. This creates a great deal of distress for participants:

> It was a tremendous argument in my head many times I spent my time thinking in my head for hours and hours stretched out on my bed and crying, asking why this happened to me, why if I was born with a masculine identity do I feel more attraction for feminine things and I like boys? (*trans*, 25)

This participant describes how her socially assigned gender conflicts with her feminine tendencies and sexual preferences. Social norms have taught her that there is something profoundly wrong with stepping outside the boundaries defined at birth by her genitalia.

In the following quote, one participant describes why a *travesti* can never *be* a woman:

> Being a woman is a very different thing ... we'll never become women, no matter how much I have my sex changed, and if I have a vagina made, I'll never be a woman. We seem to have the shape, even the looks of a woman, but unfortunately we'll never be that, the truth must be admitted. (*travesti*, 24)

While not stated explicitly, it is likely that female reproduction is 'that' which can never be achieved by this participant and will prevent her from ever *being* a woman. Not being born a woman, this participant feels that she can only achieve successive approximations, constantly limited by a heteronormative social discourse that fails to recognise an authentic female transgender identity.

Body transformation

Body transformation through hormone use and silicone injection, while not universal, is a pervasive aspect of the *travesti* experience. Industrial silicone, called *aceite de avion* (airplane oil), is injected into the butt, hips, breasts, forehead, and chin to give a more feminine appearance. Silicones are desired to pass as a woman, earn more in sex work, be more attractive to men, and because attractive *travestis* are more socially accepted.

> ... *Trans* friends who I know who don't look as good femininely ... get harassed ... for a *trans* who still hasn't fixed herself up physically to be more feminine but dresses as a woman, lets her hair grow out or uses makeup but her features still look a little masculine, there is this type of rejection toward them. (*trans*, 25)

A *travesti* who wants to be desired and accepted needs a curvy womanly figure. The fastest, cheapest way to achieve a feminine body is through silicone injections.

> In order to attract someone else, that's the most important thing in us, because we are aware that we're not women, especially in ourselves, that we weren't born women. Then, how can we make it up? We have nose jobs, silicones. The others get silicones, and then it's like, Oh, I'm going to get them, too! Because I want to look good, because I like myself, I'm proud, I want to meet a man some day along the way. I want to be loved, to be touched, to be liked, not because of my body, but at least to be liked for who I am. (*travesti*, 37)

For this participant, silicones are necessary for her to be who she is, to 'make up' for not being born a woman. While it is understandable that she wants her appearance to match her identity, she struggles to integrate the exterior and the interior, unable to find a category for her true 'normal' female self.

Despite all of this work to change the body, only one participant wants to have bottom surgery to remove her penis and construct a vagina. In fact, many participants mention getting pleasure from her penis, either through masturbation or through insertive sex. Many sex work clients even pay more to be penetrated by a *travesti*. The participant quoted below discusses both the pleasure she gets from her penis and also her frustration that, in her view, having a vagina still will not make her a woman.

> What would be next to be completely identified as a woman? You'll need to be able to get pregnant, to have a family, and that just won't happen…. On the outside I'd like to look like a woman, but I wouldn't have a sex change… being a woman is the sum of many things, it's the sum of physical, psychological and emotional characteristics, which can't be achieved in practice, because I… I look at my DNI [national identification card] and I'm still [my male name], and your DNI says masculine sex, and that creates a psychological struggle… I can't marry, It's frustrating. I can't be called ma'am, that's frustrating, that will result in psychological disaster. (*trans*, 35)

In this quote it is clear that the socially defined category of 'woman' necessitates female reproduction. In this sense, it is not the vagina that makes a woman, but the ability to have children. Within a society that does not allow any alternative constructions of womanhood, and that will not even recognise *travestis* as female on official documentation, a *travesti* can never achieve a fully integrated sense of self and full realisation of her femininity.

Sexual relationships

Two important mirrors can validate a *travesti*'s femininity. One is a literal mirror – seeing her reflection and feeling that the image reflected matches her feminine self-perception and makes her feel good. The second, often more important, mirror is the male gaze. Many of the participants talk about the first time they 'became *travesti*' or the first time they dressed as a woman:

> Seeing myself dressed as a woman and made up, I'd never used makeup before, having the long hair which I'd never had … I liked seeing myself like that and I felt really good and I felt like I was more attractive for the masculine sex because they didn't come on to me as a *gay*, instead they came on to me as a woman, so I liked that. (*trans*, 25)

Being desired as a woman, instead of as a gay man, is affirming. But there is a deeper meaning in this quote that comes across in many of the interviews: men find it easier to approach a potential partner when that partner is or appears as a woman, thus not undermining his own heterosexual masculinity.

> I've had the need to be *travesti*, in order to get guys… there are more opportunities for us girls to have a partner…. If I don't dress well, if I don't put on make-up, I won't be able to get a partner easily… that's why the other gay guys, they want to become *travestis*, to be more attractive. (*travesti*, 37)

This is not to imply that *travestis* adopt a feminine appearance only to attract men, but rather that the reactions from men gauge a *travesti*'s success in achieving femininity.

> You'll be more attractive to men, you'll get more clients [if you get silicone injections to change your body]. Besides, you will feel more fulfilled. They'll look at you, you'll look prettier, sexier. Men will .... I'll do it because I want to feel good about myself, not for other people. I'll look prettier, I'll feel good about myself, not just for other people. (*travesti*, 28)

Discussions of sexual relationships also demonstrate the rigidity and strength of heterosexuality normativity, such that it comes to define *travesti* desire. The participant quoted below reiterates the assumption that every partnership must have a 'man' and a 'woman'.

> I don't see anything nice about it [men who openly go out with other men], I don't know who is the man, nor who is the woman. If one person, how can I explain it, has a form, a body, has a feminine appearance, then you can differentiate .... (*travesti*, 24)

Within this context of societal and internalised homophobia, some of the participants report that being *travesti* is more acceptable than being *gay*.

> I get treated better, let's say, I get into better places ... when I get to the discothèque, they open the door for me, I know that as a man since I'm not made up, with my hair like this, they'll look at me like a *mariconcita* (little queer). (*transformista*, 28)

This is likely because feminine appearance can at least be understood as female, whereas an effeminate man who is looking to have sex with men does not fit into any culturally legible gender category.

Participants invariably describe their partners as 'real men', 'heterosexual men', or 'machos', distinguishing them from homosexuals, gays, or effeminate men, reflecting another way in which their relationships are structured within a heteronormative standard. *Travestis* and their partners reproduce exaggerated 'traditional' gender relations: jealousy and violence as a sign of masculinity and masculine desire; forgiveness and submission as a sign of femininity and feminine desire.

> When he saw me [after I got silicones], he went crazy on me. He wouldn't let me go out into the street, and well, with him I'm fine, now he doesn't let me go out, I'm holed up in here [laughs] .... Now he's more attached to me. (*travesti*, 24)

This participant views her partner's control of her as a reflection of his desire for and attachment to her. His increased jealousy is a sign that she must be doing something right as a woman. In this sense, *travesti* identity is built in relation to sex partners in an interaction process framed within a *machista* environment regarding the perceived dynamics of gender roles. Both the *travesti* and her partner need each other to become what they are.

Participants forgive their partners for many transgressions out of 'love', or 'because I liked him,' returning again and again to violent partners.

> Because I loved him, I still felt I loved him, I left with him, and I didn't care about leaving everything behind. I'd suffered so much, so many months and I left with him, despite everything he'd done to me .... He treated me like a woman. He beat me up, he beat me up like a woman. (*travesti*, 40)

Violence reaffirms the dominant masculinity of the male partner and, therefore, the submissive femininity of the *travesti* partner. In addition to replicating a heteronormative script, this dynamic also suggests very low self-esteem, a severe lack of potential partners, and a feeling that she does not deserve any better.

Violence and discrimination

Violence and discrimination impact most aspects of the *travesti* experience. *Travestis* are subjected to harassment, rape, and physical violence in their homes from family and primary partners; in their neighbourhoods from complete strangers; and in the street from clients, police, pimps, and other characters in the social milieu of sex work. The following quote describes a situation where a participant's partner wanted to force her to have sex without a condom:

> I'd always behaved like a lady with him … but when I told him 'No!' he grabbed my hands strongly, and he wanted to force me, I mean like rape. The man came out in me, I started to curse, the macho came out in me, and I threw him back. (*travesti*, 40)

Attacks like this one are disturbingly commonplace, and the *travesti* have no recourse. In fact, the city officials who should be offering protection are themselves a threat: 'Even the police patrol, they insult you, the *serenazgo* (city patrol), the same, they hit you' (*travesti*, 28).

Many of the participants' families have rejected them based on their sexuality or femininity, throwing them out of the house, threatening to disown them, or resorting to violence.

> My mom's words, they hurt more than a blow, didn't they? When someone hits you, the pain is over soon, but the words stay here in your heart and that's it. Now my mom hates me, she doesn't want to see me. That's why I ran away when I was 15. (*travesti*, 24)

A few participants, fortunately, had found acceptance from their families, which was instrumental in raising their self-esteem: 'My mom mentioned it to my dad and my dad supported me just the same. Their support has helped me so much to find fulfillment as *trans*' (*trans*, 25).

Work-related discrimination often prohibits fully adopting a feminine role day and night. Making permanent or visible changes to one's body, even growing one's hair out, explicitly means not being able to work a 'normal' job. A participant who works in party planning fears that no client would hire her if she had a feminine appearance. 'I mean, let's say I get breast implants … I'll have to leave the job that I'm at. It's good for me as a person; as a worker it's better to be without breasts, dressed like a boy' (*transformista*, 28). Thus, she hid her long hair under a cap during the day. On the other hand, for those involved in sex work, *travestis* with a more feminine appearance can earn more money: 'They picked up all the girls with silicones, they didn't pick me up … you've gotta have at least hips and butt' (*travesti*, 28).

Discussion

In Lima, individuals born male but with a female public appearance and identity primarily socially identify as *travesti*, with more recent adoption of the term *trans* or transwoman in more activist circles. *Travesti* identity entails social and sexual roles, which incorporate feminine, masculine, and uniquely *travesti* attributes. The non-normative *travesti* identity is constructed and validated within a heteronomative and homophobic framework that defines womanhood and relationships.

The *travesti* participants in this study do not have a frame that allows them to conceptualise a fully interior transgender identity. They are forced to define their femininity based on how it is reflected back to them, in the form of sexual interest and, unfortunately, intimate partner violence. Like cis-gendered individuals, *travestis* are constantly adapting aspects of themselves so that other people will perceive them as they want to be perceived. When these adaptations fail or are met with violence or discrimination, this rejection becomes re-incorporated into the individual's self-perception Butler (2006) argues that the physical markers of sex only become meaningful and powerful as marks of sex in the course of the body's reiterated performance of gender. Violence and discrimination, when enacted against a *travesti* as a 'woman' is affirming; when enacted against a 'feminine appearing man' it furthers a cycle of low self-esteem and internalised homophobia.

Unfortunately, for the majority of *travestis* in Lima, there is no socially recognised way to 'become' a woman. There is also no established legal procedure for changing one's name and sex. These individuals face marginalisation, exclusion, rejection, and violence on a daily basis as they strive to find an 'acceptable' femininity. A *travesti* can be a hairdresser or a sex worker, but cannot be a businesswoman or a mom. She can be a kept mistress, but cannot be a wife. She can get black market silicone implants and perform in a gay discotheque, but cannot get an identification card with her female name and gender. If she attempts to fight back, it is only through a crack in her femininity that allows her 'macho' side to show through. Although *travestis* seek relationships in which they are loved and valued for who they are, and which reaffirm the gender identity they feel, these relationships are difficult to achieve, and most sexual and romantic relationships are mediated by an economic component (Salazar et al., 2006, 2010). This context forces *travestis* underground into illicit transactional economies that increase their risk of harm, including an increased risk of HIV.

Implications for HIV prevention

Transgender women are the population most affected by the HIV epidemic in Peru and Latin America (Baral et al., 2013), the result of additive problems rooted in social exclusion. *Travestis*, with their feminine identity and appearance, distinguish themselves from gay and bisexual men, and face a unique set of challenges. This study provides useful data to identify the limits and scope of the categories usually used as MSM and transvestite in the region. This population must be disaggregated from MSM in HIV prevention and surveillance efforts in Peru, to support effective programmes and interventions. *Travestis* face a tremendous amount of discrimination, homophobia, and transphobia, much of which is so pervasive and deeply felt that it is internalised. Every day is a struggle to meet basic needs and avoid violence. Preventing HIV and seeking treatment once infected is far from the top of the hierarchy of needs. Additionally, gender enhancement procedures occur outside the health system in a parallel system embedded into *travesti* culture, linked to sex work and the expression of female identity (Kulick, 1998; Silva Santisteban et al., 2012). This perpetuates exclusion and decreases access to HIV prevention programmes and information, as well as health care for other needs. Health personnel at clinics who provide HIV testing and treatment need to be sensitive to the specific needs of the *travesti* population, including using correct names and pronouns, and avoiding discriminatory or discourteous practices.

We have described vulnerability at the individual level contributing to an increased risk to HIV. If the full realisation of feminine identity implies submissiveness in a relationship, it will remain very difficult for *travestis* to effectively negotiate for condom use. The majority of *travestis* describe having male partners (Silva Santisteban et al., 2012). Therefore, any effective HIV prevention intervention must include the men who have sex with *travestis*. For this, we need to better understand this elusive and hidden population. Additionally, interventions aimed at behavioural change need to acknowledge that *travestis* do engage in insertive anal intercourse, both out of economic necessity and for pleasure. There is urgent need for multilevel culturally tailored interventions, addressing broader issues such as the right to health, identity, and housing, among other basic human rights. Overcoming exclusion remains a huge challenge for *travestis* and HIV prevention has to be framed in this context.

Conclusion

Hopefully by now it has become clear why we have chosen to employ the term *travesti* rather than an English equivalent. The term *travesti* is frequently translated as 'transvestite', although this is not entirely accurate. First, the term 'transvestite' implies dressing in women's clothes only some of the time, whereas *travestis* have full-time female dress and feminine identification. Second, the *travesti* identity entails much more than just dress. *Travesti* identity is defined primarily by full-time adoption of feminine dress by individuals born male who feel a sexual attraction for men and a deep-rooted internal sense of femininity. *Travesti* also implies a cultural concept; the construction of an identity within a specific heteronormative context, with its attendant discrimination and rejection. Peruvian activists have recently adopted the term *mujer trans* (trans woman), as an umbrella term that includes *travesti*, importing a discourse of acceptance and destigmatisation. At the same time, they attempt to invert the meaning of *travesti* to do the same, without losing its specific cultural context.

Work is needed to change many contextual aspects of the *travesti* experience, to increase self-esteem and decrease the pervasive violence, stigma, and discrimination. To accomplish this, public health and human rights workers need to recognise transgender identity as separate from gay and bisexual men, not only to account for unique challenges and risk factors, but also as one important step towards recognising transfemininity as authentic femininity. One very thoughtful trans leader was passionate about helping other *travestis* come to the realisation that they are not reducible to just their bodies. She discussed the self-objectification that happens among *travestis* – that they internalise how others define them by their bodies and appearance and neglect to cultivate other aspects of their lives and personalities:

> You should build yourself up as a whole product, you won't just be a pair of tight jeans, some long hair or a pair of little boobs, no, sweetie, you must have something in here ... [that] starts with the love one creates here and which needs to be for one's self. You need to find the way, if this door is closed, I'll look for another one to open, if they close this door, I'll get in through the window, we need to move on, always, always ... it's never too late, the question is to stand up on your feet and to start to walk. (*trans*, 25)

Limitations

Like most qualitative work, this study does not aim to include a representative sample. This work represents the perceptions and identity constructions of a particular group of *travestis* in Lima. All interviews were conducted in Spanish by a female investigator from the United States, for whom Spanish is a second language. The complicated dynamics of being a foreign investigator, and representing a renowned Peruvian university could have affected participant responses.

Note

1. Misogynist, privileging traditional masculinity.

Acknowledgements

We would like to thank all of the study participants and everyone at la Unidad de Salud, Sexualidad y Desarrollo Humano at UPCH who contributed to this work. Special thanks to Carlos Cáceres and Jeffrey Klausner for their support, which made this work possible.

Disclosure statement

No potential conflict of interest was reported by the authors.

References

Baral, S. D., Poteat, T., Strömdahl, S., Wirtz, A. L., Guadamuz, T. E., & Beyrer, C. (2013). Worldwide burden of HIV in transgender women: A systematic review and meta-analysis. *The Lancet Infectious Diseases*, *13*(3), 214–222. doi:10.1016/S1473-3099(12)70315-8

Barreda, V. (1993). Cuando lo femenino está en otra parte. *Revista De Antropología Publicar*, Año 2 (3), 29–32.

Bockting, W. O., Robinson, B. E., & Rosser, B. R. S. (1998). Transgender HIV prevention: A qualitative needs assessment. *AIDS Care*, *10*(4), 505–525. doi:10.1080/09540129850124028

Butler, J. (2006). *Gender trouble: Feminism and the subversion of identity*. New York: Routledge.

Cáceres, C. F. (1996). Male bisexuality in Peru and the prevention of AIDS. In P. Aggleton, & P. Aggleton (Eds.), *Bisexualities and AIDS: International perspectives* (pp. 136–147). London: Taylor and Francis.

Cáceres, C. F., Konda, K. A., Salazar, X., Leon, S. R., Klausner, J. D., Lescano, A. G., ... Coates, T. J. (2008). New populations at high risk of HIV/STIs in low-income, urban coastal Peru. *AIDS and Behavior*, *12*(4), 544–551. doi:10.1007/s10461-007-9348-y

Crabtree, B. F., & Miller, W. L. (1999). *Doing qualitative research* (2nd ed.). Newbury Park, CA: Sage.

Instituto Nacional de Estadística e Informática. (2014). *Perú: Encuesta Demográfica y de Salud Familiar*. Retrieved from https://www.inei.gob.pe/media/MenuRecursivo/publicaciones_digitales/Est/Lib1211/index.html

Kulick, D. (1998). *Travesti: Sex, gender, and culture among Brazilian transgendered prostitutes*. Chicago, IL: The University of Chicago Press.

Melendez, R. M., & Pinto, R. (2007). 'It's really a hard life': Love, gender and HIV risk among male-to-female transgender persons. *Culture, Health & Sexuality*, *9*(3), 233–245. doi:10.1080/13691050601065909

Operario, D., Nemoto, T., Iwamoto, M., & Moore, T. (2011). Unprotected sexual behavior and HIV risk in the context of primary partnerships for transgender women. *AIDS and Behavior*, *15*(3), 674–682. doi:10.1007/s10461-010-9795-8

Reisner, S. L., Mimiaga, M. J., Bland, S., Mayer, K. H., Perkovich, B., & Safren, S. A. (2009). HIV risk and social networks among male-to-female transgender sex workers in Boston, Massachusetts. *Journal of the Association of Nurses in AIDS Care*, *20*(5), 373–386. doi:10.1016/j.jana.2009.06.003

Salazar, X. (2005). *Resultados de los Grupos Focales con Trabajadores Sexuales Travestis Sobre el Trabajo Sexual y los Clientes.*

Salazar, X., Cáceres, C., Maiorana, A., Rosasco, A. M., Kegeles, S., Coates, T., & NIMH Collaborative HIV/STI Prevention Trial Group. (2006). Influencia del contexto sociocultural en la percepción del riesgo y la negociación de protección en hombres homosexuales pobres de la costa peruana [Influence of socio-cultural context on risk perception and negotiation of protection among poor homosexual males on the Peruvian coast]. *Cadernos De Saúde Pública/Ministério Da Saúde, Fundação Oswaldo Cruz, Escola Nacional De Saúde Pública, 22*(10), 2097–2104.

Salazar, X., & Villayzán, J. (2009). *Lineaminetos para el trabajo multisectorial en población trans, derechos humanos, trabajo sexual y VIH/SIDA.* Lima: IESSDEH, REDLACTRANS, UNFPA.

Salazar, X., Villayzán, J., Silva Santisteban, A., & Cáceres, C. (2010). *Las personas trans y la epidemia del VIH/SIDA en el Perú: Aspectos sociales y epidemiológicos.* Lima: IEESSDEH, UPCH, UNOSIDA, AMFAR.

Sevelius, J. M. (2013). Gender affirmation: A framework for conceptualizing risk behavior among transgender women of color. *Sex Roles, 68*(11–12), 675–689. doi:10.1007/s11199-012-0216-5

Silva Santisteban, A., Raymond, H. F., Salazar, X., Villayzán, J., Leon, S., McFarland, W., & Cáceres, C. F. (2012). Understanding the HIV/AIDS epidemic in transgender women of Lima, Peru: Results from a sero-epidemiologic study using respondent driven sampling. *AIDS and Behavior, 16*(4), 872–881. doi:10.1007/s10461-011-0053-5

Vieria Garcia, M. R. (2008). Care of the body among low-income travestis. *Sexualidades, 2*, 1–15.

HIV vulnerability and the erasure of sexual and gender diversity in Abidjan, Côte d'Ivoire

Matthew Thomann

ABSTRACT

In the fight against concentrated HIV epidemics, men who have sex with men (MSM) are often framed as a homogeneous population, with little attention paid to sexual and gender diversity and its impact on HIV vulnerability. This article draws on ethnographic research conducted in Abidjan, Côte d'Ivoire among les branchés – a local term encompassing several categories of same-sex desire and practice. In the context of increased HIV prevention programming targeting Ivoirian sexual and gender minorities, such diversity is effectively erased. This obfuscation of difference has particularly negative impacts for travestis, who may be at higher risk for HIV infection, though research and prevention efforts in which they are grouped with 'MSM' render them underrepresented and make their vulnerability difficult to quantify. Branchés whose class and/or ethnic backgrounds compound their stigmatised status as sexual and gender minorities also bear the burden of this exclusion. Furthermore, some branchés deploy 'MSM' as a form of self-identification, further complicating who such categories represent. By highlighting the ways in which constructions of gender and sexuality within HIV/AIDS programming obscure complex social realities, I aim to reorient thinking around the development of purposeful HIV programming that engages the complexity of sexual and gender minority experience.

Introduction

In this article, I offer an ethnographic examination of the ways in which constructions of gender and sexuality within HIV/AIDS programming obscure the complex social realities of sexual and gender minorities in Abidjan, Côte d'Ivoire. Drawing on research conducted in Abidjan among *les branchés* – a local term encompassing several categories of same-sex desire and practice including *travestis* and *transgenres*, *woubis*, *yossis*, and increasingly 'MSM' – I explore the erasure of difference and the creation of new boundaries of belonging and exclusion in the context of increased HIV prevention programming targeting Ivoirian sexual and gender minorities. Throughout this article, I focus on the category of 'men who have sex with men' (MSM), a term often assumed to be apolitical and 'outside' of culture because of its relationship with evidence-based interventions and an unyielding focus on identifying risk practices and behaviours. I argue that such uncritical use of language in HIV/AIDS programming and research overlooks the diversity of sexual and gender minority experience and fails to address the ways in which complex, intersecting and overlapping social realities may shape HIV vulnerability. In fact, this language effectively erases certain populations from the category of MSM, thus excluding them from HIV care and prevention. In Abidjan, this exclusion is perhaps most felt among travestis and transgender persons, whose vulnerability to HIV is shaped by both the state-sponsored violence and victimisation that they experience as gender trangressive sex workers, as well as their exclusion from branché spaces and broader society (Thomann, 2014; Thomann & Corey-Boulet, 2015). Other branchés whose class and ethnic backgrounds are stigmatised within broader cosmologies of belonging in Côte d'Ivoire (Akindès, 2001, 2004; Cutolo, 2010; Konate, 2004; Marshall-Fratani, 2006; McGovern, 2011; Newell, 2006, 2012) also feel this exclusion. Thus, certain branches find themselves excluded from the institutional spaces and programmes, and thus the resources and 'community', intended to serve them.

Many branchés further identify themselves and others according to 'local' categories such as *woubi*, *yossi*, and *travesti*. These seemingly local identifications are complicated by and run parallel to the term MSM, which is claimed and deployed by some sexual minority men in Abidjan, particularly those with ties to local non-governmental organisations (NGOs). These branchés deploy MSM not only as a bio-behavioral risk category in their community-based HIV prevention work, but also as an emic identity category with a set of symbolic meanings of its own. This political and strategic negotiation of the MSM category by some is not to suggest that all branchés deploy this identification when referring to their same-sex practice, desire, or identities, nor that other terms are not available and in wide circulation in Abidjan (indeed this article will discuss many of them). However, I argue that the deployment of the MSM category by branchés in Abidjan destabilises the assumed coherence of epidemiological and evidence-based perspectives that imagine sexual and gender minorities as a universally comparable subpopulation and argue that enumerative regimes articulate with local identity politics to create new and unexpected forms of sociality.

Following recent anthropological scholarship (Boellstorff, 2011; Lorway & Khan, 2014; Aggleton & Parker, 2015), I do not advocate for purging the acronym MSM or any of its derivatives from our vocabulary. For all of the label's shortcomings, this article will not outline a plan for eschewing the MSM category in favour of one or a few other emic categories. Such a substitution would not guarantee more inclusive depictions of gender and sexual subjectivities and may enable the reification of cultural categories, as they are 'fed back into HIV and AIDS research as seemingly culturally inherent forms of sexuality …' (Boyce, 2007, p. 176). In Abidjan, a turn to emic categories in HIV prevention and programming would entail its own set of erasures because not all branchés have the same operational definitions for and lived experiences of local identifications. Furthermore, these identifications overlap with other social realities, including class and ethnicity, in meaningful ways.

Thus, this article tackles the following questions: How are the specific cultural categories used in HIV prevention programming locally interpreted and embodied? How should public health practitioners and researchers understand travestis, who may or may not identify as transgender and whose risk factors overlap with but are distinct from most gender normative men? Who does 'MSM' represent as a culturally 'neutral' risk category if it has been transformed into a culturally loaded form of identification? What are the ideological aims of MSM 'body counts' (Nguyen, 2010, pp. 178–180) and how are they shaping the landscape of HIV/AIDS prevention? What new forms of sociality are produced by evidenced-based interventions and global health research targeting gender and sexual minorities?

Methods

Between 2010 and 2012, I conducted eight months of ethnographic fieldwork in Abidjan, primarily in two community-based NGOs – Alternative-Côte d'Ivoire (Alternative) and Arc-en-Ciel+ (Arc-en-Ciel) – as well as a clinic with which the HIV peer educators and activists in both NGOs collaborated. Other than Claver, who, as the Executive Director of Alternative, is a highly visible public figure and who insisted that I use his real name, I have assigned research participants pseudonyms to ensure their anonymity. At the request of leadership at Alternative and Arc-en-Ciel, which have been highly publicised in both the local and foreign press (Corey-Boulet, 2012, 2013, 2014; Fioriti, 2014; Kouassi, 2011), I have retained the real names of both organisations.

Research participants

The findings presented in this article are not representative of all sexual and gender minorities in Abidjan. As Patrick, the former Head of Monitoring and Evaluation for Arc-en-Ciel, explained to me in 2012 – the branché milieu touched by HIV prevention programming is only the 'tip of the iceberg'. This is perhaps most evident in the relative absence of women in leadership positions within the local nonprofit industrial complex (Rodriguez, 2007; Smith, 2007; Spade, 2011), which marginalises and overlooks the particular vulnerabilities of sexual minority women through its focus on counting and enrolling MSM into research and interventions.

Though on the periphery of the homosocial milieu, the lives of my branché research participants were deeply tied to a diverse set of individuals identified as female from birth. Some had developed close friendships with lesbian-identified women and joked about marrying such women to please their families, while maintaining romantic connections with other branchés. Other branché research participants had or previously had intimate, sexual relationships with women and a few had married and/or had children with women. Most of these men identified as bisexual but also as branché. As the branchés that I came to know explained to me, bisexual practice and desire did not preclude inclusion in the branché milieu.

Interviews

I conducted interviews with HIV peer educators, activists, and branchés who frequented these milieus. Interviews were conducted in French and touched on a variety of themes about the experiences of gender and sexual minorities in Abidjan. Perhaps most pertinent for the purposes of this article, I asked branché research participants questions about their subjective experiences of sexual and gendered identifications and how they are or are not related to the HIV/AIDS programming in which they participate to varying degrees. I also asked research participants to discuss their experiences with violence, broadly defined, and the divisions that exist within the community and within NGO spaces in particular. In total, I conducted, audiotaped, and transcribed interviews with 45 members of Arc-en-Ciel and Alternative, as well as branchés who used their services or regularly hung out in their headquarters. Of these interviews, 24 were conducted with peer educators and activists employed by Alternative and/or Arc-en-Ciel, 10 identified as travestis or transgender (one of whom was also a peer educator at Arc-en-Ciel), and 12 were members or 'clients' of Alternative and/or Arc-en-Ciel.

Participant observation

My participant observation at the headquarters of Alternative and Arc-en-Ciel were filled with the quotidian activities of the organisations. I recorded field notes, observed, and asked questions as staff prepared for last-minute audits conducted by foreign donors and intermediary NGOs, sat in on organisational meetings, translated reports and budgets, and participated in support groups and weekly discussions activities. I also spent several hours per week socialising with branchés outside of the NGOs. My daily participant observation in NGOs and other 'safe spaces' (mostly bars, restaurants, and branchés' apartments) was also guided by questions concerning the relationship between how branchés understood and organised themselves in relation to the ideas, norms and values promoted by HIV prevention programming and by Ivoirian society more generally. I supplemented participant observation with a mapping project (Thomann, 2016) and archival research, including analysis of US President's Emergency Plan for AIDS Relief (PEPFAR) Country Operational Plans, organisational documents and budgets, and national and international media coverage pertaining to issues of homosexuality.

'MSM', foreign interventions and sexual and gender minority organising in Abidjan

A basic, university library search will turn up nearly 50,000 results when queried for 'men who have sex with men' The ubiquity of the MSM category in public health is tied to epidemiological and evidence-based logics and the imperative to generate data that can be analysed statistically, with the aim of uncovering some 'truth' about a population. This logic situates qualitative work as anecdotal and unscientific. Like the randomised controlled trials described by anthropologist Vincanne Adams, the MSM category 'eliminates the need for data collection about complex social realities' (Adams, 2013, p. 71), and supplants qualitative evidence on sexual identity rather than being used alongside it (Young & Meyer, 2005, p. 1144). In an effort to scale up testing among 'most at risk populations' the MSM category is used to identify and group a population and to document their coverage in interventions, the results of which may then be quantified (Nguyen, 2010, p. 180). However, as I will show, some gender and sexual minorities 'do not count' as MSM. And though the MSM category has been internalised and reappropriated by some sexual and gender minorities in Abidjan, it remains a deeply normative category and a means by which branchés establish boundaries for group membership (Lorway & Khan, 2014, p. 52).

RETHINKING MSM, TRANS* AND OTHER CATEGORIES IN HIV PREVENTION

From an epidemiological perspective, the push towards a category of practice that is culturally universal and therefore measurable and quantifiable is understandable. Globally, MSM shoulder a much greater HIV-burden than the general population. In sub-Saharan Africa, approximately 5% of the general population is living with HIV, compared to nearly 18% of MSM (Beyrer et al., 2012). This distribution is strikingly similar in Abidjan, where 5.1% of the general population is HIV+ (PEPFAR, 2013), while 18% of MSM in Abidjan are living with HIV (Aho et al., 2014, Hakim et al., 2015; Vuylsteke et al., 2012). However, this universalising category of practice, which eschews identity in favour of behaviour, erases a significant amount of heterogeneity. Furthermore, the enumerative rationality of epidemiology and evidence-based interventions is more complex than the desire to save lives. Sexual and gender minorities have become part of an industry wherein continued financial support is contingent upon counting and enrolling them into international programming.

When I first arrived in Abidjan in the summer of 2010, Alternative and Arc-en-Ciel ran their programmes on small budgets funded by French NGOs and had few paid staff. Arc-en-Ciel was housed in a bare, one-room office and the newly formed Alternative had no official headquarters and held its meetings in private homes. A PEPFAR-implementing partner had begun working with Arc-en-Ciel activists in 2007, employing them as peer educators to provide counselling in the clinic. Despite this progress, controversy over governance and leadership and rumours of financial misconduct had begun to divide the staff members at Arc-en-Ciel. Feeling that the organisation's reputation had taken a major hit and after repeated disagreements over leadership, Claver and a few other key members of Arc-en-Ciel left to create Alternative in 2010, shortly before I arrived.

By the time I returned to Abidjan in 2012, PEPFAR was financing a $1.7 million project aimed at improving access to HIV prevention and care for MSM and female sex workers. And there was a new player in town. Heartland Alliance International (Heartland), the global arm of a nearly $82 million Chicago-based NGO, had responded to PEPFAR's (2010) call for a new 'primary partner' to work with 'highly vulnerable populations' (PEPFAR, 2010). Their project provides technical and financial support to 12 clinics across Côte d'Ivoire and to three community-based NGOs in Abidjan, including Alternative and Arc-en-Ciel. Both organisations acquired large headquarters, well equipped with computers, office furniture, LCD projectors, and Wi-Fi capabilities and employed government-certified HIV peer educators with different titles, responsibilities, and pay scales. This outsourcing of HIV prevention programming and testing is part of broader trends in the commodification of testing (Fan, 2014, p. 86) and came with the expectation that these 'community members' would recruit an ever increasing number of MSM into intervention programming, data which they can then use to prove a 'return' on donor investments.

When Heartland arrived in Abidjan in 2010, they entered a complex network of advocacy and organising around issues faced by branchés. In 1994, militant travesti activists, who later formed an organisation called *Association de Travestis de Côte d'Ivoire* (Travesti Association of Côte d'Ivoire), stormed the headquarters of an Ivoirian newspaper that had published an inflammatory report about the community, assaulting journalists and breaking windows (Nguyen, 2010, p. 165). A few years later, a French-documentary entitled *Woubi Cheri* (Brooks & Bochaut, 1998) chronicled their work and was aired in Abidjan on Canal +. After its leader, an outspoken travesti named Barbara, emigrated to France, the organisation lost momentum. Despite this setback, a homosocial milieu has flourished in Abidjan for over four decades (Broqua, 2012; Nguyen, 2010; Le Pape & Vidal, 1984) and the milieu have long used a coded language, known as *woubi-can*, in order to identify one another in social and intimate settings and to remain discreet. Understanding this language, its limitations, and the politics of its use is imperative to ensuring fuller representation of sexual and gender minorities in Abidjan in current research and programming.

Branchés in focus: the language and politics of 'MSM health' in Abidjan

In Abidjan, sexual and gender minorities identify themselves and one another as *les branchés,* a euphemism long used in place of words such as homosexual and gay (Nguyen, 2010, p. 163). The literal English translation of the French verb *brancher* is 'to connect' or 'to plug in', as in an electrical cord. Though likely seen as dated in the contemporary French context, the adjective branché can be used as slang to identify an individual as 'hip' or 'trendy', and thus 'plugged in' or 'connected' to popular culture. In Abidjan, sexual minority men and travestis employ this identification in public settings, without passersby comprehending its hidden meaning.[1] However, whom exactly the branché identification constitutes is hardly agreed upon. When I asked HIV peer educator Alain about the identifications he used to describe himself, he first stated that he used the French *homo* to connote his sexuality identity. When I asked him if he also employed the word branché, he admitted to using it, adding,

> It means more, though [than *les homos*]. I would say that a branché is someone who is *homo* and someone who knows a lot more. There are people who are *homo* but who aren't branché. That means they don't go out. They don't go to the branché bars. They are at home. They stay camouflaged in their corner.

Within the localised category of practice of branché, there exists a diverse set of identifications. This form of in-group identification forms part of a 'flexible language' (Leap, 2004), whereby branchés sometimes self-identified using North Atlantic terms such as the English 'gay' and the French *homo* while other times employing woubi-can, which allowed them to have discreet discussions about broad sexual preferences, specific sexual acts, penis size, and preferred sexual position. During one meeting, Jean, an HIV peer educator and proud woubi explained:

> We use woubi only between branchés. All the branches know what woubi and yossi are. You know what it means to *gnazri* [to fuck]. You know what *gbali* [dick] means. You know what *tchapa* [rectum] means. It's our language. If you are branché you should know all of that. If you don't know what they mean, you are not branché. We call it woubi-can.

I first learned of woubi-can in 2009 while watching *Woubi Cheri*, the 1998 documentary that followed Barbara the leader of Association de Travestis de Côte d'Ivoire. In one of the opening scenes, Barbara discussed the coded language with a woman whom she identified as heterosexual:

> We have our own dictionary, our own way of talking. So, for example, when we say woubi, woubis are boys who play the role of the woman, who aren't necessarily travesti, who remain boys and who love men. Me, I am a travesti, it's special. Well, they call me woubi too because despite everything, I am a boy but I behave like a woman. And then there are the yossis. They are boys who sleep with women, travestis, and homosexuals. They are boys who keep their

role. They play the role of the boy. They are the ones who behave like boys. They are the husbands of the woubis.

As Barbara highlighted, and as was confirmed by nearly every branché with whom I spoke, woubis played the role of *les femmes* (women) and yossis of *les hommes* (men). As Barbara pointed out, travestis deserve special consideration. Branchés use the category of travesti to refer to individuals born anatomically male who live their lives as women on a full or part time basis. Some travestis undergo hormonal therapy to produce secondary sex characteristics associated with women, such as breast growth, fat redistribution and the thinning of body hair (Thomann & Corey-Boulet, 2015). Still, travestis should not be uniformly considered to be transgender women. Like the Brazilian travestis described by anthropologists Don Kulick, many travestis 'did not conform to standard northern Euro-American sexologies' (Kulick, 1998, p. 12) and most of those I came to know were only marginally aware of 'transgender' as a social and political category. In Côte d'Ivoire, the definition of a travesti varies widely, even among travestis themselves. Points of contention include how often one must dress and present as a woman to qualify as a travesti as well as whether sex work is an essential component of travesti identity. Julie, a young branché peer educator who had recently began taking hormones and living as a woman after leaving her parents home, explained this diversity:

> There are transgender women (*transgenres*) who live strictly as women as often as possible. Like me, like Sarah [another travesti]. There are also travestis who are professional sex workers, some of whom change just at night to do sex work. During the day they are dressed as men. There are also transgender women who are sex workers, like Sarah, who live strictly as women and who are sex workers. And there are occasional transgender women who do it maybe just two times each year.

Thus, while Barbara suggested that she is 'despite everything, a boy', in contemporary Abidjan, branché definitions of who constitutes a travesti vary widely (Thomann & Corey-Boulet, 2015).

Despite the ubiquity of terms like woubi, yossi and travesti, they are not recognised as salient categories by major donor institutions and the international NGOs that act as intermediaries between these donors and Arc-en-Ciel and Alternative. In their recent summary of their cross-sectional, bio-behavioural surveillance study on MSM, Aho et al. (2014) do not explore the woubi/yossi distinction or how it may shape vulnerability to HIV. Though they did ask survey respondents whether or not they identified as travestis, only 2% of the sample identified as such, providing little evidence about how their experience might differ from that of gender normative branchés. Descriptive statistics of these categories were only presented in the original report (Semde-Abla, 2012) but were ignored entirely in subsequent publications (Aho et al., 2014; Hakim et al., 2015; Vuylsteke et al., 2012). Furthermore, questions posed about the gender of respondents' sex partners did not include travestis or transgender persons as an option, providing minimal information about the extent to which gender normative MSM engage sexually with travesti and transgender partners. These and other questions assume that respondents understand travestis as 'men who have sex with men', though perhaps more effeminate versions of themselves, an assumption that does hold true for some branchés (Thomann & Corey-Boulet, 2015) but also miss an opportunity to engage the complexity of sexual and gendered identifications and the reality of their practice.

It is worth considering, though, what the wholesale adoption of terms like woubi, yossi and travesti would add to current HIV prevention efforts in Abidjan. Cultural competence advocates might argue that adopting the woubi/yossi dichotomy into HIV prevention programming makes sense. If researchers had clear and culturally specific roles then they would be able to envision two discreet risk groups, while having the added benefit of resonating with the local population. Like those gendered homosexualities in rural South Africa discussed by anthropologist Graeme Reid, the categories of 'woubi' and 'yossi' reveal a 'sharp distinction between masculine and feminine, with a marked hierarchical aspect that resonates with a heterosexual model' (Reid, 2012, p. 59). However, my branché research participants described these as idealised categories, suggesting that they offer little insight into the lived experience of sexual and gender minorities. Many of the branchés that I came to know during my research suggested that there is more fluidity in branché relationships than the dichotomous terms woubi and yossi imply.

Thus, integrating emic categories into current prevention efforts runs the risk of the same kind of reification and oversimplifications that the MSM category is guilty of, when in fact, those who practice these identifications recognise them as anything but. Merely integrating woubi-can terms into HIV prevention language without a critical understanding of the ways in which other social realities complicate lived experience would lead to the same kind of homogenisation as the category of MSM. In the following section, I turn to the ways in which issues of gender normativity, class, ethnicity, and even religion shape lived experiences of these categories.

NGOs as sites of social ordering

When Alternative and Arc-en-Ciel were chosen as subcontractors on the PEPFAR-funded project in 2011, their new headquarters became spaces in which increasingly large numbers of branchés gathered to celebrate national holidays, hold dance parties, and attend HIV prevention and identity workshops. Because of the deeply heteronormative context in which they live, branchés came together in these spaces to socialise, to learn, and to build relationships. But while NGO spaces seemingly disrupted Abidjan's heteronormativity, they were also sites for the reproduction of various forms of social exclusion. HIV peer educators and activists asserted moral orders that reflected their assumptions about what kinds of branchés belong – and where. In this section, I show that inclusion in community-based, HIV prevention programming for branchés is circumscribed by other social realities which create 'zones of exclusions' (Lorway & Khan, 2014, p. 60) and raise questions about the extent to which branchés are covered by current HIV research and prevention programming.

Branchés who come from the northern regions of Côte d'Ivoire, who are Muslim or were raised in Muslim families, and/or who have a sub-standard level of education found it difficult to fit into the new milieus that have emerged around NGOs like Claver's Alternative. Stigma *within* the community has resulted in low participation from branchés living in Abidjan's northern neighbourhoods and a rift between branchés in communities like the northern Ivoirian and Muslim-dominated neighbourhood of Abobo and those residing in neighbourhoods that NGO activists and peer educators deemed 'gay friendly', creating a moral geography of belonging to Abidjan's branché milieu (Thomann, 2016). On numerous occasions, I witnessed HIV peer educators and activists single out branchés from Abobo for being too loud, too flamboyant, and too aggressive. They claimed that branchés from Abobo were less versed in proper social decorum and etiquette and unconcerned with their visibility in neighbourhoods that were not their own. Even branchés who did not work as peer educators or activists confirmed the existence of such stigma and its links to cosmologies of modernity and belonging in broader Ivoirian society. Ibrahim, himself *un gen du nord* (a person from the north), but born in Abidjan, provided his own explanation of such stereotypes:

> It's sad but there is truth to the stereotypes about branchés from Abobo, like that they like fights and that they are poorly raised and all of that. In my opinion, it's because people from Abobo are mostly from the north of Côte d'Ivoire, where I am also from. And we, the people from the north, we are said to be hot-blooded ... So they don't know how to behave well in society.

These branchés were often ridiculed for their ethnic, linguistic, or cultural backgrounds in the same spaces they sought tolerance on the basis of their sexual orientation and/or gender identity. HIV peer educators, activists and members of the organisations saw branchés residing in northern districts as drawing unwanted attention with their uncouth behaviour, as victims of a culture of poverty that made them prone to aggression, and as unable or unwilling to become 'modern' Ivoirian branches (Thomann, in press).

Travestis also confronted stigma from gender normative branchés, compounding their vulnerability to state-sponsored violence in the wake of Côte d'Ivoire's brief, but all too familiar, political conflict. A month after the Ivoirian government recognised Alternative as a legal NGO, Ivoirians went to the polls to elect a new president, only the third election in Ivoirian history. When incumbent President Laurent Gbagbo refused to cede power to the internationally recognised victor Alassane Ouattara, the country erupted into bloody violence. Following the 2010–2011 post-election crisis and regime change, a new military presence rendered branchés, and travesti sex workers in particular, more vulnerable. The *Forces Républicaines de Côte d'Ivoire* (FRCI) are former-rebel members of the Ivoirian armed forces with a reputation for being violent, hostile, and extortive. During my research in 2012, the FRCI attacks on travesti sex workers had been the subject of much discussion at Alternative and Arc-en-Ciel. And yet, travestis rarely frequented, nor were they particularly welcomed at, the community-based NGOs. Indeed, throughout my research, travestis' presence at Alternative and Arc-en-Ciel was a subject of much controversy. There were numerous occasions on which gender normative HIV peer educators and activists discouraged travesti participation in events sponsored by the NGOs. For example, when planning for one of their 'mass HIV sensitization' events, Kouadio, a 23-year-old peer educator, organised a small faction of the staff to instil an unofficial policy of not giving out invites to travestis and to telling those lucky enough to receive one not to bring anyone 'who would dress like a queen'. Furthermore, at weekly 'identity workshops', HIV peer educators and activists relayed messages concerning a variety of gender non-normative behaviours that could attract unwanted attention to the individual and to the milieu more broadly, highlighting the behaviour of travestis as particularly problematic. Even the Executive Director of Alternative, Claver, told me unabashedly when asked,

> If you have to dress as a travesti, that's going to cost you your family. It's not worth doing it. I call those things that aren't necessary … I can't keep people who feel like they are women from doing it [living as a travesti]. But if you think that you can wear a dress and walk in front of a mosque and they are not going to stone you, go right ahead. Because you know that's going to cost you your life.

Increased vulnerability for travestis extends beyond their vulnerability to state-sponsored violence and exclusion from NGO programming – there are also important and underexplored differences in their sexual behaviour. While exceptions exist, all but a few of the travestis I have interviewed since 2012 currently support themselves primarily through sex work or have engaged in sex work at some point in their lives. When I asked Jocelyn, a travesti sex worker, if most of the travestis she knew engaged in sex work, she stated simply, 'Yes, they are travestis!' Jean, one of the few HIV peer educators who was friendly with many travestis, suggested that sex work is an essential part of their lived experience. He explained,

> I think that travestis are very different from gays, the other gays. A travesti doesn't have the spirit of someone who is not travesti. You see? They have their separate thing. That is the *trottoir* [stroll]. The travesti is the stroll. They don't have time to insert themselves in activities that don't bring them anything.

Thus, travestis and branchés from the northern districts of Abidjan were not only vulnerable to violence and discrimination because of their sexual and gendered identifications, but also because they faced discrimination and exclusion from the same organisations meant to improve their conditions. Furthermore, there are important differences in behaviour to consider. Travesti's involvement in sex work rendered them more vulnerable to HIV and violence. Excluded from the very spaces meant to provide inclusion based on sexual orientation and gender identity, northern branchés and travestis were effectively cut off from the interventions, resources, and 'community' intended to serve Abidjan's sexual and gender minorities. These networks offer political inclusion and new opportunities for self-fashioning to only certain members of Abidjan's branché milieu, while further entrenching existing forms of exclusion. In the following section, I examine the deployment of the identification 'MSM' and consider the new social boundaries enabled by MSM interventions.

'We're an industry': the making of MSM

Anthropologist Tom Boellstorff has suggested that the term MSM 'may be on its way to becoming a globally dominant identity category' (Boellstorff, 2011, p. 288) that is altogether different from what public professionals had in mind when they began employing the acronym to connote sexual behaviour instead of identity. In this section, I argue that interventions targeting MSM do more than describe sexual and gendered subjectivities, 'rather they are one of the discourses available through which people might conceive what they understand their sexuality to be' (Boyce, 2007, p. 184). Institutions like Alternative and Arc-en-Ciel become those in which gender and sexual minorities come to understand, identify and organise themselves and one another, producing new social relations and entrenching existing ones. I argue that the deployment of MSM as an identity category by local HIV peer educators and activists challenges the widely accepted notion that the category is purely behavioural and demonstrates that MSM interventions are part of a broader industry which shapes new forms of sociality among sexual and gender minorities.

The first time I heard someone say *Je suis MSM* (I am MSM) was in 2010. I was seated in the offices of Arc-en-Ciel, taking field notes and participating in a staff meeting, when Marius, a young HIV peer educator explained, 'We're all MSM, right?' Later, I asked him why he had said 'MSM' and not branché, or any of the other linguistic choices sexual minority men held in their repertoire. Marius rolled his eyes, laughed, and said, 'MSM, branché, it's all the same'. In Abidjan, many HIV peer educators and activists – and to a lesser extent the branchés served by local NGOs – self-identified as MSM both to me and to one another. During a conversation with Felix, a 28-year-old peer educator and certified HIV tester, he explained its use in local NGO networks: 'It's [the use of MSM] in the NGO milieu. It's a language that those who hang out in the NGOs understand. If I say MSM to you and you are not in a MSM NGO, you'll say 'MSM, what's that?' If you were in the NGO you would know what that means. It's a technical term. If you are on the inside.'

Branchés also used the term MSM to be discreet in public settings, which woubi-can could also have accomplished. For example, Antoine, the Head of Communications at Alternative described it as follows:

> It's a word that you can say everywhere without looking to see if someone is watching. If you say, 'I am gay', everyone is going to look at you. While in the middle of the street you can say 'I am MSM' and no one knows what that means.

Not all of the branchés whom I met in Abidjan identified as MSM, indeed most of them did not, but many of the peer educators and activists discussed in this article drew on the MSM category as a form of self-fashioning, whereby they discreetly indexed their same-sex desire, as well as their position within local NGOs.

This dynamic use of the MSM category is tied to shifts in the industry of global public health. MSM are one of several marginalised populations (in addition to sex workers and intravenous drug users) on which the global health community has increasingly focused, as its strategy has shifted towards addressing concentrated HIV epidemics. This recently acquired exceptionality is perhaps most evident in the growing industry of donor institutions and NGOs from the global North targeting the HIV epidemic among sexual and gender minorities throughout the global South. As subcontractors in this system, HIV peer educators and activists are charged with doing the 'on the ground' work of reaching MSM, while staff at Heartland engage in monitoring and programme evaluation and conduct financial audits that carry with them the threat of funding cuts. In our discussions about their relationships with foreign donors and intermediary NGOs, peer educators and activists at Alternative and Arc-en-Ciel complained of a relentless focus on numbers-based results. Taped to the wall of Claver's office were poster-board sized Post-Its with 'new MSM' targets to be reached that year. These numbers were a constant source of anxiety and frustration for the staff at Alternative. In 2011, Heartland set the target at 1570 MSM reached. In 2012, the target jumped to 2153 *new* MSM. The staff often joked about the enormity of these targets, noting that if targets continued to rise this way in 2013 they would have to start 'making MSM'.

In October of 2012, Heartland proposed a performance-based pay system for HIV peer educators working at Alternative and Arc-en-Ciel, which would pay them 500 CFA (approximately 1 USD) per 'new MSM reached'. This performance-based pay model draws on business models of development that creates competition (between organisations and between staff within the same organisation), while turning branchés and other sexual and gender minorities into (single) dollar signs. The proposed programme would have effectively removed long-term social support for HIV positive branchés from the organisation's formal objectives. Heartland's strategy would also have defunded transportation and activity costs for the HIV support groups and compromised other long-term relationships that peer educators and activists had worked to cultivate with some of the most vulnerable members of the community. Many peer educators and activists voiced these concerns during internal meetings that Claver held to discuss the suggested plan and they coordinated a coalition-based response with other community-based organisations to reject it. Speaking to me hours before that meeting, Claver explained:

> With Heartland, if you are a new person, that's great. But if you already came and we already wrote your name down, that means that you are not eligible to take any more condoms. If that's the case, then you can't come back for more. Because they put [in the action plan] that you have to reach 2000 *new* people. But just because someone is not a new person doesn't mean that you are going to leave him. With Heartland, it's not like that. Because it's only numbers that interest them.

This enumeration-based programming assumes that data can be generated and analysed statistically to measure the impact of prevention programming. But who is actually counted among these thousands of MSM? This terminology, intended to lump people together, distracts from other complex social realities and lived experiences, including those of ethnicity, gender performance and class. Furthermore, it threatened to erode social support for HIV positive individuals and reimbursements that HIV peer educators needed in order to continue service provision. Thus, an increasing number of 'new MSM' enrolled in interventions did not ensure that the most vulnerable were reached.

As Claver suggested, financial interests are served by this audit culture (Strathern, 2000). Heartland, via its PEPFAR grant, puts pressure on HIV peer educators and activists to reach the largest sample of MSM possible. However, this drive for an adequate statistical power belies other forms of diversity that shape HIV vulnerability in the Ivoirian context. In their conversations and actions, activists and peer educators regularly challenged the fundamentally unequal donor/recipient relationship that existed between them and Heartland, between them and PEPFAR, and ultimately between the Ivoirian and US governments. Eric, a 23-year-old peer educator at Alternative said:

> In Africa, we [branchés] have become a bit like AIDS. We're an industry. Meaning that most people are taking more care of what is going back in their pockets than the lives of branchés. Organizations care about branchés insofar as they can fill their pockets. They don't care about the health of branchés.

Conclusion

In this article, I have argued that the diversity of sexual and gender minority experience is obscured by the uncritical and reductive language used in HIV research and interventions, resulting in their failure to address the complex and intersecting social realities that shape HIV vulnerability. In Abidjan, this has resulted in questionable coverage of branchés in current research and programming, as the assumption of a homogeneous population of MSM entrenches the invisibility and exclusion of travestis and Ivoirians of stigmatised ethnic and/or class backgrounds. While I have argued that recent research and prevention ignore the salience of emic identity categories in their work, I have also suggested that the mere integration of local identifications, such as woubi and yossi, would be inadequate to ensure greater inclusion and representation. Researchers and practioners concerned with the health and well-being of sexual and gender minorities should not take local identifications to be self-evident. Rather, they must acknowledge the diversity of lived experience within terminologies, and investigate, in local contexts, other social realities that may shape HIV vulnerability.

I have also argued that these shallow conceptualisations of sexual and gender minority experience are linked to the culture (and business) of public health itself, which prioritises quantitative evidence and considers qualitative knowledge to be anecdotal at best. In order for HIV prevention programming to reach those most in need, it is paramount that researchers begin to think about the development of programming that engages the complexity of sexual and gender minority experience. This includes thinking about the ways in which interventions shape identity. Importantly, as Fan points out in her work on the outsourcing of HIV testing among MSM in China (Fan, 2014), much of the current international HIV funding for key populations requires that NGOs continually redefine themselves in order to exist. Heartland needs HIV peer educators at Alternative and Arc-en-Ciel to produce these numbers in order stay relevant. It is essential to question normative identifications in public health, whether they are imposed by outside forces or developed from within, and to interrogate the goal of using, promoting, and accepting them.

Increased research on the intersections of critical public health and sexuality studies will allow researchers to engage with novel and fluid sexual and gender subjectivities and their impact on HIV vulnerability. Ethnographic research provides a powerful tool for studying both the complexity of the lived experience of sexual and gender minorities and the impact of interventions in shaping new form of social reality and may lead to greater insight into the 'broader politics that enmesh and shape global health priorities' (Fan, 2014, p. 95). Ethnographic data that engages both the complexity of lived experience and the impacts of interventions that almost always overlook those complexities could serve as a starting point for rethinking the assumptions inherent in the culture of public health itself. An engagement with this kind of complexity requires a movement away from the logic that devalues qualitative research, prioritises generalisability and eschews individual experience, as well as a deeper reflection on the ways in which public health culture itself may be contributing to and further entrenching vulnerabilities.

Note

1. A similar system of in-group identification has been documented in Senegal (Dramé et al., 2012) and Mali (Broqua, 2013).

Disclosure statement

No potential conflict of interest was reported by the author.

Funding

Research reported in this publication was supported by the National Institute of Allergy & Infectious Diseases of the National Institutes of Health [grant number T32AI114398]. The content is solely the responsibility of the authors and does not necessarily represent the official views of the National Institutes of Health.

References

Adams, V. (2013). Evidence-based global public health: Subjects, profits erasures. In J. Biehl and A. Petryna (Eds.), *When people come first: Critical studies in global health* (pp. 54–90). Princeton: Princeton University Press.

Aggleton, P., & Parker, R. (2015). Moving beyond biomedicalization in the HIV response: Implications for community involvement and community leadership among men who have sex with men and transgender people. *American Journal of Public Health*, 105(8), 1552–1558. doi:10.2105/AJPH.2015.302614

Aho, J., Hakim, A., Vuylsteke, B., Semde, G., Gbais, H. G., Diarrassouba, M., ... Laga, M. (2014). Exploring risk behaviors and vulnerability for HIV among men who have sex with men in Abidjan, Côte d'Ivoire: Poor knowledge, homophobia, and sexual violence. *PLOS ONE*, 9(6), e99591. doi:10.1371/journal.phone.0099591

Akindès, F. (2001). *Dynamique de la politique sociale en Côte d'Ivoire*. Genève: Institut de recherché des Nations Unies.

Akindes, F. (2004). *The roots of the Political Military crisis in Côte d'Ivoire*. Research Report. Uppsala: Nordiska Afrikaininstitutet.

Beyrer, C., Baral, S. D., van Griensen, F., Goodreau, S. M., Chariyalertsak, S., Wirtz, A. L., & Brookmeyer, R. (2012). The global epidemiology of HIV infection among men who have sex with men. *The Lancet*, 380(9839), 367–377. doi:10.1016/S0140-6

Boellstorff, T. (2011). But do not identify as gay: A proleptic genealogy of the MSM category. *Cultural Anthropology*, 26(2), 287–312. doi:10.1111/j.1548-1360.2011.01100.x

Boyce, P. (2007). 'Conceiving Kothis': Men who have sex with men in India and the cultural subject of HIV prevention. *Medical Anthropology: Cross-Cultural Studies in Health and Illness*, 26(2), 175–203. doi:10.1080/01459740701285582

Brooks, P.(Producer) & Bochaut, L. (Director). (1998). *Woubi Cheri*. San Francisco: California Newsreel.

Broqua, C. (2012). L'émergence des minorités sexuelles dans l'espace public en Afrique. *Politique Africain*, 126, 5–23. doi:10.3917/polaf.126.0005

Broqua, C. (2013). Male homosexuality in Bamako: A cross-cultural and cross-historical comparative perspective. In S. N. Nyeck & M. Epprecht (Eds.), *Sexual diversity in Africa: Politics, theory, citizenship* (pp. 109–128). Montreal: McGill-Queen's University Press.

Corey-Boulet, R. (2012). Transgender prostitutes face abuse in ivory coast. *Associated Press*. Retrieved December 11, 2012, from http://bigstory.ap.org/article/transgender-prostitutes-face-abuse-ivory-coast

Corey-Boulet, R. (2013). Ivory Coast: A fragile tolerance. *Caravan Magazine*. Retrieved June 1, 2013, from http://www.caravanmagazine.in/letters/ivory-coast-fragile-tolerance

Corey-Boulet, R. (2014). Ivory Coast: Mob attacks gay rights group office. *Huffington Post*. Retrieved January 28, 2014, from http://www.huffingtonpost.com/huff-wires/20140127/af–ivory-coast-gay-attack-1st-ldwritethru/

Cutolo, A. (2010). Modernity, autochthony, and the Ivoirian nation: The end of a century in Côte d'Ivoire. *Africa*, 90(4), 527–551. doi:10.3366/E0001972010000756

Dramé, F., Peitzmeier, S., Lopes, M., Ndaw, M., Sow, A., Diouf, D., & Baral, S. (2012). Gay men and other men who have sex with men in West Africa: Evidence from the field. *Culture Health and Sexuality*, 15(1), 7–21. doi:10.1080/13691058.2012.748935

Fan, E. (2014). HIV testing as prevention among MSM in China: The business of scaling-up. *Global Public Health, 9*(1–2), 85–97. doi:10.1080/17441692.2014.881520

Fioriti, J. (2014). Gay in Côte d'Ivoire find haven on hostile continent. *Africa Review*. Retrieved February 15, 2014, from http://www.africareview.com/Analysis/Gays-in-Cote-dIvoire-find-haven-on-hostilecontinent/-/979190/2199628/-/3d0oo6z/-/index.html

Hakim, A. J., Aho, J., Semde, G., Diarrassouba, M., Ehoussou, K., Vuylsteke, B., ... SHARM Study Group. (2015). The epidemiology of HIV and prevention needs of men who have sex with men in Abidjan, Côte d'Ivoire. *PLoS ONE, 10*(4), e0125218. doi:10.1371/journal.pone.0125218

Konate, S. (2004). The politics of identity and violence in Côte d'Ivoire. *West Africa Review, 5*, 1–15.

Kouassi, S. M. (2011). Côte d'Ivoire: Is Abidjan becoming a gay El Dorado? *Radio Netherlands Worldwide*. Retrieved September 21, 2011, from http://www.rnw.nl/africa/article/ivory-coast-abidjan-becoming-a-gay-eldorado

Kulick, D. (1998). *Travesti: Sex, gender and culture among Brazilian transgendered prostitutes*. Chicago, IL: University of Chicago Press.

Leap, W. (2004). Language, belonging, and (homo)sexual citizenship in Cape Town, South Africa. In W. Leap & T. Boellstorff (Eds.), *Speaking in queer tongues: Globalization and gay language* (pp. 134–152). Urbana: University of Illinois Press.

Le Pape, M., & Vidal, C. (1984). Libéralisme et Vécus Sexuels à Abidjan. *Cahiers internationaux de sociologie, 1*(26), 111–118.

Lorway, R., & Khan, S. (2014). Reassembling epidemiology: Mapping, monitoring, and making up people in the context of HIV prevention in India. *Social Science and Medicine, 112*, 51–62. doi:10.1016/j.socscimed.2014.04.034

Marshall-Fratani, R. (2006). The war of who is who: Autochthony, nationalism and citizenship in the Ivoirian crisis. *African Studies Review, 49*(2), 9–43. doi:10.1353/arw.2006.0098

McGovern, M. (2011). *Making war in Côte d'Ivoire*. Chicago, IL: University of Chicago Press.

Newell, S. (2006). Estranged belongings a moral economy of theft in Abidjan, Côte d'Ivoire. *Anthropological Theory, 6*(2), 711–737. doi:10.1177/1463499606065034

Newell, S. (2012). *The modernity bluff: Crime, consumption and citizenship in Côte d'Ivoire*. Chicago, IL: University of Chicago Press.

Nguyen, V. K. (2010). *The republic of therapy: Triage and sovereignty in West Africa's time of AIDS*. Durham: Duke University Press.

PEPFAR – The United States president's emergency plan for AIDS relief. (2010). Côte d'Ivoire operational plan report.

PEPFAR – The United States president's emergency plan for AIDS relief. (2013). Côte d'Ivoire operational plan report.

Reid, G. (2012). *How to be a real gay: Gay identities in small-town South Africa*. Scottsville: University of KwaZulu-Natal Press.

Rodriguez, D. (2007). The political logic of the non-profit industrial complex. In Incite! Women of Color Against Violence (Ed.), *The Revolution will not be funded: Beyond the Non Profit Industrial Complex* (pp. 21–40). Cambridge: South End Press.

Semde-Abla, G. (2012) *Etude sur le VIH et les facteurs de risqué associés chez les hommes ayant des rapport sexuels avec des hommes à Abidjan*, Côte d'Ivoire. Rapport final. Family Health International.

Spade, D. (2011). *Normal life: Administrative violence, critical trans politics, and limits of the law*. Brooklyn: South End Press.

Smith, A. (2007). Introduction: The Revolution will not be funded. In Incite! Women of Color Against Violence, (Ed.,). *The Revolution will not be funded: Beyond the Non Profit Industrial Complex* (pp. 1–20). Cambridge: South End Press.

Strathern, M. (2000). Introduction: New accountabilities. In Marilyn Strathern (Ed.), *Audit cultures: Anthropological studies in accountability, ethics and the academy* (pp. 1–18). London: Routledge.

Thomann, M. (2014). *The price of inclusion: Sexual subjectivity, violence and the nonprofit industrial complex in Abidjan, Côte d'Ivoire* (Ph.D. diss.). Department of Anthropology, American University.

Thomann, M. (2016). Zones of difference, boundaries of access: Moral geography and community mapping in Abidjan, Côte d'Ivoire. *Journal of Homosexuality*, 63(3). doi:10.1080/00918369.2016.1124706

Thomann, M., & Corey-Boulet, R. (2015). Violence, exclusion and resilience among Ivoirian travestis. *Critical African Studies*. Advance online publication. doi:10.1080/21681392.2015.1087323

Vuylsteke, B., Semde, G., Sika, L., Crucitti, T., Traore, V. E., & Buve, L. M. (2012). High prevalence of HIV and sexually transmitted infections among male sex workers in Abidjan, Côte d'Ivoire: Need for services tailored to their needs. *Sexually Transmitted Infections*, 88, 288–293. doi:0.1136/sextrans-2011-050276

Young, R. M., & Meyer, I. (2005). The trouble with 'MSM' and 'WSW': Erasure of the sexual minority person in public health discourse. *American Journal of Public Health*, 95(7), 1144–1149. doi:10.2105/AJPH.2004.046714

Gender identity, healthcare access, and risk reduction among Malaysia's *mak nyah* community

Britton A. Gibson [ID], Shan-Estelle Brown, Ronnye Rutledge, Jeffrey A. Wickersham, Adeeba Kamarulzaman and Frederick L. Altice

ABSTRACT

Transgender women (TGW) face compounded levels of stigma and discrimination, resulting in multiple health risks and poor health outcomes. TGW identities are erased by forcing them into binary sex categories in society or treating them as men who have sex with men (MSM). In Malaysia, where both civil and religious law criminalise them for their identities, many TGW turn to sex work with inconsistent prevention methods, which increases their health risks. This qualitative study aims to understand how the identities of TGW sex workers shapes their healthcare utilisation patterns and harm reduction behaviours. In-depth, semi-structured interviews were conducted with 21 male-to-female transgender (*mak nyah*) sex workers in Malaysia. Interviews were transcribed, translated into English, and analysed using thematic coding. Results suggest that TGW identity is shaped at an early age followed by incorporation into the *mak nyah* community where TGW were assisted in gender transition and introduced to sex work. While healthcare was accessible, it failed to address the multiple healthcare needs of TGW. Pressure for gender-affirming health procedures and fear of HIV and sexually transmitted infection screening led to potentially hazardous health behaviours. These findings have implications for developing holistic, culturally sensitive prevention and healthcare services for TGW.

Introduction

In public health research, a number of frequently conflated terms serve as significant barriers to truly understanding and addressing a population's health needs. For instance, there is a common misclassification of the terms 'sex', 'gender', and 'sexual orientation' as synonyms, which perpetuates a heteronormative structure with binary classifications for: (1) a person's biology as male or female; (2) socio-sexual identity (i.e. masculine or feminine); and (3) sexual orientation (i.e. opposite-sex or same-sex attraction) (Valdes, 1996). For many transgender persons, this structure creates dissonance between their social identification and their biological sex, as well as sexual orientation. Not surprisingly, many researchers perpetuate this incorrect conflation of terms, which causes misunderstanding in service provision for diverse groups of people (i.e. gay or bisexual men, other men who have sex with men [MSM], and transgender women [TGW]) by virtue of inadequate targeted services and/or data granularity. Male-to-female transgender persons, or TGW, are individuals who are born biologically male but identify as women and may or may not have undergone gender-affirming surgery (e.g. vaginoplasty, breast augmentation, facial reconstruction, etc.) (Beemyn, n.d.); this term is distinct from sexual orientation. TGW, however, are often grouped with MSM, largely because of similar biological risk, resulting in a lack of specific data on health concerns within this specific population worldwide (UNAIDS, 2014). In one qualitative study, TGW expressed being socially excluded from MSM groups and that outreach efforts were largely focused on MSM and sex workers, but not targeted to TGW (Logie, James, Tharao, & Loutfy, 2012). Thus, TGW remain a vulnerable population with inadequate representation in HIV programming and insufficient data quantifying their burden of disease.

Where data on TGW are available, HIV burden is extremely high, with prevalence rates reaching 49% in some contexts (UNAIDS, 2014). A meta-analysis on the global burden of HIV among TGW found pooled HIV prevalence at 19.1%, with HIV prevalence in TGW being 48.8-fold higher compared with reproductive age adults (Baral et al., 2013). Despite excess burden, HIV prevention strategies lack specificity for TGW programming, with only 43% of countries reporting in 2012 that they targeted TGW (UNAIDS, 2014). Consequently, TGW are both socially and medically marginalised, including from traditional healthcare settings and from HIV/AIDS prevention and treatment services.

The disproportionate HIV rates seen in TGW are related to mutual HIV risk and increased vulnerability. 'Risk' and 'vulnerability', however, represent another set of frequently conflated terms relating to HIV in TGW. 'Risk' refers to an individual's likelihood of acquiring HIV infection, which is determined by engagement in behaviours that may result in transmission, such as unprotected sex or sharing needles (UNAIDS, 1998). It is rooted in the concept of 'vulnerability', which refers to social and structural factors that influence the likelihood that a person will contract HIV when they engage in elevated HIV risk behaviours, such as their social network, legal and economic structures, accessibility of prevention and treatment services, and societal marginalisation (Sumartojo, 2000; UNAIDS, 1998). While some TGW have similar biological risk as MSM, they may experience social vulnerabilities similar to cisgender females and structural vulnerabilities that are unique to them, given dichotomous gender structures (Daryani, 2011; LeBreton, 2013; Logie et al., 2012; Nemoto, Luke, Mamo, Ching, & Patria, 1999).

Several studies have highlighted the structural and social factors that stigmatise and marginalise TGW. Transphobia and societal discrimination are common experiences for TGW, which contribute to high rates of depression, suicidal ideation, substance abuse, and other mental illnesses within this population (Clements-Nolle, Marx, & Katz, 2006; Nemoto et al., 1999). Increased stigma and discrimination also impacts TGW's ability to find and maintain employment, leading many to turn to sex work to support themselves financially and increasing their risk for HIV and sexually transmitted infections (STI) (Nemoto et al., 1999; Reisner et al., 2009).

Gender-based health needs of TGW are also inadequately addressed in healthcare settings, due in part to individual and structural factors. Stigma, discrimination, and erasure (the lack of recognition of gender identity outside a male/female binary system) may restrict TGW's health-seeking behaviours for prevention, treatment, and care (Bauer et al., 2009). Additionally, TGW are often overtly stigmatised by or discriminated against in healthcare settings, ranging from incorrect pronoun use, insensitive treatment, judgmental statements, and unwillingness to provide care (Logie et al., 2012; Lombardi, 2010). While most research on TGW health assessments focus on HIV and STI risk, it is evident that healthcare providers lack the crucial knowledge and cultural sensitivity regarding other important and relevant health concerns, including gender-affirming care, like hormone replacement therapy (HRT) and cosmetic surgery. In this context, we explore the importance of holistically integrating HIV/STI prevention with culturally relevant and contextually affirming healthcare to address the complex needs that are crucial to longitudinally engage TGW in care.

Background on Malaysia

Malaysia is a high, middle-income country of 29.7 million people located in Southeast Asia. Predominant ethnic groups include Malays and indigenous persons (67.4%), Chinese (24.6%) and Indians (7.3%). While Islam is the country's major religion, a sizeable portion of the population practices Buddhism (19%), Christianity (9%), or Hinduism (6%) (Department of Statistics Malaysia, 2011).

Though TGW are historically significant in Southeast Asia and Malaysian culture, the legal and public attitudes toward TGW have been tumultuous. TGW could access gender-affirming surgery and change their national identification cards to match their gender through the early 1980s. By 1983, however, mounting Islamic conservatism resulted in a *fatwa* that banned Muslims (and consequently all others) from genital-altering surgery, further increasing stigma and discrimination. In 1996, even surgically affirmed non-Muslim TGW were unable to change their sex designation on their identification card (Suresh, n.d.).

Despite Malaysia's overarching secular government, religious (Sharia) law is also present and influences policies and practices. In this system, Muslim TGW risk imprisonment for publically expressing their gender identity and are charged as 'men dressing as women', an offence punishable by fine and imprisonment. Secular laws also continue to criminalise 'carnal intercourse against the order of nature', including oral and anal sex, which may uncommonly be invoked to fine or imprison TGW of any ethnicity (Attorney General's Chamber of Malaysia, 2006; Ghoshal, 2014).

The TGW community coined the term *mak nyah* ('*mak*' means 'mother' in Malay) in 1987 to refer to TGW as a way to counteract growing discrimination of derogatory labels that grouped them as 'effeminate males' (Slamah, 2005). Thus, the term *mak nyah* dually distinguished TGW from MSM, while also preserving their dignity. Though the total number of TGW in Malaysia is unknown, an estimated 21,000 TGW engage in sex work, with 37.5% of them residing in greater Kuala Lumpur (Lim, Ang, & Teh, 2010); HIV prevalence among all TGW is estimated at 10% (Ministry of Health Malaysia, 2013). While some literature has highlighted the need for HIV prevention and advocacy services for *mak nyah* (Teh, 2008a), there is otherwise limited recent research available, particularly surrounding how their identity influences access to and engagement in healthcare generally and specifically for HIV prevention and treatment services.

Methods

Data from 21 *mak nyah* sex workers were analysed from a larger study that included an additional 19 female sex workers (FSWs) in greater Kuala Lumpur.

Data collection

Semi-structured, in-depth interview guides were developed to explore the topics of health behaviours, healthcare access, substance use, violence, and discrimination among FSW and *mak nyah* sex workers, recruited through convenience sampling at community-based organisations and through peer referral with the aim of targeting ethnic and geographic variation, as well as diversity in sex work involvement. Interviews (60-90 minutes) were conducted between September 2013 and January 2014 in English, Malay, or Tamil.

Definitions

For the purposes of this paper, we use TGW as a global or general term, *mak nyah* for TGW specifically in the Malaysian context and *mak nyah* sex workers as TGW who met inclusion criteria for this study, encompassing those who traded sex for money, rent or services.

Data analysis

All interviews were recorded, transcribed, translated into English and back-translated (Brislin, 1970). Key findings from interviews were discussed between interviewers and investigators to understand broad themes. Transcripts were reviewed and thematically coded (BAG) and then collectively reviewed and discussed (BAG, SB, RR, FLA) to understand the prominent themes that emerged. After finalising coding structure, interviews were reviewed again to ensure accuracy of all codes. Coding and analysis were done using Atlas.ti software (ATLAS.ti, 2014). Institutional Review Boards at Yale University and the University of Malaya approved the study.

Results

A description of the 21 *mak nyah* sex workers can be found in Table 1 and linked to selected quotes. Overall, mean age was 41.5 years, including ethnic Malays (47.6%), Indians (42.8%), and other (9.5%). No significant differences emerged between ethnicities. Three prominent and connected themes emerged from the data: gender identity, healthcare utilisation, and HIV prevention priorities[1].

Gender identity

Gender identity, central to all discussions, was of prime importance, which participants clarified was not defined by their biological sex designation. Concerns were raised about how their lives were commonly influenced by societal gender norms in relationships, behaviours, and occupational choice. Most participants focused on their childhood and

Table 1. Participant references with demographics.

Participant	Age (years)	Ethnicity	Healthcare utilisation site	Gender-confirmation surgery?	Ever tested for HIV?	Ever tested for STIs?	HIV/STI screening within last year?	Reported condom use during SW
1	50	Malay	Transgender-sensitive provider	No	Yes	Yes	No	Consistent
2	50	Malay	Transgender-sensitive provider	No	No	No	No	Consistent
3	43	Malay	Private clinic	No	Yes	Yes	Yes	Consistent
4	50	Malay	Governmental hospital	No	Yes	Yes	No	Inconsistent
5	37	Malay	Private clinic	No	Yes	No	No	Consistent
6	43	Indian	Governmental hospital	No	Yes	No	No	Consistent
7	57	Indian	Governmental hospital	Yes	No	No	No	Consistent
8	40	Indian	Transgender-sensitive provider	No	Yes	Yes	Yes	Consistent
9	47	Indian	Governmental clinic	No	Yes	No	No	Consistent
10	55	Indian	Governmental clinic	No	Yes	Yes	Yes	Consistent
11	33	Indian	Private clinic	Yes	Yes	Yes	Yes	Consistent
12	44	Indian	Governmental clinic	Yes	Yes	Yes	Yes	Consistent
13	40	Indian	Governmental clinic	Yes	Yes	Yes	Yes	Consistent
14	35	Malay	Private & governmental clinics	No	No	No	No	Inconsistent
15	33	Bidayuh	Private clinic	No	No	No	No	Inconsistent
16	26	Malay	Private clinic	No	No	No	No	Inconsistent
17	35	Malay	Transgender-sensitive provider	No	Yes	No	No	Inconsistent
18	50	Iban/Chinese	Transgender-sensitive provider	No	Yes	Yes	Yes	Consistent
19	38	Malay	Governmental clinic	No	No	No	No	Consistent
20	40	Indian	Transgender-sensitive provider	Yes	Yes	Yes	Yes	Inconsistent
21	26	Malay	Governmental hospital	No	No	No	No	Inconsistent

Note: STI= Sexually transmitted infection; SW=Sex work.

gender transition. Common to these stories was the conflict in childhood that their inner gender awareness did not match their biological sex.

> When I was in school at kindergarten, my late father dressed me in girl's clothes. When I was 12 years old, I was close to girls, not guys. In Form 3 [age 15], I would [pretend to be a] super-model in the school's hall. Until now, I still act like this. It has come from my soul since I was small. – [4]

Many participants recalled displaying similar effeminate behaviours from a young age, often referring to themselves as 'soft' and noting their inclination towards traditionally feminine activities. These behaviours were commonly met with resistance and abuse from family, teachers, and peers.

> From the time I was small, I have been very soft. I used to wear my mother's sari. My mother would beat me but it is not like I wanted to be [like this]. God made me to be like this. I didn't like to play football with the boys; I cooked for fun like a girl. I only played volleyball like a girl. I only liked to be friends with girls. [8]

Participants also felt their gender identity was not their choice. They often discussed the inevitability of their gender identity in the context of violence and discrimination.

> In the world, there is male, female, and after that is transgender. We did not want be transgender but that is how God created us. [20]

> Of course I feel sad. People discriminate against you because you are transgender. It's not that you want to be like this. [14]

As participants began to recognise and identify themselves as transgender, the transgender community played an important role in assisting them with transitioning and teaching them how to be a *mak nyah*.

> I was born as a guy who is soft. I started to socialize [with other mak nyah] when I was 12 and I was already 'doing drag' when I was in Form 1 [age 13]. At that time, I was still confused about myself ... [Then], around 15 to 16 years old I started having long hair. [16]

> We knew [mak nyah]. They wear women's clothing. They also wear wigs. We also want to look like those people. After that, [the mak nyah] gave us clothes. After one or two days, we also liked to dress like that. Before I came to KL (Kuala Lumpur), I always dressed like a male. Even though I was soft, I dressed like a male. I never took hormones. I just started doing that [in Kuala Lumpur]. I started dressing like a woman here. They taught me how to dress, also. [8]

It should be noted that with gender transition, *mak nyah* participants did not necessarily identify as female. Participants seemed to find their gender identity across a spectrum, with some feeling fluid in masculine and feminine expression, others feeling they are strictly women, and most identifying as transgender.

> When [people] come to talk [to me], they always ask why can't I be a woman, a perfect woman or a perfect man. I say there is no perfect person in this world. If you tell me a woman is perfect, why are they killing their babies? Why does a man rape his daughter? Is there a perfect person in this world? No, sorry to say that ... I was born to be a she-male and I didn't change myself to be like that. I didn't change myself to be a woman. [18]

As part of the discussion on their identity, participants spoke about systemic discrimination embedded in the political and religious climate of Malaysia that marginalised them.

> The government doesn't give any support for transgenders. In Singapore, India, and other countries, they support transgender [persons]: employment, housing, identity. Like in Singapore, they get female identity after [vaginoplasty]. They can get married and live. In Malaysia, it is a Muslim country, [there are] so many problems. Overseas [countries] have everything but here in Malaysia, we don't have [anything]. We only have ourselves. [20]

> As an Islamic country, we know we can't have equality. I just want no discrimination, to have my own rights, open minded organisations, companies that can accept transgender [women]. Most of the companies that accept transgender [women] are retail, hotels, shopping complex and [jobs are] very limited. Most transgender [women] are not stupid, but because of

restrictions, they can't join government jobs. There are a lot of boundaries. It's because we have no chance that we are doing sex work. We don't want to do sex work. [14]

The multiple levels of discrimination faced by *mak nyah* cause many to turn to sex work as their primary source of income, as they are unable to obtain and maintain formal employment (Teh, 2008b). As *mak nyah* help support each other, sex work is taught as a substantial source of income in a society that marginalises them. All participants mentioned that other members of the transgender community introduced them to sex work.

> My friend was working in Singapore. She told me, 'You suffer with problems. You [should] come and work here. We are born as transgenders. We can work at a company but ... that is too difficult. If you work at a company, you will not be satisfied. The guys will tease you. Here you will find some money and when you become stable, you will see.' After she recommended that, I started working there. [20]

> I knew of one Indian [*mak nyah*]. She asked me, 'You want money? Accompany me to [the red light area].' I noticed a lot of beautiful [*mak nyah*] and I became excited and wanted to be like them ... She said if I want to get more money after work, I need to work here [as a sex worker]. Since then, I have gone to [the red light area]. [5]

Although a high proportion of *mak nyah* are sex workers (Teh, 2008b), the community is not defined by participating in sex work and camaraderie is much more dependent on gender than occupation. (Note: *Though mak nyah are not legally allowed to marry a male, several participants referred to their long-term intimate partners as 'husbands', supporting their identification as women*).

> I have a husband. We stay together. I'm a dancer. I come [to the red light area] to meet transgenders. Sometimes [I also come] to meet my regular customers for sex. Once they call me, then I come. [13]

> The transgender community is quite close. We always meet, mix up with each another once in a while. We know people from other places and other cities also. [3]

There remains considerable competition between *mak nyah* who sell sex, as they try to solicit customers to support themselves. This is largely based on appearance, with substantial emphasis placed on beauty and femininity to attract customers.

> [Competition] is quite strong ... they say beauty is number one. Actually, breast is number one and second is beauty ... the third, we call it 'services.' [3]

> There are so many she-males who are bad looking, so they can't work as a sex worker because when you talk about sex work, you need 'the package.' If you are not beautiful, you can't earn and if you can't earn, what will you do? I am so lucky I am beautiful so that I can make money ... I thank God that I have this 'package' for me to work on the streets and get easy money. [18]

For *mak nyah* sex workers, feminisation procedures play a dual role in both affirming an individual's gender with their appearance and also helping them to solicit more customers. HRT is common and many had also undergone surgery for cosmetic procedures, with five participants having received vaginoplasty. Because of the religious climate, regulation, and cost in Malaysia, *mak nyah* usually travel outside the country, generally to Thailand, to receive gender-affirming surgeries.

> I started taking hormones when I was 15. Now still take them but with my age being 37, the doctor advised me to reduce it. So, I just get extra vitamins. [I got] breast implants in Thailand because in Thailand the cost is a bit lower than Malaysia, RM4000 (USD$1100). In Malaysia, it may be a bit expensive. [5]

With such pressure for feminisation, widespread societal discrimination, and difficulty in accessing gender-affirming procedures, several practices have emerged that pose health concerns.

Healthcare access and utilisation

While *mak nyah* often experience stigma and discrimination in healthcare settings, they also must navigate through a system that largely does not recognise or accept their gender identity. Many healthcare providers are unaware of the health risks faced by *mak nyah* who self-regulate the transition of their bodies. There may also be a lack of clarity and comfort in discussing medically assisted gender transitions, sexual organs, and high-risk behaviours between providers and their *mak nyah* patients who are sex workers.

A common practice among participants included HRT without prescription by a supervising physician. Often, HRT pills were purchased at pharmacies or obtained from friends and multiple pills would be taken daily, with the aim of 'speeding up' their transition. Participants spoke to their independence with HRT.

> Sometimes, I inject hormones. I will accompany a friend to do an operation in Thailand and I will buy hormones there. Then, I will inject it here. [17]

> I take hormone injections. I will go to clinic only if my blood pressure goes up. I give myself injections once a week. Then, I take [hormone] capsules in the morning and at night. [16]

Despite mostly non-supervised treatment, some participants mentioned receiving HRT from doctors at private, 'for profit' clinics who were friendly toward *mak nyah* and offered HRT, which allowed some monitoring of their transition. Beyond monitoring the gender transition, these *mak nyah* -friendly doctors also seemed to provide a safe, non-judgmental environment where some *mak nyah sex workers* would discuss sexual behaviours and receive screening for HIV and STIs.

> I used to go and see my doctor at the clinic. My doctor really understands me and really understands she-males. She is very good with me and she always gives good advice. Even if I'm itchy, I go to her, [she asks] 'Do you need injections? Cream?' I don't simply go to the pharmacy and buy the medicine. I believe I need to consult a doctor. [18]

> Sometimes I'm afraid to go to government hospital because my body is a 'hormone body.' Sometimes they inject a different injection. I'm scared about that. If we go to a clinic that knows we are transgender, they give medicine, take care and give results. That's why we go there. [20]

> For blood tests … there is a special doctor for us. There's [a private] clinic. They know we are [transgender] and doing this job [sex work]. [17]

Other participants mentioned receiving care from private doctors because they felt by paying more money, they would receive better care. While these providers were not labelled as transgender-friendly, they were seen as a way to maintain privacy and confidentiality.

> At a private [clinic], they cost more money. If you pay, they will do their jobs. If we go to a government [clinic], they will treat us, but very poorly … If at a private clinic, we don't have any issue. It's because we pay for it, right? If we pay for government clinic, we get less service. [5]

While the government healthcare system is free, many reported avoiding it due to past discriminatory experiences. Participants who used government clinics recounted being denied care, mistreated, asked to change their appearance, or felt they had to present as male in order to receive proper care.

> [The government clinic] staff is rude. When I say, 'Doctor, I am [HIV-positive],' they start thinking negatively and act uncomfortable towards me. When asked for bathing assistance, they got mad and asked me to clean myself … When my CD4 dropped, I was admitted to the ward for 5 days, 4 nights. They asked me to cut my hair … I had long hair but I accepted it. [6]

> When I'm sick, I go to my friends. My biggest worry is that I am infected with any virus. I'm very, very worried about that. I go to my friends and ask them first. Then, I go to the clinic. I will go to government clinic as a boy. Every time I go to the clinic, I camouflage myself as a normal male. [They don't say anything] because I came as a male. [19]

To avoid discrimination, participants often withheld their sexual history from healthcare providers. For some, however, this meant that they were unable to be tested for HIV and STIs because they were not willing to share high-risk behaviours.

> Oh. I do not tell [that I do sex work]. I hide everything. [The doctor] has asked, 'Do you have anal sex?' I said no because I'm afraid of disclosing my 'taboo' behaviours. [I don't know] if they can accept it or not. [19]

> I wanted to [get tested for HIV]. I have wanted to do it but I went to a government clinic and asked for it. The staff asked whether I am at risk for HIV and [if I told them], only then they would do a test. [15]

Participants were asked about their mental health and while several responded that they often felt sad and depressed, they preferred keeping their feelings to themselves or turned to religion, friends, or substance use.

> [When I'm depressed], I pray to God. I cry. He listens to me. He loves me. That is the only person I believe. He is the only person who can listen to me and he is the only one who can understand me. [18]

> After I separated with my husband, the first thing I wanted to do is commit suicide. I climbed to the 9th floor and stood. I wanted to jump but my friend grabbed me. When I was at home, I tried to play with knives … [My friend] took leave from work for a week to take care of me and it took me about 3 months to stop crying. [19]

Risk reduction behaviours

As *mak nyah* sex workers are at increased risk for HIV and STIs, it is important that they utilise evidence-based prevention strategies. Condom use is the most commonly used risk reduction strategy for sex workers, but not fully effective without proper lubricants or if expired. To avoid healthcare systems, participants chose alternative and ineffective methods for preventing and treating HIV/STIs, such as self-medication with antibiotics, inspecting clients, and washing with antibacterial soap.

Testing for HIV/STIs was neither regular nor typical, partly due to healthcare-related stigma and discrimination, but additional fears emerged about learning they are HIV-positive and how they would be treated.

> I have not tested. I'm afraid. HIV is not something like cancer or ... if you ask me, I'm more worried about myself. HIV is not something that you easily get support from doctors, family or someone else. If you know you have HIV, your life will change immediately. This is not something easy and it's very serious. Definitely, it will change your life. [14]

Despite reporting high-risk behaviours, they feared being HIV-positive but perceived themselves at low risk for HIV.

> I feel I haven't had the chance [to test for HIV] and I'm scared. I know its important [but] I'm scared of the result. But my heart says strongly that I'm still clean. [2]

Risk perception appeared to be mitigated by viewing condoms as fully protective against HIV/STIs. Multiple contradictions about condom use occurred, including use with paying but not regular customers and negotiated non-use situations. However, some participants were insistent on using condoms with all customers.

> Yes, [customers] offer to pay more, RM50 (USD$14) or RM20 (USD$6). I won't do that. I advise them that in one day, ten customers have sex with me. So, if a customer has HIV, that means you will get it. It will spoil your life. [20]

> Of course I use condoms. All the time. Of course [customers request no condom], but normally I discuss this at the beginning and if the customer says he doesn't want to wear condom, its ok. I don't want your money. [2]

Despite knowing that water-based lubricants with condoms were important, a few used a variety of lubricants that are incompatible with condoms.

> When I was teenager, I used saliva, lotions, and K-Y [for lubricant]. The funniest thing I have used is mayonnaise. My K-Y finished, I saw mayonnaise so I took it for an instant fix ... it's better than lotion because lotion has alcohol, right? [But] K-Y is better than mayonnaise. [15]

Paradoxically, when probed, many participants did not use condoms with some customers, and instead inspected their customers and/or self-medicated with antibiotics.

> I am doing sex work, and it impossible to use condoms for everyone, right? It depends, if he is good-looking and handsome, I will not use [condoms]. [16]

> Honestly, no, sometimes I am not using [condoms]. I do my personal check to the person I am not using condoms with to see whether he has gonorrhoea or not. I pull from the [penis] base to tip. If he doesn't have anything, I will begin sex. [15]

> When I have sex with someone that I like without condoms, I will shower and clean myself. After that, I will take the antibiotic. I am also worried, so we need to prevent [infections]. [17]

With non-paying partners, condom use was much lower regardless of whether it was with a regular partner or a casual partner. In long-term relationships, no participant reported consistently using condoms.

> [For customers], I use condoms. I only won't use condoms for my husband. Sometimes, I use condoms with my husband also. He works in Singapore and I don't know what happens there. If I feel something happened, then I use a condom with my husband. When we are drunk, sure, no condoms for my husband. [13]

Discussion

Findings from this qualitative assessment provide important insights into how gender shapes not only past and current experiences within society, but also within healthcare establishments, especially surrounding gender-affirming treatments and HIV/STI prevention. Findings here build on a previously published legal framework for *mak nyah* in the Malaysian context and how it impacts sex work, other criminal behaviour, and societal engagement. Figure 1 represents how the trajectory of a *mak nyah*'s identity influences their health risks and HIV risk behaviours in an environment with high levels of stigma and discrimination. While recognition of gender incongruence happens internally, it is typically with integration into the *mak nyah* community that individuals begin their gender transition. Sex work is generally introduced by key members of the *mak nyah* community but also is uniquely tied to gender transition. Transitioning often leads to workplace discrimination and a lack of other employment options, but sex work is also commonly used to finance gender-affirming procedures. *Mak nyah* who engage in sex work are thus subjected to increased levels of stigma and discrimination based not only on their gender identity and community affiliation, but also heightened by their engagement in illegal sex work. The synergy of these factors requires focused and concerted efforts to holistically create a supportive environment to meet the unique prevention and healthcare treatment needs of the *mak nyah* community.

Gender identity among *mak nyah* is similar to existing literature on TGW globally, especially in the shared experience of recognising the incongruence of their gender and biological sex early in childhood, and also in how they are treated. In Malaysia, however, the transition process happens later and importantly, with the support and guidance of the *mak nyah* community through trusted insights, friendship, and a strong community network. These same *mak nyah* also provided guidance about survival and initiated them into sex work.

The *mak nyah* community creates a de facto ethnic enclave that is not geographically restricted, demonstrating strong social cohesion. However, this is not always positive (Caughy, O'Campo, & Muntaner, 2003). While the community is supportive, it also promotes competition between *mak nyah sex workers* through guidance that accelerated and exaggerated the transitional process by endorsing self-regulation and overuse of HRT and medical tourism to Thailand for HRT and surgical gender-affirming activities (breast implants, etc.), all of which resulted in lack of supervision by licensed doctors locally.

Healthcare utilisation for *mak nyah sex workers* was rarely normative, despite multiple health risks that could be effectively addressed by holistic and comprehensive services. Healthcare use generally fell into three categories: (1) private and expensive 'for-profit' care, from a transgender-sensitive doctor in some cases; (2) acute and erratic care from free governmental settings; or (3) care from free governmental clinics, but disguised physically as male. Neither HRT, other gender-affirming care, nor HIV/STI prevention or treatment was accessed at free clinics. Those seeking gender-affirming care at transgender-friendly clinics often still avoided HIV/STI prevention and treatment. Fear and stigma of positive test results often further restricted participants from seeking screening procedures. Though 14 of 21 participants had ever received HIV testing and 10 had ever received STI screening, only 8 were regularly screened for either HIV and/or STIs. Several

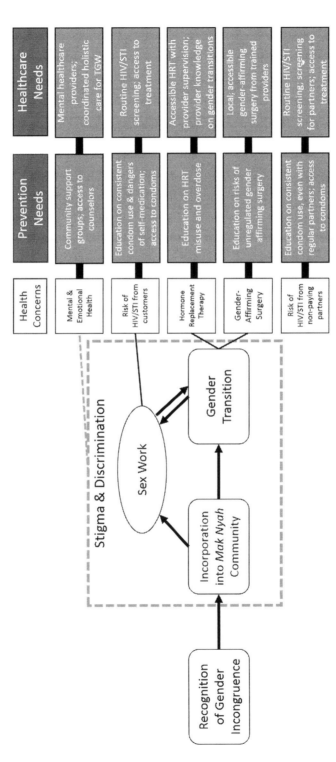

Figure 1. Model for understanding and holistically addressing health concerns relevant to *mak nyah*.

participants reported commonly feeling sadness or depression, but mental health was never discussed or addressed in clinical or professional settings.

Not surprisingly, despite high HIV and STI prevalence among *mak nyah* sex workers, low perceived risk may have contributed to low screening levels, potentially due to denial given the contradictory statements about condom use. Moreover, most associated HIV with symptoms that they did not have, thereby assuming they were not infected and did not need to test routinely. Self-medication with antibiotics as a means to avoid HIV and not undergo testing is also concerning. Despite all participants recognising the importance of condom use, only 15 of 21 participants reported consistently using condoms with customers and none of them consistently used condoms with non-paying, intimate partners.

Until funding ended in 2012, a sexual minority clinic (Safe Clinic) that provided tailored services for *mak nyah* and MSM was available. Since then, culturally sensitive HIV prevention and treatment for *mak nyah*, aligned with HRT, are no longer routinely available in a single setting. Moreover, the Malaysian government does not provide funding for targeted HIV prevention or clinical care services for *mak nyah*. Such integrated services are likely to have the highest yield for retaining *mak nyah* in care, especially in Malaysia where gender identity for *mak nyah* is criminalised and where stigma and discrimination prevail. Routine and regular HIV/STI testing and other prevention services linked to gender-affirming care are urgently needed.

Additionally, *mak nyah* face legal barriers that prevent the recognition of their gender identity and instead criminalise it. This contributes to the widespread stigmatisation and marginalisation of *mak nyah* and prevents them from accessing adequate health and social services. It also perpetuates harmful practices, such as self-medication with antibiotics and the overuse of HRT, which can have detrimental health effects when not provided in a treatment setting.

Ultimately, evidence-based HIV treatment and prevention would greatly benefit from removing the existing structural barriers that perpetuate stigma and discrimination for *mak nyah* and specifically, *mak nyah* sex workers. Decriminalisation of gender expression and ability to change sex markers on national registration cards are crucial first steps. Given the community cohesiveness, social-network-based prevention and healthcare engagement strategies should be considered and if efficacious, expanded more broadly. Culturally sensitive education and supportive services are also necessary and should include providers in healthcare settings. It has been proposed that such cultural training should start during medical and nursing training (Earnshaw et al., 2014; Jin et al., 2014) and extend to current clinical providers.

Limitations

While a sample of 21 participants was sufficient for qualitative research (Mason, 2010), this data is descriptive and cannot be extrapolated to the entire TGW sex worker population nor the TGW population as a whole. Though a substantial proportion of *mak nyah* reside in Kuala Lumpur, these findings may not be representative of the experience of all *mak nyah* who may not have access to clinical services, HIV prevention and/or related education. Moreover, Kuala Lumpur is an urban and more secular area of Malaysia and *mak nyah* may be more repressed, stigmatised and discriminated against elsewhere, resulting in less engagement in services and HIV prevention strategies. Lastly, our sample consists of predominately Malay and Indian *mak nyah* and thus, these results may not be characteristic of other ethnic communities in Malaysia, such as the Chinese.

Conclusion

This qualitative assessment adds to the limited information on identity and healthcare utilisation of *mak nyah* sex workers in Malaysia, who are even further marginalised in society, but remain at higher risk for HIV/STIs than *mak nyah* who do not engage in sex work. Importantly here, the healthcare and prevention system is poorly equipped to provide targeted HIV prevention and treatment, which would be optimised if aligned with gender-affirming treatments, such as HRT and other gender-affirming procedures. Ultimately, decriminalisation of both gender identity constraints and homosexuality will contribute to improved HIV prevention and treatment strategies, especially when provided in a culturally sensitive and supportive environment.

Note

1. The terms for transgender women used in the quotations below reflect the exact term used by the participants and include trangender, mak nyah, ladyboy, and she-males.

Acknowledgements

We thank our community partners at the Pink Triangle (PT) Foundation, Pertubuhan Wanita dan Kesihatan Kuala Lumpur (WAKE), and Pertubuhan Advokasi Masyarakat Terpinggir (PAMT) for their assistance in this project.

Disclosure statement

No potential conflict of interest was reported by the authors.

Funding

This research was supported by the University of Malaysia's High Impact Research Grant [E000001–20001] and the National Institute on Drug Abuse [R01 DA025943 and K24 DA017072].

ORCID

Britton A. Gibson http://orcid.org/0000-0003-0058-4272

References

ATLAS.ti (7.1.8) [computer software]. (2014). Berlin: Scientific Software Development GmbH
Attorney General's Chamber of Malaysia. (2006). Laws of Malaysia: Act 574, Penal Code, 377a, The Commissoner of Law Revision, Malaysia, p. 148. Retrieved from http://www.agc.gov.my.
Baral, S. D., Poteat, T., Stromdahl, S., Wirtz, A. L., Guadamuz, T. E., & Beyrer, C. (2013). Worldwide burden of HIV in transgender women: A systematic review and meta-analysis. *The Lancet Infectious Diseases*, *13*(3), 214–222. doi:10.1016/S1473-3099(12)70315-8

Bauer, G. R., Hammond, R., Travers, R., Kaay, M., Hohenadel, K. M., & Boyce, M. (2009). "I don't think this is theoretical; this is our lives": How erasure impacts health care for transgender people. *Journal of the Association of Nurses in AIDS Care*, 20(5), 348–361. doi:10.1016/j.jana.2009.07.004

Beemyn, G. (n.d.). Transgender Terminology. Retrieved from http://www.umass.edu/stonewall/uploads/listWidget/8758/trans%20terms.pdf

Brislin, R. W. (1970). Back-translation for cross-cultural research. *Journal of Cross-Cultural Psychology*, 1, 185–216. doi:10.1177/135910457000100301

Caughy, M. O., O'Campo, P. J., & Muntaner, C. (2003). When being alone might be better: Neighborhood poverty, social capital, and child mental health. *Social Science and Medicine*, 57(2), 227–237. doi:10.1016/S0277-9536(02)00342-8

Clements-Nolle, K., Marx, R., & Katz, M. (2006). Attempted suicide among transgender persons: The influence of gender-based discrimination and victimization. *Journal of Homosexuality*, 51(3), 53–69. doi:10.1300/J082v51n03_04

Daryani, P. (2011). Differentiating the vulnerability of Kothis and Hijras to HIV/AIDS: A case study of Lucknow, Uttar Pradesh. *Independent Study Project (ISP) Collection*. Paper 1144. Retrieved from http://digitalcollections.sit.edu/isp_collection/1144

Department of Statistics Malaysia. (2011). Population distribution and basic demographic characteristics, 2010. *Population and Housing Census of Malaysia*. Retrieved from http://www.statistics.gov.my

Earnshaw, V. A., Jin, H., Wickersham, J., Kamarulzaman, A., John, J., & Altice, F. L. (2014). Exploring intentions to discriminate against patients living with HIV/AIDS among future healthcare providers in Malaysia. *Tropical Medicine and International Health*, 19(6), 672–679. doi:10.1111/tmi.12306

Ghoshal, N. (2014). I'm scared to be a woman: Human rights abuses against transgender people in Malaysia. *Human Rights Watch*. Retrieved from https://www.hrw.org/report/2014/09/24/im-scared-be-woman/human-rights-abuses-against-transgender-people-malaysia

Jin, H., Earnshaw, V. A., Wickersham, J. A., Kamarulzaman, A., Desai, M. M., John, J., & Altice, F. L. (2014). An assessment of health-care students' attitudes toward patients with or at high risk for HIV: Implications for education and cultural competency. *AIDS Care*, 26(10), 1223–1228. doi:10.1080/09540121.2014.894616

LeBreton, M. (2013). The Erasure of Sex and Gender Minorities in the Healthcare System. *Bioethique Online*, 2(17). Retrieved from: http://hdl.handle.net/1866/9811

Lim, H. E., Ang, C. L., & Teh, Y. K. (2010). *Size estimation for local responses in Malaysia for HIV prevention in sex work*. Unpublished manuscript.

Logie, C. H., James, L., Tharao, W., & Loutfy, M. R. (2012). "We don't exist": A qualitative study of marginalization experienced by HIV-positive lesbian, bisexual, queer and transgender women in Toronto, Canada. *Journal of the International AIDS Society*, 15(2), 17392. doi:10.7448/IAS.15.2.17392

Lombardi, E. (2010). Transgender health: A review and guidance for future research-proceedings from the summer institute at the center for research on health and sexual orientation, University of Pittsburgh. *International Journal of Transgenderism*, 12(4), 211–229. doi:10.1080/15532739.2010.544232

Mason, M. (2010). Sample size and saturation in PhD studies using qualitative interviews [63 paragraphs]. *Forum Qualitative Sozialforschung / Forum: Qualitative Social Research*, 11(3), Art. 8. Retrieved from http://nbn-resolving.de/urn:nbn:de:0114-fqs100387

Ministry of Health Malaysia. (2013). *IBBS 2012 Preliminary Results*. [PowerPoint Presentation] Unpublished manuscript.

Nemoto, T., Luke, D., Mamo, L., Ching, A., & Patria, J. (1999). HIV risk behaviours among male-to-female transgenders in comparison with homosexual or bisexual males and heterosexual females. *AIDS Care*, 11(3), 297–312. doi:10.1080/09540129947938

Reisner, S. L., Mimiaga, M. J., Bland, S., Mayer, K. H., Perkovich, B., & Safren, S. A. (2009). HIV risk and social networks among male-to-female transgender sex workers in Boston, Massachusetts. *Journal of the Association of Nurses in AIDS Care*, 20(5), 373–386. doi:10.1016/j.jana.2009.06.003

Slamah, K. (2005). The struggle to be ourselves, neither men nor women: Mak Nyahs in Malaysia. This is a chapter. In G. M. A. R. Chandiramani (Ed.), *Sexuality, gender, and rights: Exploring theory and practice in South and South East Asia* (pp. 99). New Delhi: Sage.

Sumartojo, E. (2000). Structural factors in HIV prevention: Concepts, examples, and implications for research. *AIDS, 14*(Suppl 1), S3–S10. doi:10.1097/00002030-200006001-00002

Suresh, S. (n.d.). *The importance of sex reassignment surgery and other medical treatments for transgender people in Malaysia.* Retrieved from http://isean.asia/elibrary/the-importance-of-sex-reassignment-surgery-and-other-medical-treatments-for-transgender-people-in-malaysia-2/

Teh, Y. K. (2008a). HIV-related needs for safety among male-to-female transsexuals (mak nyah) in Malaysia. *SAHARA-J: Journal of Social Aspects of HIV/AIDS, 5*(4), 178–185. doi:10.1080/17290376.2008.9724917

Teh, Y. K. (2008b). Politics and Islam: Factors determining identity and the status of male-to-female transsexuals in Malaysia. This is a chapter. In P. A. J. Fran Martin, M. McLelland, & A. Yue (Eds.), *AsiaPacifiQueer: Rethinking genders and sexuality* (pp. 85–97). Champaign, IL: University of Illinois Press.

UNAIDS. (1998*). Expanding the global response to HIV/AIDS through focused action: Reducing risk and vulnerability: Definitions, rationale, and pathways.* Retrieved from http://data.unaids.org/Publications/IRC-pub01/jc171-expglobresp_en.pdf

UNAIDS. (2014). *Guidance note: Services for transgender people.* Retrieved from http://www.unaids.org/sites/default/files/media_asset/2014unaidsguidancenote_servicesfortransgenderpeople_en.pdf

Valdes, F. (1996). Unpacking Hetero-Patriarchy: Tracing the conflation of sex, gender, and sexual orientation to its origins. *Yale Journal of Law and the Humanities, 8*(1), Article 7. Retrieved from www.lexisnexis.com/hottopics/lnacademic

The limitations of 'Black MSM' as a category: Why gender, sexuality, and desire still matter for social and biomedical HIV prevention methods

Jonathan Garcia, Richard G. Parker, Caroline Parker, Patrick A. Wilson, Morgan Philbin and Jennifer S. Hirsch

ABSTRACT

The USA faces disproportionate and increasing HIV incidence rates among Black men who have sex with men (BMSM). New biomedical technologies such as pre-exposure prophylaxis (PrEP) have been developed to address their HIV risk. Very little consideration, however, has been given to the diversity obscured by 'BMSM' as a category, to how this diversity relates to men's sexual partnering strategies, or to the relevance of these issues for new HIV prevention methods. We conducted a community-based ethnography from June 2013 to May 2014 documenting factors that affect the acceptance of and adherence to PrEP among BMSM. We conducted in-depth interviews with 31 BMSM and 17 community stakeholders, and participant observation. To demonstrate the diversity of social identities, we present a taxonomy of indigenous categories organised along the axes of sexual identity, sexual positioning, and gender performance. We analyse how HIV prevention strategies, such as PrEP, may be more effective if programmes consider how gender, sexuality, and sexual desire shape sexual partnering strategies. This article underlines the importance of attending to the diversity of sexual and social subjectivities among BMSM, of bringing the study of sexuality back into HIV prevention, and of integrating biomedical prevention approaches into community-based programmes.

Introduction

In the context of rising HIV incidence rates among non-heterosexual and racial-ethnic minorities in the USA, HIV research and intervention efforts frequently employ the epidemiological category Black men who have sex with men (BMSM), without giving due consideration to how this category obscures diversity. This article highlights the importance for rolling out new HIV prevention methods of addressing (1) diversity in gender, sexuality, and desire among BMSM and (2) power inequalities that operate within sexual networks in this category. We begin by describing the historical creation of the category of BMSM and by discussing its key limitations. We then draw on our community-based ethnographic research to present a taxonomy of indigenous cultural ('emic') categories organised along the axes of sexual identity, preferred sexual position, and gender performance. The emphasis on social processes that contextualise sexual partnerships provides important insights for understanding the HIV epidemic in many places throughout the world where sexuality and gender performance shape HIV vulnerability at the same time that they are fluid and negotiable.

In the USA as in many parts of the world, HIV prevention began through safer sex education efforts that were both initiated and disseminated at the grassroots level (Parker, 1996; Patton, 1996; Watney, 1990); early prevention efforts were heavily grounded in local expertise about community organisation and sexual cultures (Parker, 1996; Patton, 1996; Watney, 1990). In the 1980s, amid concern that non-heterosexual men who did not identify with the gay community were not engaging with prevention efforts, grassroots community groups turned their attention to homosexually active *other* men who have sex with men (Aggleton & Parker, 2015; Patton, 1996). In the 1990s, epidemiologists appropriated the category 'MSM'. Although the category was originally created to refer to *non*-gay identified men, its public health appropriation transformed MSM into a catch-all category, lumping together all MSM, independent of social identities or sociocultural and community ties (Boellstorff, 2011; Kippax, Stephenson, Parker, & Aggleton, 2013; Young & Meyer, 2005). The remaking of this category into 'MSM' erased the initial concern with social identities and obscured the social organisation of sexuality (Altman et al., 2012).

The ways public health research and practice have attempted to include MSM who do not identify as gay or bisexual into this category have sometimes failed to address the range of variation in how stigma and discrimination affect those aggregated within it (Altman et al., 2012; Young & Meyer, 2005). Furthermore, the category itself became a source of stigma (Malebranche, Arriola, Jenkins, Dauria, & Patel, 2010), as both popular culture and research literature hold 'hard-to-reach' MSM responsible for HIV transmission to heterosexual populations. Researchers have argued that the stigma generated by the discussion about men on the 'down low' (Ford, Whetten, Hall, Kaufman, & Thrasher, 2007; Malebranche, 2008; Saleh & Operario, 2009) may make the men to whom it refers even more vulnerable to HIV, by rendering them less willing to participate in research and interventions.

As the epidemic in the USA shifted towards socioeconomically disenfranchised racial-ethnic minority men, researchers and policy-makers generated further subcategories, such as BMSM, that aimed to capture health disparities associated with race and ethnicity. However, this continued to erase potentially important differences between diverse kinds of BMSM (gay identified or not, behaviourally bisexual, gender variant, etc.). There are, to be sure, vital reasons to focus on the undeniable epidemiological trends towards increased and disproportionate infection among non-heterosexual and racial-ethnic minorities. While BMSM represented only 2% of the US population from 2008 to 2010, they accounted for nearly 75% of new HIV infections (CDC, 2012). A recent study of BMSM in six US cities reported an HIV prevalence of 21% (Koblin, 2012). Our fieldsite, New York City has one of the highest HIV infection rates in the USA. In 2011, 66.1% of all new HIV diagnoses in NYC were among Black men, of whom 56.2% were MSM (NYCDOHMH, 2012). Compared to other racial-ethnic groups, HIV-infected BMSM are less likely to know their HIV status (Centers for Disease Control and Prevention, 2005; MacKellar et al., 2005; Millett, Peterson, Wolitski, & Stall, 2006).

A significant body of literature underlines contextual factors (i.e. structural, social, and cultural) as key drivers of the epidemic (Maulsby et al., 2014; Millett et al., 2012). However, most medical and public health responses to increasing incidence and barriers to linkage to care have de-emphasised the sociocultural and economic drivers of HIV vulnerability, and instead focused on more proximal biomedical prevention approaches (Aggleton & Parker, 2015). In addition to structural, social, and cultural issues, some researchers have argued that the response to HIV itself, through its erasure of meaningful social differences – for example, men's notions of 'selfhood', community affiliation, and experiences of stigma – has perhaps itself contributed to the rising rates of HIV among BMSM (Altman et al., 2012; Arnold, Rebchook, & Kegeles, 2014; Boellstorff, 2011; Garcia et al., 2015a).

Stigma is a critical element of this broader social context that shapes the disproportionate rates of HIV infection within the epidemiological category of BMSM. Stigma heightens HIV vulnerability by creating relationships of unequal power among BMSM (Jones, Wilton, Millett, & Johnson, 2010; Parker & Aggleton, 2003; Wilton, 2009), challenging engagement with healthcare (Eaton et al., 2015) and contributing to sexual risk behaviours (Radcliffe et al., 2010). The consequences of stigma for the health of Black MSM are particularly severe because Black MSM experience multiple forms of stigma along the intersecting social axes of marginalisation, including sexuality, race, gender, and class (Bowleg, 2013; Earnshaw, Bogart, Dovidio, & Williams, 2013) and HIV status (Arnold et al., 2014; Radcliffe et al., 2010). Although ethnographic research has begun to reveal considerable sexual diversity (Miller, Serner, & Wagner, 2005) as well as gendered diversity (Fields et al., 2014) among BMSM, there remains an urgent need for empirical research documenting how this heterogeneity in social subjectivities may affect the acceptance and uptake of emerging HIV prevention methods.

This article (1) identifies meaningful subcategories that we found within the BMSM category to note the diversity in 'local' or 'emic' organisation of social and sexual experience; (2) problematises local categorisations, noting the fluidity that exists in navigating sexual relationships and gender expectations; and (3) describes how recognising diversity and fluidity can potentially shape and inform the use of the expanding HIV prevention tool kit, especially with the introduction of pre-exposure prophylaxis (PrEP) and other emerging prevention technologies.

Methods

A community-based ethnography conducted in New York City from June 2013 to May 2014 examined how these intersectional identities and strategies may affect engagement with various methods of HIV prevention, including PrEP. The goal of the study was to describe and analyse the connections between the sociocultural and economic context of BMSM's lives, including but not limited to their vulnerability to HIV, and their desire for, acceptance of, and adherence to PrEP.

Selection of participants

We recruited 31 BMSM for in-depth interviews through recruitment cards that provided brief information about the project and a phone number. The cards described the study as focused on the life stories of Black men ages 15 and older, and had the name of the ethnographic component of the study: 'Your Life, Your Words', but did not mention sexual identity/behaviour or HIV. Cards were available at health centres, community-based organisations, bars, and online. Eligibility criteria included (1) being born as and identifying as biologically male, (2) identifying as Black or African American, (3) having had anal or oral sex with a man in the past 12 months, and (4) being 15 years or older. The average age in our sample was 29.0 years (SD, 12.3), with 17 men between ages 15 and 24 and 16 men ages 25–54. The majority self-reported as HIV negative ($N = 23$), while a few did not know their status ($N = 3$) or were HIV positive ($N = 5$). We used participant observation and the assistance of our Community Advisory Board to identify community stakeholders who were involved in service provision for BMSM in New York City. Twenty-one potential key informants were contacted by phone/e-mail and invited to participate. Four did not respond to those messages; the 17 who responded agreed to participate. In accordance with the protocol approved by the Columbia University Medical Center Institutional Review Board, the study was granted a waiver of parental consent to protect the sexual identity of men under 18. All participants were read a verbal informed consent form. Because participants were asked sensitive questions that could potentially reveal information about sex work and drug use, verbal consent provided a higher level of confidentiality than written consent. Participants were made aware that a Certificate of Confidentiality granted by the National Institute of Mental Health protected data collected. Their understanding was assessed with a series of follow-up questions about the content of the consent form. This assessment of understanding was audio-recorded and data collection began following participants' recorded declaration of verbal consent.

Procedures

Interview guides for community stakeholder and in-depth interviews were developed by the research team and then discussed with and validated by our Community Advisory Board. In-depth interview guides were divided into three sessions as described in Table 1.

In-depth interviews (3 sessions, each roughly 90 minutes) and community stakeholder interviews (1 session, 60 minutes) were conducted face-to-face. Participant observation took place twice per week over the course of 11 months in spaces recommended by our Community Advisory Board or that emerged in interviews. Participant observation consisted of 'community observation' and 'short-term observation' with in-depth interviewees. In community observation, we participated in weekly community events and public forums (e.g. weekly happy hour at Black LGBT groups and mobilisation discussions at community-based organisations). In 'short-term observation', the lead ethnographer accompanied five in-depth interviewees to places where the in-depth interviewees agreed to invite the ethnographer (e.g. private house parties, gay family dinners, police precincts, public cruising in parks among other situations). Participant observation was recorded in jottings, fieldnotes, maps, and analytic memos. The lead ethnographer's (first author) own subjectivities and sensibilities as a gay Latino man may have facilitated 'hanging out' with other men who were also racial-ethnic and sexual minorities.

Data analysis

Interviews were digitally recorded, transcribed verbatim and entered into Atlas.ti 7.0, the qualitative analysis software used for coding and organising qualitative and visual data.

Table 1. Methods.

Data collection method	Specific data elicited	Sample description
Participant observation	Organizational behaviour, group composition, ways people discuss sexuality, race, gender, age, class; /interaction, spoken rules of conduct and implicit cultural norms expressed, enforced, followed and navigated	11 months of observation in: private spaces (homes, parties); public spaces (parks, streets, events); virtual spaces (chat rooms, blogs, social media); and institutions (community organisations, health centres, religious institutions)
Key informant interviews	Organisational mission; role in organisation/group/community; knowledge and attitudes about black MSM, HIV vulnerability, institutions and networks available to Black MSM; views on PrEP and other for HIV/STI prevention	17 informants, including 2 physicians; 3 mental health providers; 4 community organisation programme administrators; 5 outreach workers; 3 community mobilisers
In-depth interviews	*Session 1*: History of family relations, coming of age, education, housing, making money, friends; community, recreation *Session 2*: Sexual history, including desire, casual and steady relations, sexual identity and racial identity *Session 3*: Perceptions of health and risk; practices and attitudes about medications and seeking health services; knowledge and attitudes about HIV prevention	31 participants

Data were analysed using an approach that drew on a range of ethnographic and qualitative research strategies, including aspects of extended case method (Burawoy, 1998) in relation to the interrogation and extension of existing theoretical frameworks in relation to HIV among MSM, as well as aspects of grounded theory (Corbin & Strauss, 2008), which helped to problematise the ways in which existing research has theorised the question of MSM. In particular, we sought to extend this methodological point of departure by emphasising aspects of an interpretive approach to cultural and linguistic meanings (Geertz, 1973), and to highlight the analysis of sexual categories and classifications (Parker, Herdt, & Carballo, 1991) that were found to operate social interaction and sexual practice on the part of the BMSM community where our research was carried out. This emphasis on the cultural and linguistic categories that organise the lived experience of sexuality on the part of different communities has long been used in HIV research, especially in cross-cultural studies of sexual practices in different social contexts, but has less frequently been employed in the investigation of key populations and communities in the USA. This hybrid approach allowed for theory modification, based on narrative and observation data, which problematised the way that existing work has theorised the category of MSM and drew on new insights from empirical data (men's sexual and gender presentation and lived experience). The use of multiple methods allowed for data triangulation during the analysis; this involved comparing the perspectives of community stakeholders with BMSM, as well as with observed behaviour. We presented data analysis reports to the clients and providers in CABs to validate salient themes and perform member checking. These analyses employed a codebook that was developed based on domains (code families) derived from the interview guides and through open coding. Here we draw on several code families, including 'identity', 'community', 'stigma', 'masculinity', and 'sex position'. Two members of the research team (first and third authors) coded the data set after arriving at an adequate level of inter-coder agreement (over 80%).

Results

Multiple dimensions of identity: sexual identity, sexual position, and gender performance

Drawing on social interactions revealed through participant observation and described in narrative data, we came upon three interrelated axes that were central to men's understanding of who they were, as well as their partnering strategies (i.e. ways in which men seek sexual encounters while negotiating between erotic ideals and social presentation): sexual identity, preferred sexual position, and gender performance. Table 2 describes the local categories that constituted these three axes.

As shown in Table 2, men in our sample identified their sexuality as gay ($N = 15$), straight ($N = 3$), bisexual ($N = 4$), discreet ($N = 4$), same-gender-loving ($N = 3$), or preferred no sexual identity ($N = 2$). Although approximately half of the sample identified as gay, the meaning of this identity varied. Some men felt more comfortable than others in feeling 'part of' the gay community. In fact, several gay men were consciously resistant of the gay community because they felt discriminated because they were Black. A few men identified as same-gender-loving, an identity that politicised the inherent need for more attention to racial inequalities within the gay community. In addition, nearly half of the sample identified as straight, discreet, bisexual, or preferred no sexual identity. Most straight and bisexual men reported currently having long-term (more than one year in a relationship) girlfriends, while they had sex with men in casual relationships. Men who chose to identify as discreet focused on 'not being out of the closet', as the main characteristic of their sexuality. Similar to a preference of no sexual identity, this sexual description allowed for men seeking sex with men to be 'up front' about not wanting to be sexually labelled as gay.

Even though sexual identity labels began to tell a story about men's social self-representation, Table 2 also shows how men preferred to label themselves when negotiating sexual intercourse. Some had very strict notions of what sexual position they preferred (e.g. total tops, total bottoms, and power bottoms), while others were willing to be both insertive and receptive in anal sex to varying extents (e.g. vers-tops, vers-bottoms, and vers). In many ways, men's preferred sexual roles set the boundaries for their expected gender performance: men seeking partners who were solely receptive in anal sex often presented themselves as more masculine, and vice versa. In short, other aspects of their sexual and erotic preferences – what might perhaps better be described as their gendered sexual 'subjectivity' – appeared to be far more important than identity in terms of shaping specific sexual practices (Dowsett, 1996; Lorway, Reza-Paul, & Pasha, 2009; Weeks, 1998)

For this reason, the third axis of the taxonomy in Table 2 depicts how men qualify their gender performance or expression using a range of labels. Men who were perceived as hyper-masculine were described as 'trade' (Bowleg, 2013; Ford et al., 2007). Approximately a third of the sample was versatile during anal sex and gay identified, many of whom identified as 'butch queens' to denote self-acceptance of the feminine and masculine aspects of their social presentation. In addition, there were those who were proud of their femininity, enjoyed being bottoms (sometimes finding power in being anally receptive). Among these men there was a meaningful play on normative notions of gender and sexuality.

Many of them identified as 'the cunts'. They used intentionally vulgar or transgressive language to represent their 'sassy' and 'stylish' feminine gender performance and to

Table 2. Taxonomy of sexual identities, sexual roles, and gender performance.

Term/phrase	Meaning	Representative narrative	HIV prevention practice
2.1 Sexual identity			
Gay (N = 15)	Most believed the gay 'label' has a racially White connotation, leading many times to feeling doubly excluded from gay and black communities	'Gay is a lifestyle. It definitely is. It's a way of life. A lot of people don't understand the terms and things of that nature'. (24-year-old)	More than half of these men had condomless sex, although they expressed remorse about it. Many practised sex work, were homeless, and many had links to CBOs. A few of them (N = 5) had private health insurance and saw staying healthy as a life project
Same-gender-loving (SGL) (N = 3)	A few used the counter-hegemonic term to undercut feelings of exclusion through solidarity based on sexuality and race	'Same-gender-loving, me being an African American man, means that I am in fact that of a man who just happens to love the same sex'. (39-year-old) 'We kind of use the term 'same-gender-loving,' which kind of burst out of the black gay community ... We'd have these conversations, anything from politics or what's happening specifically in the black gay or black homosexual community'. (31-year-old)	All three were very critical of HIV campaigns that equated African American with 'at-risk' for HIV; some knew about PrEP, and thought it was a good idea. They saw racial mistrust of medication and medical institutions as a major barrier to PrEP uptake
Bisexual (N = 4)	A few self-identified as bisexual, although for the most part they did not disclose homosexual desire or behaviour with friends, family, and other social networks	'But there is no denial I have sex with men, but it's just the culture is the part that I can't reconcile myself with and so when approaching people and dating and seeing a cavalier approach around sex and health and wellbeing, initially it was hard to understand and I didn't understand'. (32-year-old)	Some of these men used condoms with men and women; two men were open to male and female partners about their sexuality to establish honest relationships
Straight (N = 3)	Men who had steady relationships with women as primary partners identified socially as straight	'So some of the guys who might consider themselves straight, once they get high, they'll get fucked too or suck some dick. It's all good. I don't judge nobody'. (45-year-old)	For the most part did not use condoms; expressed using condoms with men but not with women. All of these men used drugs to overcome dissonance between sexuality and identity. Participant observation in public cruising spots (e.g. parks) indicated heavy drug and alcohol and sex among men engaged in secretive sexual encounters.
Discreet (N = 4)	Those who identified as discreet could be strictly homosexual or bisexual in behaviour; Discreet identity and discretion independent of identity were associated with feelings of shame and social risk	'And I kept it discreet, if I went to the studio I had on a hoodie just trying to blend in ... which was still uncomfortable because they could still see – because I used to get my eyebrows arched'. (26-year-old) 'I let him walk in front of me, you know, because where I used to work at, sometimes it'd be the trucks would be delivering stuff, and I don't want them to think I'm with him, you know? Yeah, he dressed differently. He don't wear high heeled shoes or anything, but he likes buying feminine clothes'. (47-year-old)	These men had more sexual partners than others, met men online more often, had sex with and without condoms, and two were superstitious or afraid of HIV/STI testing; key informants mentioned that discretion was a challenge for enrolling men in prevention programmes

(Continued)

Table 2. Continued.

Term/phrase	Meaning	Representative narrative	HIV prevention practice
Other (N = 2)	A couple of men had either no sexual identity or preferred to be called MSM. Both were used to reject gay stereotypes	'I normally don't like to refer to myself as gay … I think me just being a black male, I like to identify with being a black male. Gay always referred to being white, you know what I mean? When you're a black man I think for me it's so important to identify with that first, right?' (45-year-old)	They displayed greater concerns for the harmful effects of political sexual identities; and HIV prevention was important to both stemming from life experiences and formal education

2.2 Preferred sexual position

Term/phrase	Meaning	Representative narrative	HIV prevention practice
Bottom (N = 10)	Receptive in anal sex, also refers to enjoying giving oral sex. Some bottoms reframed this sexual position as a source of power (see power bottoms and 'the cunts'). Some bottom men complained that men on hook-up smart phone apps were too often bottoms, although several discreet tops preferred this venue	'When I was younger, I wasn't a top neither. The guy he was topping me I guess because I was young and kind of dumb and whatever. So he was doing that to me so imagine if that would have gotten out to my grandmother that would have been embarrassing … She always raised me to be a boy, she always raised me to be a man, and if she would have found that out it probably would have just crushed her. You're doing what; she always raised me to be a man, none of that girly, sissy stuff. So those are all the roles that play with that.' (24-year-old)	Men expressed that bottoms were more at-risk for HIV infection; and self-identified bottoms were more open to using PrEP
Total top/dominant (N = 9)	Many men described being strictly insertive partners in anal sex, sometimes misconstruing that for not having anal sex	'I don't know. I guess that would be it. I haven't been – I haven't had anal sex. I'm always the top, never bottom. And – so you're always on top, never the bottom with the man… At 54 I haven't tried it … It would put me on the other end, and I don't want to be on the other end. I enjoy being the dominant one. I don't want to be submissive one … Power and control. It could be that'. (54-year-old)	This is associated with both sexual and social domination; tops being better 'men' than bottoms. Guys who identified as 'dominant' were more often straight or bisexual, although several were gay. The sense of control associated with this sexual position kindled HIV stigma, placing complacent tops who perceive less risk vulnerable to HIV
Vers-top (N = 12)	Mostly Top, prefers being insertive partner in anal and/or oral sex but would bottom for the right person (if they are emotionally into them or if the other person is a Total Top)	'I'm a vers-top … I just put that on me because I'm a top, but I'm a verse/top. It depends on the boy I really like. Like the one I was talking to, he was a top. The one that I was telling that we kept texting each other and then it just changed after a while … I was compromising because I like him, and that's what it is when you like somebody when you're willing to compromise … I just feel like compromising is good'. (22-year-old)	Perceived less risk than men who were mostly bottoms, used strategic positioning to reduce HIV risk, and sometimes reported not using condoms when they are bottoms because they only bottomed when they love or trust someone

(Continued)

Table 2. Continued.

Term/phrase	Meaning	Representative narrative	HIV prevention practice
Power bottom ($N = 2$)	A receptive partner in anal sex that exhibits control/dominance in intercourse	'We're like the fun in the sex game, because we're in control like when … the guys just are pumping. That's basically what – that's all they do. They're pumping. They're doing this … But like the ones, basically in controlling. Like I said, we choose the positions, how fast we want to – like we – it's like we lead them on, really. If the guys – if we didn't communicate with the guys, it would just be like sex. We're like, 'Oh, yeah, daddy, give it to me harder,' or, 'oh, no, we take it slow,' like we control them. Bottoms are like the females. We do the scratching, the sucking, the fucking, the kissing. It's just – it's amazing. I love being on the bottom. [*Laughter*] … I am a power bottom'. (22-year-old)	Having a sense of power as a receptive partner in anal sex counters stigma and indicates more ability to negotiate condom use
2.3 Gender performance			
Trade ($N = 10$)	Highly masculine men, 'hood but not ghetto', mostly a top in sex; term also refers to the penis ('his trade'), or to sex work ('the trade') depending on context	'Trade, which is the guys you wouldn't really expect to be gay, but they look straight. That's what we call trade … I find trades more attractive. I don't know … I see a guy that looks straight. I feel like it's more attractive because if he's feminine, I feel like the whole effeminate thing though wouldn't fit some guys … . It's not really attractive'. (16-year-old)	Key informants that referred to 'trade', described men who had concurrent relationships with men and women; feeling that dominance was protective increased HIV vulnerability because men perceived less risk
Butch queen ($N = 11$)	Refers to masculine presentation, but versatile sexual role performance	'Then you have the butch queen … the sort of effeminate but still masculine man. But he can still walk on the street and be identified as a normal male, so you have that. And the butch queen trades generally go for trades'. (18-year-old)	Men described ability to navigate as tops and bottoms, used condoms inconsistently and more often when they were bottoms; had some difficulty negotiating condoms with trade men
Boy ($N = 2$)	Some 'signs' of being homosexual, but masculine enough to pass as a 'regular' man or not be immediately pegged as gay; attracted to other 'boys' or masculine guys	'We're way too girly, too effeminate. They just weren't boy-boy about it … .I'm not saying you got to be macho and play sports and all this shit. Let's just be a boy'. (46-year-old)	Similar to butch queen in gender performance and sexual partnering strategies; being 'a boy' also meant these men showed strength by avoiding health services
Femme queen ($N = 2$)	A term for gender performance and identity; sometimes referred to as 'chicks with dicks' by 'straight' men in this sample who prefer them sexually	'Femme queens are Trannies … they're femme queens, like they're girls, yeah. Or they wear really girly clothes where they look like women. Like they just look like women … Or they look like boys in drag'. (26-year-old)	Several men and key informants talked about a lack of focus of research and prevention for transwomen, even though they are highly vulnerable to violence and HIV

(*Continued*)

Table 2. Continued.

Term/phrase	Meaning	Representative narrative	HIV prevention practice
The cunts (N = 6)	Several gay identified men identified as 'the cunts'. They were in their early 20 and teens. The term connotes solidarity in androgyny; other young men who were not 'the cunts' had heard of the term and meaning	'I would be considered a cunt. That's the gay term. The cunts are basically … Pretty gay boys who dress fashionable, basically. They always cute. Always pretty and always on point. They dress nice and yeah. You have a certain androgyny feel to them because they're boys, but they're femme, but they're not trans. So I think I would like to identify as more with that … But yeah, that's the general meaning of what the cunts are and I hang around probably two other cunts'. (18-year-old)	These men tended to be socially incorporated in HIV prevention, CBOs, some but not all in the house ball scene; although they were knowledgeable about HIV prevention, some had occasional unprotected sex

undercut ways that they felt discriminated or undermined due to their femininity. In categorising themselves as 'feminine', these men were not seeking to reproduce symbolic patterns associated with 'normative femininity', but rather emphasise a transgressive version of femininity – that is, what is viewed as a transgressive performance of prohibited female sexuality – being sexually aggressive as 'power', etc. At the same time, their sexual objects of desire were normatively masculine, often 'straight' or 'trade' men. Gender transgression is thus multiple (or at least double): biological males acting like females, and normative female sexual behaviour transformed into transgressive female sexuality – the 'play on' gender seems to be on male fantasies (or at least symbolic representations) about female sexuality. The kinds of local identities men adopted along these three axes reveals how much notions of gender and sexuality were intertwined.

Thus, beyond looking at these local identities as static or independent of each other, we found that the ways in which these axes were interrelated and sometimes fluid revealed critical insights for culturally nuanced HIV prevention strategies. As discussed below, this fluidity and interrelation were particularly evident in relation to partnering strategies and community formation.

How sexual identity, sexual performance, and gender performance are fluid and intertwine

There was a real fluidity to these categories of identity over time and space; the way men presented and understood themselves shifted depending on where they were and with whom they were socialising. Nonetheless, despite the ways in which gender and sexuality were performative and intentional, there was some consistent social patterning regarding sexual identity, preferred sexual position, and gender performance, as follows.

Group 1 (N = 8): Men in this group identified as straight, discreet, or bisexual, had a masculine gender performance and most were 'total tops' (only insertive) in anal sex:

These men always sought to keep their homosexual behaviour a secret from family, friends, and religious communities. Nearly all of these men had girlfriends and children, and prized discretion as a strategy that preserved their access to heterosexual privilege.

This group of men understood competent gender performance to be constituted in part by sexuality, and as a result, these men often perceived their homosexual behaviour as shameful or experienced guilt. Their understanding of what was expected of a man extended beyond appearing heterosexual, however, to include having children, resolving problems through anger and violence, providing for the family, and being (or at least presenting themselves) as self-sufficient.

For men in this group, belonging to what they considered important aspects of the Black community and complying with what was expected of Black men was more important than disclosing their homosexuality. For this reason, some strategically partnered with male sex workers (found in the streets, parks, online, or through gay-magazine ads), carefully negotiated discretion with male partners before meeting them, and preferred feminine men or transgender women. These men saw themselves as being 'controlling' and 'dominant', often choosing male sexual partners (sometimes referred to as 'bitches') with whom they could establish unequal sexual partnerships, especially if partners were sex workers or very feminine. Choosing men who were feminine, but whom they could control and keep private, allowed discreet and straight men to manage their heterosexual social privilege while fulfilling sexual desire.

In addition, these men preferred Black and Latino sexual partners. A 54-year-old, straight-identified man explained, 'Hispanic and Black chicks with dicks [who] are more of a turn on than Caucasians for some reason:'

> [In White transgender women,] their hormone level is not as strong. And that may have something to do with the melanin in the system. I don't know, but when I see them, they never as busty as derriered as the Hispanic or the Black chicks with dicks … and well, the larger the penis is, the better.

His narrative suggests that men or 'chicks with dicks' who have accentuated feminine features (being 'busty' or having large 'derrières') and masculine features (a large penis) are more erotically desirable and that possession of these characteristics is seen as racialised. Thus, racialised sexual desire (i.e. finding Black and Latino men sexier) also shaped these men's partnering strategies.

Juggling their masculine and heterosexual social appearance with their homosexual behaviour shaped this group's engagement with health services and how these men perceived HIV risk, which in turn translated into their HIV prevention strategies. Seeking health services for routine check-ups was a sign of 'weakness' and femininity, and adherence to HIV testing was among other 'emergency' reasons for health-seeking (i.e. others included breaking a bone, being shot, and extreme pain). Many of these men felt 'in control' and less vulnerable because they were tops in anal sex and because they were not gay. Some reported always using condoms with men or 'chicks with dicks' but not with their girlfriends. Nearly all men in this group recognised that they used condoms inconsistently, and because of this they perceived themselves at risk and got tested regularly. Reflecting on his own sexual identity, a discreet 46-year-old explained that men who feel they are not part of the gay risk 'subgroup' would not even consider PrEP as applicable to them:

> 'Cause I'm not gay, that nigga's gay – he's suckin' my dick', or 'I don't do that', but you don't know what your partner's doing, and I think that a lot of people are just in denial about their

existence. And if you're in denial about your existence, why would you wanna seek any help? '[HIV infection] is not gonna happen to me, or anybody I know'.

In fact, none of these men thought PrEP was a prevention tool that would work for them because of their association of HIV with gay men, taking medication as a sign of weakness and because of fear that if someone found their pills, they would be labelled 'gay'.

Group 2 (N = 7): Men in this group identified as gay, were bottoms in anal sex, and felt a sense of pride about their femininity:

These men, most of whom adopted the identity of 'the cunts', found masculine partners sexually desirable, and sought to hook-up with butch queens and trade men. They felt they belonged to a particular niche in the Black gay community, and often hung out with other men who were proud of their femininity. As a 22-year-old gay man explained, some of them called themselves 'power bottoms', expressing their feeling that they controlled their partners' sexual pleasure and contradicting notions that bottoms had no power.

Identities such as 'the cunts' and 'power bottoms' reflect these men's efforts to construct a powerful femininity, to resist stigmatisation, and to counteract the gender power inequalities they experience in relationships with trade or straight men. They generally felt a sense of belonging to a community of similar men, which afforded them social support. This was important to them because many of them described experiencing stigma and discrimination because of their feminine gender performance. When these men also hooked up with men who were hyper-masculine and discreet, they could not hang out with their sexual partners in public, meeting furtively in hotel rooms, parks, and other discreet spaces. Although they resisted perceived gendered power imbalances, many of these men had experienced sexually violent situations (forced unprotected sex) with more masculine-appearing men, and they felt emotionally hurt by their partners' inability to acknowledge them socially.

Sexual desire and gender inequalities led to power dynamics that sometimes made it difficult to negotiate condom use. Some of these men used condoms inconsistently when their potential partners were 'trade' (hyper-masculine) because they found the masculinity of these partners to be highly desirable. Many of these men saw PrEP as a good prevention strategy. For example, a 22-year-old gay man, who describes himself as one of 'the cunts', explained 'Yes, I would use it [PrEP] if it's to help keep me healthy and safe'. The greater willingness to use PrEP that characterised men in this group seemed to reflect their sense of belonging to a community of similar Black gay men that attempted undercut masculine norms, including power imbalances when having sex with 'trade' men and the notions of 'weakness' that dissuaded other men from seeking health services.

Group 3 (N = 8): Men in this group were gay and same-gender-loving men, were versatile in anal sex, and expressed both feminine and masculine gender performance:

The diverse partnering strategies of men in this group, many of whom identified as 'butch queens', varied depending on the relative masculinity and sexual identity of prospective sexual partners. Although the performance of an exaggerated version of masculinity made potential partners highly desirable for most men in our sample, for men in this group the value of masculine performance depended on whether their partners were open about their non-normative sexual identity. In fact, some men stigmatised straight-identified men, even though they were extremely masculine, referring to them as 'DL' (down low) and blaming them for sexual transmission to women.

Men in this group often saw themselves as belonging to the Black gay community. Some were also explicitly critical of the White gay community because they felt it 'hyper-sexualised' Black men and that they did not fit in unless they 'queened out' for white men. Several had a strong sense of community as 'same-gender-loving' men, as opposed to gay men, because this label was started in the Black community. Like several others in our sample, one 45-year-old man rejected the label 'gay' because racial solidarity among Black same-gender-loving men was a 'political' act:

> I normally don't like to refer to myself as gay. I think I just being a Black male; I like to identify with being a Black male. Gay always referred to being white, you know what I mean? When you're a Black man I think for me it's so important to identify with that first, right?

Their sense of racial community also affected their partnering strategies, as many of them only dated Black men. Although a few referred explicitly to political dimensions of racial solidarity, many men explained preferring other Black men as sexual partners in terms of sexual desire. Whereas several men affirmed stereotypes about a Black man having a large penis, for others – such as a 26-year-old gay man who, 'love[s] Black men' because he 'like[s] the swag' or 'the way they carry themselves' – sexual desire for Black men was fuelled by a shared sense of style and sensibility, social presentation, and cultural beliefs about sexuality.

Moreover, many of these men reported using condoms consistently and were apt to see a doctor regularly at community-based clinics and for routine HIV testing. However, some claimed they had condomless sex with men in the last year to pay bills or to have a place to stay for the night. Men sometimes chose their sexual positions strategically to reduce the risk of acquiring HIV. As a 31-year-old same-gender-loving man explained, he is 'not just a top' and believes 'risks are lower with HIV' when he tops, so he is more careful when bottoming. He attributes tops becoming infected to 'some of them eventually being penetrated at one point in time'. In fact, vers-tops perceived less HIV risk than men who were mostly bottoms, and sometimes reported not using condoms when they were bottoms because they only bottomed when they loved or trusted someone. Our findings about how men chose sexual position strategically depending on the kind of partnership (i.e. casual/one-time versus steady with affective bonds) corroborate findings in the literature about strategic positioning in gay minority men and Black MSM (Marks et al., 2010; Van De Ven et al., 2002).

Thus, because of their sexual versatility (as bottoms/tops) and gender-awareness, these men thought critically about how strategic sexual roles and partnering strategies affected their willingness to take PrEP. Some of these men thought PrEP was a good idea for others (e.g. serodiscordant couples) but not for themselves because, as a 41-year-old gay man put it, taking a daily pill was 'crazy', 'a big commitment other than just putting a rubber on', although, 'raw sex is nice'. Many men did not think condoms would be used with PrEP, as a 29-year-old gay man explained: 'people are just absolutely fascinated with just raw sex. So they would be like the first ones probably in line for PrEP. Like, oh my god, I can take this pill and have raw sex'. In fact, very few men would use PrEP and condoms for the added protection and in case the condom broke. In addition to being 'real' about the possibility that men would not use PrEP and condoms, men in this group were also very reflexive about how masculinity and femininity could affect PrEP acceptance. Several likened taking Truvada daily to 'the pill' for contraception, and as one 22-year-old man suggested, messaging should, 'call it "The Pill for Men"', to capitalise on gender ideology.

Although key informants thought that PrEP was best for 'bottoms' and people who already have 'raw sex', they thought that more community-based education was necessary, like a social worker at an HIV prevention CBO explained:

> They should have a professional ... also want somebody that they can relate to, who are versed in PrEP and hear the good and the bad and the ugly, and then they'd be allowed to make a decision as to whether it's for them. I think a lot of the times they don't have much information or it's rushed.

Thus, for men who are open to consider PrEP as a prevention tool, community stakeholders thought clear messaging and community engagement would 'demystify' this new prevention tool and its proper use.

Group 4 (N = 8): Men in this group had fluid sexual identity, versatile sexual role preference, and their gender performance largely depended on their social context or situation:

This group includes men whose sexual identity is gay or openly bisexual in some contexts, such as bars, whereas it is straight or discreet in others. These men also visited different venues strategically when they wanted to be tops or bottoms in anal sex. For example, a 26-year-old man explained that he could choose to present themselves as 'trade' and seek to be the insertive partner through hook-up applications and online, whereas he was more of a 'butch queen' or 'cunts' at parties or clubs. A 47-year-old discreet man maintained a long-term relationship with an older man, but also had casual sex with men he met on hook-up websites. Thus, several men displayed strategic ways to fulfil their desire to be a top by adhering to masculine gender norms on smart phone apps, and more feminine (through their clothing, dancing, flirtatious character) in bars or parties.

The greater degree of sexual and gender fluidity in this group was associated with men's socioeconomic disadvantage, including employment insecurity and being uninsured. Socioeconomic disadvantage led many of the men we interviewed to survive through sex work, which challenged their ability to negotiate condoms. A 24-year-old sex worker, for example, expressed his need to be the provider for his grandmother and 'put food on the table'. For sex workers, their sexual identity, gender performance, and sexual position depended on their clients. Male sex workers could charge more for bottoming if they presented themselves as masculine.

Socioeconomic disadvantage challenged condom negotiation and the importance of staying HIV-negative. Because these men had context-dependent gender presentation and sexuality, they participated in the gay scene and several were tested through HIV community-based organisations. An 18-year-old gay man, explained:

> PrEP is more like a want. It's not something you need. PrEP is more expensive than PEP (post exposure prophylaxis). I was told by ... a youth counsellor at the Harlem Prevention Center. And he told me that PrEP can be up to thousands of dollars ... We educate people to have protected sex, safe sex with condoms, safer sex, so if you are having safer sex and you just depend on PrEP ... You don't really need it. You want it ... It's like cable. You don't need cable.

Many men in this group thought PrEP could be an effective tool for sex workers, but they were concerned about the cost, since many of them did not have health insurance. From key informant interviews with service providers at CBOs, it was clear that some providers believed PrEP was too expensive considering other available prevention methods and the cost of care for those with HIV and AIDS. Overall, some of the men who were at-risk (e.g. sex workers, socioeconomically disadvantaged men) encountered resistance about PrEP from providers because it was 'too expensive' and 'unnecessary'.

Discussion

This study lays out numerous local or emic categories that exist within the externally created, etic category BMSM. By examining the meanings associated with these categories, and analytically grouping men into configurations constructed in relation not only to sexual identity, but also preferred sexual position and gender performance, we were able to unpack some key differences in social and cultural experiences that organise significant diversity within the otherwise undifferentiated category of BMSM – and that may ultimately affect the possibilities for advancing the use of PrEP and other methods in the HIV prevention toolkit. Like all prevention techniques and technologies, use of PrEP requires a complex set of ideas and practices to be put in place within the context of broader cultural meanings and social relationships, and its effective incorporation into the broader range of prevention options needed for diverse BMSM will only be possible if greater attention is given to this social reality. Advancing the use of PrEP for those who might benefit from it will only be possible if it is truly embedded within this social context and becomes meaningful within it. To accomplish this, our research suggests that a number of key considerations will be crucial: (1) recognising the importance of understanding local social and sexual subjectivities; (2) bringing a meaningful discussion of sexuality, sexual subjectivities, and sexual practice back into the response to HIV through community-based prevention efforts; and (3) reinforcing community-based prevention programmes, even in times of constrained resources, and integrating biomedical prevention approaches into these services.

The importance of social and sexual subjectivities

First, we want to emphasise the importance of shifting the focus of our attention from broad, undifferentiated epidemiological categories, such as BMSM, and even from the more nuanced categories such as the diverse sexual identities that this broad category largely conceals, to a deeper understanding of the social and sexual subjectivities that shape the lives of these men. In fact, these configurations – which are intersectional in their inclusion not just of race and sexual identity but also through their inclusion of gender performance and sexual practices as axes of social diversity – tell us more about HIV vulnerability than broad (or even local) categories. The importance of these categories became more evident as plays on gender and sexuality were used strategically in seeking sexual partners, in deploying stigma, and in delimiting boundaries for belonging to the gay and/or Black communities.

Our results indicate that HIV, sexuality, and gender-related stigma may affect HIV prevention among men in each of these groupings differently. The most vulnerable group seems to be comprised of men with straight or discreet sexual identities, who report being tops in sex with men, and who have masculine ideologies and gender expectations. This group would be the least likely to take PrEP, especially because of the strongly held association of HIV with gay-identification among these men, the priority they give to being discreet about their sexual desires, and their disengagement with health care services because they deem health-seeking weak or feminine. Meanwhile, in seeking to secure their preferred sexual position as tops and feel dominant, straight-identified, and discreet men interact sexually with sexually versatile men, femme queens, transwomen, and partners who were often sex workers. The group of more feminine men and those who were sex workers were more open to the idea of taking PrEP and less mistrustful of health institutions.

Thus, understanding partnering strategies reveals important ways in which various prevention tools may function in a sexual scenario: one partner (e.g. a man who describes himself as straight and only assumes the insertive role) could choose to use condoms and an anally receptive partner may choose to be on PrEP. Men most affected by gender-related inequalities because of their feminine presentation may have less leverage to negotiate condom use and may thus benefit significantly from the option of taking PrEP. Studies that have begun to uncover ways in which PrEP affects sexual partnering through processes such as 'biomed matching' (Newcomb, Mongrella, Weis, McMillen, & Mustanski, 2015) also need to consider the gendered dimension of sexual sorting processes.

Rather than stigmatising non-gay identified men as a 'bridge population' and as unfaithful 'cheaters' 'on the down low' – potentially as a response to unequal gendered power dynamics – our findings support research that calls for community approaches to reduce stigma among this 'hidden population'. In fact, HIV prevention may reach hidden populations as well as address multiple forms of sexuality and gender-related stigma experienced by both openly gay men and discreet/straight men by understanding these sociocultural dimensions of sexual partnering, opening ways to engage potential sexual partners in different forms of community outreach.

To consider the 'social reality' of HIV prevention methods, it was therefore important to explore how gender performance and sexual practice together operate as organising principles of social life that generate social divisions and differentiations among BMSM. Gender is often discussed as a way to distinguish biological difference rather social differentiation, and thus public health fails to recognise that gender is not reducible to male or female bodies but rather is continuously performed and enacted (Bridges & Pascoe, 2014; Connell, 2005). Few scholars have considered strongly 'hybrid masculinities': the distinct melding of masculine and feminine gender norms and expectations independent of sexuality or biological sex (Bridges & Pascoe, 2014; Bowleg, 2013; Connell, 2005). Ethnographic research has illuminated how normative expectations of masculinity lead some BMSM to monitor their gender performance (Balaji et al., 2012; Bowleg, 2013; Miller et al., 2005). We found that gender performance differences shaped key aspects of sexual practices and sexual cultures, but these differences were masked by the catch-all category of BMSM. Categorical lenses such as BMSM do not allow us to see what is actually going on in men's sexual experiences and gendered realities. This may have important implications for packaging HIV prevention to address the social factors that shape risk situations.

This study goes further to highlight the ways in which gendered performances may 'play on' or intentionally transgress normative gender expectations for what is 'successful' or 'failed' masculinity or femininity – and how this becomes critical when (within the category of BMSM) when men use gender expression as a strategy for social differentiation and as a way to navigate power dynamics and social and sexual relationships. Populations such as the ones included in this study remain 'hidden' insofar as the research is unprepared to account for them because of limitations in close-ended surveys or other methods that are less engaged with communities. Ethnographic engagement was crucial and points to the conceptual and methodological contributions of this research. Our findings indicate that the erasure of difference and diversity, the silencing of sexuality, and waning effort to engage hard-to-reach communities through grassroots approaches is precisely the set of conditions that made it almost inevitable that infections would rise in the most marginalised and stigmatised communities – which are also precisely the communities that are least served by the unilateral biomedical administration of the epidemic.

Bringing sex back into HIV prevention

The concentration of the HIV epidemic in specific subpopulations, like BMSM, in the USA has happened over much the same period when community-based prevention programmes have been scaled back and even curtailed as the result of funding cuts and a growing reliance on biomedical approaches such as test and treat and treatment as prevention. Whether intentionally or unintentionally, there has thus been a shift from more community-based approaches to more clinic-based approaches. This, in turn, has almost always been associated with a gradual process of marginalising, silencing, and sanitising the direct and open discussion and exploration of sexuality as absolutely central to the development of meaningful prevention programmes. Indeed, one of the reasons that biomedical approaches to prevention appear to have generated significant enthusiasm on the part of many public health policy-makers and practitioners may be precisely because they are incorrectly perceived to make it possible to implement HIV prevention programmes without having to engage with the lived realities of sexuality on the part of affected populations – realities that are almost always very distant from those of the policy-makers and practitioners who supposedly serve them.

These tendencies run directly counter to many of the key lessons learned over the history of the HIV epidemic, both in the USA and globally: that it is only by engaging with local realities, and in particular with local sexual meanings and sexual practices, that we can effectively address the epidemic (Aggleton & Parker, 2015). It was precisely because of this that community-based approaches to HIV emerged in the first place – and because of this that for more than three decades they have continued to be the most important settings for developing meaningful programmes to address the epidemic among marginalised and excluded communities and populations. It was in these settings that sexuality could be openly addressed and discussed in meaningful ways, and that safer sex could be invented and reinvented 'as community practice' (Watney, 1990).

Our research underlines the fact that understanding local cultures of sexual desire still matters in what has come to be called the science of HIV prevention, even when we consider biomedical prevention methods, such as PrEP. In fact, sexual desire was linked to plays on domination and submission, among other sexually enacted power dynamics that reflected and affected men's social relationships and their ability to negotiate HIV prevention strategies. Unless there is a new emphasis on, and a renewed approach to prevention that recognises the complexity of sexual communities and the need for community-based, community-owned, and community-led prevention programmes, new approaches to HIV prevention will be destined to fail precisely because they will never be integrated into meaningful sexual and erotic practice. Such integration, on the contrary, will depend on identifying how best to apply new prevention tools within vulnerable populations, and to strengthen a kind of 'treatment/prevention literacy' at the local level that will make it possible for these populations to effectively employ them in practice (Aggleton & Parker, 2015).

Twenty-five years later, Simon Watney's prescient understanding of safer sex as community practice continues to be as true today as it was then – precisely because it is only within the context of communities that otherwise marginalised and stigmatised sexualities can be openly discussed and addressed. In our sample, men who were more willing to consider using PrEP also showed a greater sense of belonging to a community of similar Black gay men, framed their social identities to undercut normative gender inequalities, and rejected gendered norms that they understood to dissuade other men from seeking health services (e.g. notions of health-seeking as 'weakness'). It is only within a context that brings back a focus on sexual cultures of desire and sex education as community practice that it will be possible to overcome short-sightedness of biomedical approaches that alone do not strongly consider sexual partnering strategies, stigma, and socioeconomic inequalities.

Integrating biomedical prevention approaches into community-based programmes

Finally, just as our findings emphasise the importance of bringing sex and sexuality back into meaningful HIV prevention programmes – and highlight the fact that community-based services are best positioned to be able to do this – they also underscore the fact that HIV prevention in different venues must be differentially tailored precisely because of the trust (or lack of it) that different venues are capable of generating. For important sectors of the broader BMSM population, especially for straight-identified and other non-gay identified men who are socioeconomically disadvantaged, medical institutions, and medical authority are clearly suspect. A long history of ethically questionable practices (and sometimes outright discrimination and abuse) on the part of biomedical researchers and health practitioners have left their mark on the trust that many members of this population have in health services. Even with the best of intentions, there are limits to the extent that clinical services will be able to reach all segments of this population.

For new approaches to HIV prevention, treatment and care to be accepted as legitimate and incorporated into community practice, information about such approaches needs to disseminated and appropriated at the community level – and in ways that communities can take ownership rather than rather than treating it as nothing more than 'following the doctor's order'. This sort of situational and contextual tailoring of prevention messages, and the building of confidence and trust needed to provide the social context for the adoption of new technologies, requires a reaffirmed commitment to community-based and community-led initiatives – precisely at a time when funding cutbacks and narrowing of available services appear to be pushing in exactly the opposite direction (Capacity for Health Project, 2013; Garcia et al., 2015b; Hampton, 2011; Weinberg, 2013). Taking seriously this recognition of diversity and of the relevance of community-based expertise about this diversity suggests that PrEP (or any other new technological innovation) will not be a universally efficacious magic bullet. Rather, we need to understand it, and how best to use it, as a new tool in a growing toolkit of possible prevention approaches. It will be the right tool for some people, depending on their specific circumstances, particularly when it is presented as a form of combination prevention that is sensitive to cultural nuances and differences.

Considering that the meaningful engagement of local communities has been crucial to rolling out prevention and treatment campaigns globally, biomedical prevention should seek to address social, cultural and economic vulnerabilities that drive HIV at the same time that technologies such as PrEP are offered as a prevention option. A growing body of literature has emerged on the importance of understanding sexual and gender diversity among MSM of colour and MSM in the Global South (Cáceres, Aggleton, & Galea, 2008; Johnson, Jackson, & Herdt, 2000; Nyeck & Epprecht, 2013). This study highlights the importance of recognising this diversity when making public health recommendations about the use of biomedical prevention approaches globally, which often rely on narrow assumptions about sexuality and gender in MSM. For instance, in 2014 the World Health Organization announced that PrEP is highly appropriate to combat HIV among MSM (2014). The WHO's recommendation appears to be a direct statement based on epidemiological data, but is very much in line with the focus of this special issue: the kinds of 'troubles with categories' mentioned above stirred confusion in communities throughout the world about how this overarching statement applied to the diversity of MSM, sexual practices, and partnering strategies (Heitz, 2014).

From the perspective of many clinical practitioners and biomedical institutions, the kind of local sexual categories and cultures that our research helps to illuminate are unfortunately seen more as impediments to effective prevention programmes and strategies. This is hardly a new development; it is something that has existed since the very beginning of the epidemic, evident in the long delays that characterised the implementation of organised public health responses to HIV and AIDS, and in the inability of official programmes to engage with the sexual cultures and meanings of non-normative communities and populations most at risk. It is precisely because of this that community-based venues and approaches have repeatedly shown themselves to be the most effective context for the delivery of HIV prevention information and technologies to marginalised and stigmatised populations; new approaches such as PrEP or other biomedical prevention techniques and technologies in the expanding HIV prevention toolkit are no exception (Arnold et al., 2012; Kerrigan et al., 2015; Parker, 1996).

While biomedical approaches are undeniably useful tools to prevent HIV and mitigate its effects on the most vulnerable populations, the historical importance of community-led HIV prevention indicates that the effectiveness of biomedical prevention will hinge on better understanding diversity within local cultures of sexuality and gender and addressing sociocultural vulnerabilities by leveraging local expertise. When looking to package HIV prevention, public health interventions focused mostly on biomedical approaches would benefit from looking back at the historical record to address elements of stigma associated with sexuality, gender, and HIV that also affect the acceptance of biomedical technologies such as PrEP.

In light of this, our empirical and theoretical argument is supported by the undeniable diversity in both local sexual subjectivities and sexual partnering patterns, which demonstrates the important forms of heterogeneity obscured by a category such as BMSM. Our findings suggest that identity and partnering patterns are inextricable from broader social context and shape risk behaviours and men's willingness to accept different prevention methods. Our analysis begins to explore ways that BMSM navigate through these complex social universes, as members of the various intersecting communities that cross and intersect in a social space that remain largely underexplored and undifferentiated in public health practice. It is precisely this sort of insight that serves as a point of departure for what could be truly culturally meaningful ways of responding to the epidemic, including culturally appropriate ways of making biomedical prevention available, and renewed community ownership of the premises and processes through which an expanded toolkit of prevention options might offer, to those most in need of them.

Disclosure statement

No potential conflict of interest was reported by the authors.

Funding

This research was supported by a grant from the National Institute of Mental Health (R01 MH098723, PIs: Paul Colson and Jennifer Hirsch). Additional support came from the Center for the Study of Culture, Politics and Health and the Society, Psychology, and Health Research Lab (SPHERE). Morgan Philbin is supported by an NIMH postdoctoral training [grant T32 MH019139, PI: Theo Sandfort, Ph.D] at the HIV Center for Clinical and Behavioral Studies at the New York State Psychiatric Institute and Columbia University [grant number P30-MH43520; PI: Robert H. Remien, Ph.D.].

References

Aggleton, P., & Parker, R. (2015). Moving beyond biomedicalization in the HIV response: Implications for community involvement and community leadership among MSM and transgender people. *American Journal of Public Health*, *8*(105), 1552–1558. doi:10.2105/AJPH.2015.302614

Altman, D., Aggleton, P., Williams, M., Kong, T., Reddy, V., Harrad, D., ... Parker, R. (2012). Men who have sex with men: Stigma and discrimination. *The Lancet*, *380*(9839), 439–445. doi:10.1016/S0140-6736(12)60920-9

Arnold, E. A., Hazelton, P., Lane, T., Christopoulos, K. A., Galindo, G. R., Steward, W. T., & Morin, S. F. (2012). A qualitative study of provider thoughts on implementing pre-exposure prophylaxis (PrEP) in clinical settings to prevent HIV infection. *PLoS One*, *7*(7), e40603. doi:10.1371/journal.pone.0040603

Arnold, E. A., Rebchook, G. M., & Kegeles, S. M. (2014). "Triply cursed": Racism, homophobia and HIV-related stigma are barriers to regular HIV testing, treatment adherence and disclosure among young black gay men. *Culture, Health & Sexuality*, 1–13. doi:10.1080/13691058.2014.905706

Balaji, A. B., Oster, A. M., Viall, A. H., Heffelfinger, J. D., Mena, L. A., & Toledo, C. A. (2012). Role flexing: How community, religion, and family shape the experiences of young black men who have sex with men. *AIDS Patient Care and STDs*, *26*(12), 730–737. doi:10.1089/apc.2012.0177

Boellstorff, T. (2011). But do not identify as gay: A proleptic genealogy of the MSM category. *Cultural Anthropology*, *26*(2), 287–312. doi:10.1111/j.1548-1360.2011.01100.x

Bowleg, L. (2013). "Once you've blended the cake, you can't take the parts back to the main ingredients": Black gay and bisexual men's descriptions and experiences of intersectionality. *Sex Roles, 68*(11–12), 754–767. doi:10.1007/s11199-012-0152-4

Bridges, T., & Pascoe, C. J. (2014). Hybrid masculinities: New directions in the sociology of men and masculinities: Hybrid masculinities. *Sociology Compass, 8*(3), 246–258. doi:10.1111/soc4.12134

Burawoy, M. (1998). The extended case method. *Sociological Theory, 16*(1), 4–33. doi:10.1111/0735-2751.00040

Cáceres, C. F., Aggleton, P., & Galea, J. T. (2008). Sexual diversity, social inclusion and HIV/AIDS. *AIDS, 22*(Suppl 2), S35–S43. doi:10.1097/01.aids.0000327436.36161.80

Capacity for Health Project. (2013). *HIV/AIDS ASO and CBO stability & sustainability assessment report*. Retrieved from http://www.apiahf.org/sites/default/files/2013-09-05_HIVAIDS%20ASO%20CBO%20Stability%20Sustainability%20Assessment%20Report_OCB_0.pdf

CDC. (2012). *Centers for disease control and prevention. Estimated HIV incidence in the United States, 2007–2010*. HIV Surveillance Supplemental Report 2012 (No. Volume 17, Number 4). Retrieved from http://www.cdc.gov/hiv/pdf/statistics_hssr_vol_17_no_4.pdf

Centers for Disease Control and Prevention. (2005). HIV prevalence, unrecognized infection, and HIV testing among men who have sex with men – five U.S. cities, June 2004-April 2005. *MMWR. Morbidity and Mortality Weekly Report, 54*(24), 597–601. doi:10.1001/jama.294.6.674

Connell, R. W. (2005). Hegemonic masculinity: Rethinking the concept. *Gender & Society, 19*(6), 829–859. doi:10.1177/0891243205278639

Corbin, J. M., & Strauss, A. L. (2008). *Basics of qualitative research: Techniques and procedures for developing grounded theory* (3rd ed.). Los Angeles, CA: Sage.

Dowsett, G. W. (1996). *Practicing desire: Homosexual sex in the era of AIDS*. Stanford, CA: Stanford University Press.

Earnshaw, V. A., Bogart, L. M., Dovidio, J. F., & Williams, D. R. (2013). Stigma and racial/ethnic HIV disparities: Moving toward resilience. *American Psychologist, 68*(4), 225–236. doi:10.1037/a0032705

Eaton, L. A., Driffin, D. D., Kegler, C., Smith, H., Conway-Washington, C., White, D., & Cherry, C. (2015). The role of stigma and medical mistrust in the routine health care engagement of black men who have sex with men. *American Journal of Public Health, 105*(2), e75–e82. doi:10.2105/AJPH.2014.302322

Fields, E. L., Bogart, L. M., Smith, K. C., Malebranche, D. J., Ellen, J., & Schuster, M. A. (2014). "I always felt I had to prove my manhood": Homosexuality, masculinity, gender role strain, and HIV risk among young black men who have sex with men. *American Journal of Public Health*, e1–e10. doi:10.2105/AJPH.2013.301866

Ford, C. L., Whetten, K. D., Hall, S. A., Kaufman, J. S., & Thrasher, A. D. (2007). Black sexuality, social construction, and research targeting "The down low" ("The DL"). *Annals of Epidemiology, 17*(3), 209–216. doi:10.1016/j.annepidem.2006.09.006

Garcia, J., Parker, C., Parker, R. G., Wilson, P. A., Philbin, M., & Hirsch, J. S. (2015a). Psychosocial implications of homophobia and HIV stigma in social support networks insights for high-impact HIV prevention Among black men who have sex with men. *Health Education & Behavior*. doi:10.1177/1090198115599398

Garcia, J., Parker, C., Parker, R. G., Wilson, P. A., Philbin, M., & Hirsch, J. S. (2015b). "You're really gonna kick us all out?" Sustaining safe spaces for community-based HIV prevention and control among black men who have sex with men. *PLoS ONE, 10*(10), e0141326. doi:10.1371/journal.pone.0141326

Geertz, C. (1973). *The interpretation of cultures: Selected essays*. New York, NY: Basic Books.

Hampton, T. (2011). Policy paper highlights concerns about the future of HIV care and its funding. *JAMA: The Journal of the American Medical Association, 306*(23), 2551–2552. doi:10.1001/jama.2011.1805

Heitz, D. (2014, July 16). *WHO: No, not all gay men need to take antiretroviral drugs*. Retrieved from http://www.healthline.com/health-news/not-all-gay-men-antiretrovirals-071614

Johnson, M., Jackson, P., & Herdt, G. (2000). Critical regionalities and the study of gender and sexual diversity in South East and East Asia. *Culture, Health & Sexuality, 2*(4), 361–375. doi:10.1080/13691050050174396

Jones, K. T., Wilton, L., Millett, G., & Johnson, W. D. (2010). Formulating the stress and severity model of minority social stress for black men who have sex with men. In D. H. McCree, K. T. Jones, & A. O'Leary (Eds.), *African Americans and HIV/AIDS* (pp. 223–238). New York: Springer. Retrieved from http://link.springer.com/chapter/10.1007/978-0-387-78321-5_12

Kerrigan, D., Kennedy, C. E., Morgan-Thomas, R., Reza-Paul, S., Mwangi, P., Win, K. T., ... Butler, J. (2015). A community empowerment approach to the HIV response among sex workers: Effectiveness, challenges, and considerations for implementation and scale-up. *The Lancet, 385*(9963), 172–185. doi:10.1016/S0140-6736(14)60973-9

Kippax, S., Stephenson, N., Parker, R. G., & Aggleton, P. (2013). Between individual agency and structure in HIV prevention: Understanding the middle ground of social practice. *American Journal of Public Health, 103*(8), 1367–1375. doi:10.2105/AJPH.2013.301301

Koblin, B. (2012). *Correlates of HIV incidence among black men who have sex with men in 6*. Retrieved from http://www.iasociety.org/Abstracts/A200747624.aspx

Lorway, R., Reza-Paul, S., & Pasha, A. (2009). On becoming a male Sex worker in Mysore: Sexual subjectivity, "empowerment," and community-based HIV prevention research. *Medical Anthropology Quarterly, 23*(2), 142–160. doi:10.1111/j.1548-1387.2009.01052.x

MacKellar, D. A., Valleroy, L. A., Secura, G. M., Behel, S., Bingham, T., Celentano, D. D., ... Young Men's Survey Study Group. (2005). Unrecognized HIV infection, risk behaviors, and perceptions of risk among young men who have sex with men: Opportunities for advancing HIV prevention in the third decade of HIV/AIDS. *JAIDS Journal of Acquired Immune Deficiency Syndromes, 38* (5), 603–614. doi:10.1097/01.qai.0000141481.48348.7e

Malebranche, D. J. (2008). Bisexually active black men in the United States and HIV: Acknowledging more than the "down Low". *Archives of Sexual Behavior, 37*(5), 810–816. doi:10.1007/s10508-008-9364-7

Malebranche, D. J., Arriola, K. J., Jenkins, T. R., Dauria, E., & Patel, S. N. (2010). Exploring the "bisexual bridge": A qualitative study of risk behavior and disclosure of same-sex behavior among black bisexual men. *American Journal of Public Health, 100*(1), 159–164. doi:10.2105/AJPH.2008.158725

Marks, G., Millett, G. A., Bingham, T., Lauby, J., Murrill, C. S., & Stueve, A. (2010). Prevalence and protective value of serosorting and strategic positioning among black and latino men who have sex with men. *Sexually Transmitted Diseases, 1*. doi:10.1097/OLQ.0b013e3181c95dac

Maulsby, C., Millett, G., Lindsey, K., Kelley, R., Johnson, K., Montoya, D., & Holtgrave, D. (2014). HIV among black men who have sex with men (MSM) in the United States: A review of the literature. *AIDS and Behavior, 18*(1), 10–25. doi:10.1007/s10461-013-0476-2

Miller, M., Serner, M., & Wagner, M. (2005). Sexual diversity among black men who have sex with men in an inner-city community. *Journal of Urban Health: Bulletin of the New York Academy of Medicine, 82*(1 Suppl 1), i26–i34. doi:10.1093/jurban/jti021

Millett, G. A., Peterson, J. L., Flores, S. A., Hart, T. A., Wilson, P. A., Rourke, S. B., ... Remis, R. S. (2012). Comparisons of disparities and risks of HIV infection in black and other men who have sex with men in Canada, UK, and USA: A meta-analysis. *The Lancet, 380*(9839), 341–348. doi:10.1016/S0140-6736(12)60899-X

Millett, G. A., Peterson, J. L., Wolitski, R. J., & Stall, R. (2006). Greater risk for HIV infection of black men who have sex with men: A critical literature review. *American Journal of Public Health, 96*(6), 1007–1019. doi:10.2105/AJPH.2005.066720

Newcomb, M. E., Mongrella, M. C., Weis, B., McMillen, S. J., & Mustanski, B. (2015). Partner disclosure of PrEP use and undetectable viral load on geosocial networking apps: Frequency of disclosure and decisions about condomless sex. *JAIDS Journal of Acquired Immune Deficiency Syndromes, 1*. doi:10.1097/QAI.0000000000000819

NYCDOHMH. (2012). *HIV surveillance annual report, 2012*. New York City Department of Health and Mental Hygiene. Retrieved from http://www.nyc.gov/html/doh/downloads/pdf/dires/surveillance-report-dec-2013.pdf

Nyeck, S. N., & Epprecht, M. (Eds.). (2013). *Sexual diversity in Africa: Politics, theory, and citizenship*. Montréal: McGill-Queen's University Press. doi:10.1093/afraf/adv031

Parker, R., & Aggleton, P. (2003). HIV and AIDS-related stigma and discrimination: A conceptual framework and implications for action. *Social Science & Medicine (1982), 57*(1), 13–24. doi:10.1016/S0277-9536(02)00304-0

Parker, R. G. (1996). Empowerment, community mobilization and social change in the face of HIV/AIDS. *AIDS (London, England), 10*(Suppl 3), S27–S31. doi:10.1186/1471-2458-13-234

Parker, R. G., Herdt, G., & Carballo, M. (1991). Sexual culture, HIV transmission, and AIDS research. *Journal of Sex Research, 28*(1), 77–98. doi:10.1080/00224499109551596

Patton, C. (1996). *Fatal advice: How safe-sex education went wrong*. Durham, NC: Duke University Press.

Radcliffe, J., Doty, N., Hawkins, L. A., Gaskins, C. S., Beidas, R., & Rudy, B. J. (2010). Stigma and sexual health risk in HIV-positive African American young men who have sex with men. *AIDS Patient Care and STDs, 24*(8), 493–499. doi:10.1089/apc.2010.0020

Saleh, L. D., & Operario, D. (2009). Moving beyond "the down low": A critical analysis of terminology guiding HIV prevention efforts for African American men who have secretive sex with men. *Social Science & Medicine, 68*(2), 390–395. doi:10.1016/j.socscimed.2008.09.052

Van De Ven, P., Kippax, S., Crawford, J., Rawstorne, P., Prestage, G., Grulich, A., & Murphy, D. (2002). In a minority of gay men, sexual risk practice indicates strategic positioning for perceived risk reduction rather than unbridled sex. *AIDS Care, 14*(4), 471–480. doi:10.1080/09540120208629666

Watney, S. (1990). Safer sex as community practice. In P. Aggleton, P. Davies, and G. Hart (Eds.), *AIDS: Individual, cultural and policy dimensions* (pp. 19–34). Bristol, PA: The Falmer Press.

Weeks, J. (1998). The sexual citizen. *Theory, Culture & Society, 15*(3), 35–52. doi:10.1177/0263276498015003003

Weinberg, J. (2013, August 9). *Where has all the HIV funding gone?* Retrieved from http://www.huffingtonpost.com/janet-weinberg/where-has-all-the-hiv-funding-gone_b_3733543.html

WHO. (2014). *Policy brief: Consolidated guidelines on HIV prevention, diagnosis, treatment and care for key populations*.

Wilton, L. (2009). Men who have sex with men of color in the age of AIDS: The sociocultural contexts of stigma, marginalization, and structural inequalities. In V. Stone, B. Ojikutu, M. K. Rawlings, & K. Y. Smith (Eds.), *HIV/AIDS in U.S. communities of color* (pp. 179–211). New York, NY: Springer. Retrieved from http://link.springer.com/10.1007/978-0-387-98152-9_10

Young, R. M., & Meyer, I. H. (2005). The trouble with "MSM" and "WSW": Erasure of the sexual-minority person in public health discourse. *American Journal of Public Health, 95*(7), 1144–1149. doi:10.2105/AJPH.2004.046714

Sexual identities and sexual health within the Celtic nations: An exploratory study of men who have sex with men recruited through social media

Kareena McAloney-Kocaman[iD], Karen Lorimer, Paul Flowers, Mark Davis, Christina Knussen and Jamie Frankis

ABSTRACT
Associations of sexual identity with a range of sexual and sexual health behaviours were investigated amongst men who have sex with men (MSM). Data from 1816 MSM recruited from 4 Celtic nations (Scotland, Wales, Northern Ireland and the Republic of Ireland) were collected via a cross-sectional online survey advertised via social media. About 18.3% were non-gay identified MSM (NGI-MSM). In the last year, 30% of NGI-MSM reported high-risk unprotected anal intercourse and 45% reported never having had an sexually transmitted infection (STI) test. When compared to MSM who were gay identified (GI-MSM), NGI-MSM were more likely to be older, have a female partner, fewer sex partners, fewer anal sex partners, STI diagnoses and less likely to be HIV positive, more likely to never use the gay scene and be geographically further from a gay venue. NGI-MSM were also less likely to report STI and HIV testing behaviours. The findings highlight variations in risk by sexual identities, and unmet sexual health needs amongst NGI-MSM across Celtic nations. Innovative research is required regarding the utility of social media for reaching populations of MSM and developing interventions which target the heterogeneity of MSM and their specific sexual health needs.

Introduction

In much of the developed world men who have sex with men (MSM) are disproportionately affected by HIV and AIDS (Kilmarx, 2009; McDaid, Li, Knussen, & Flowers, 2012; National Institute for Health and Clinical Excellence, 2011; Public Health England, 2013; World Health Organisation, 2011). However, MSM are not a homogenous group, with acknowledged variations in sexual identity, sexual preferences and sexual behaviours. Despite this much of our knowledge of the health, behaviours and risks of MSM is drawn from research with gay identified MSM (GI-MSM); while relatively little is known about the sexual behaviours and sexual health behaviours of non-gay (bisexual or heterosexual) identified MSM (NGI-MSM) (Lorenc et al., 2011; Lyons et al., 2012; Reback & Larkins, 2013). The existing evidence base has been impaired by long-standing challenges relating to sampling biases in relation to heterogeneous samples of MSM (see Harry, 1986) and concomitant problems in generalizability of findings. These challenges are compounded by the fluid nature of identity across contexts, environments and social situations, particularly when potential for discrimination and stigma is present (D'Augelli, 1994). Moreover, epidemiological, social and technological change further influences the transferability of evidence within these populations in relation to sexual health. HIV, for example, has been normalised, gay rights have significantly improved and new digital technologies are rapidly changing sexual networks and patterns of sexual mixing in ways which were not possible in the past. Digital forums also provide a new perspective for identity research, as they place control of self-representation information in the hands of the digital user, allowing them to construct an identity of their own choosing for consumption by the digital network (Postmes, Spears, & Lea, 2002). Within the MSM population this may permit greater freedom in self-presentation, and present an opportunity for researchers to engage with previously hard to reach groups within the wider MSM population. Little research to date has examined how the digital revolution in regard to the sexual cultures of MSM has enabled new opportunities for MSM, new risks for their sexual health and new opportunities for sexual health promotion. Here, we report an exploratory study which begins to detail for the first time key areas of emerging concern for public health with regard to NGI-MSM.

A recent meta-analysis by Friedman et al. (2014) of research published between 1946 and 2012, investigated differences among groups of MSM defined by their sexual partnering behaviours, identifying a distinct group of bisexually behaving MSM and men who have sex with both men and women (MSMW). They indicated that in comparison with MSM only, MSMW had decreased odds of a known HIV diagnosis, and reduced odds of participating in receptive, unprotected anal intercourse (UAI). In contrast, however, MSMW had significantly greater odds of a known HIV-positive diagnosis in comparison to men who have sex with women only. Although MSMW is not directly analogous with NGI-MSM, this research highlights how behaviours and risk exposure may vary across different subgroups within the larger MSM population, suggesting a need to explore and address variations in terms of behaviour and identity. There is little contemporary evidence available to gauge the impact of the social media upon the potential transformation of the sexual cultures of MSM. Arguably, new patterns of sexual mixing are facilitated and there may well be greater heterogeneity in samples of MSM than in earlier times; it is possible that recent communication technologies are decoupling identity from behaviour in new ways. Pre-social media evidence shows that comparisons of GI- and NGI-MSM have indicated that some risks and behaviours are less prevalent among NGI men (Goldbaum, Perdue, & Higgins, 1996), who report fewer sex partners than GI men (Myers, Allman, Jackson, & Orr, 1995; Pathela et al., 2006), are less likely to have ever had an sexually transmitted infection (STI) (Pathela et al., 2006) and less likely to have a known HIV-positive diagnosis (Centers for Disease Control and Prevention, 2001). However, more recent research involving social media and telephone recruitment of MSM has pointed to a greater prevalence of some risk behaviours and different patterns of risk exposure than GI-MSM; while known HIV-positive status is less prevalent, NGI-MSM are less likely to have ever been tested for HIV (Lyons et al., 2012; Margolis, Joseph, Belcher, Hirscfield, & Chiasson, 2012; Pathela et al., 2006).

Relatively recent research suggests that NGI-MSM have lower engagement in the commercial gay scene (Lyons et al., 2012; McLean, 2008) in part because they do not see themselves as gay identifying or as part of the gay community (Lyons et al., 2012). Historically, most interventions promoting safer sex and testing behaviours tend to be targeted within the gay scene and this may present a barrier to service access and information sharing among NGI men (Lorenc et al., 2011; Lyons et al., 2012). This is particularly important as Goldbaum et al. (1998) indicated that while NGI-MSM are less likely to receive HIV prevention information or interventions, those who had were significantly more likely to have used a condom during their most recent sexual intercourse. Similarly, Lelutiu-Weinberger et al. (2013) recruiting MSM both on and offline reported a protective effect of gay scene identification, whereby higher identification was associated with lower HIV risk, particularly for younger men. Heterosexual and bisexual identifying MSM, therefore, may be excluded from effective health promotion, both in terms of access and in terms of the relevance of messages. Understanding how sexual identity influences sexual health behaviours is, therefore, a central public health problem, which brings with it opportunities to reconceptualise the heterogeneity of MSM and examine the complexity of the relationships between identity and behaviour.

While previous research has focused on identifying behaviours which expose MSM to risk, comparatively little research has addressed the heterogeneity in MSM identities and subsequent influences on behaviours and risk exposure. This analysis aims to investigate differences in the characteristics and behaviours of MSM who identify as gay (GI-MSM) and those who do not identify as gay, but rather as either heterosexual or bisexual (NGI-MSM), recruited from three countries of the UK and from Ireland as part of the Social Media, MSM and Sexual Health (SMMASH) study.

Method

Design and participants

The SMMASH survey collected anonymous, self-complete questionnaires recruited online from November 2012 to February 2013 in Scotland, Wales, Northern Ireland (NI) and the Republic of Ireland (RoI). Pop up message 'blasts' and/or banner adverts invited men using gay-specific hook-up websites (Gaydar, Recon and Squirt), smartphone apps (Grindr and Gaydar) and Facebook to participate via Survey Monkey. Overall, 2668 MSM completed questionnaires from men recruited across the four targeted countries as follows: Scotland ($n = 1326$, 49.7%); Wales ($n = 459$, 17.2%); NI ($n = 301$, 11.3%); and RoI ($n = 582$, 21.8%). Given the nature of online surveys and men's multiple profiles/use of multiple sites it is not possible to calculate a response rate. The effective sample for this analysis, selected on the basis of valid responses to the items of interest was 1816 men (Scotland, $n = 896$, 49.3%; Wales, $n = 308$, 16.9%; NI, $n = 207$, 11.4%; and RoI, $n = 408$, 22.4%). Ethical approval was granted by GCU School of Community Health and Nursing Ethics Subcommittee.

Measures

Questionnaires surveyed socio-demographics (country of residence, age, relationship status, education, employment, proximity to and frequency of gay scene use within the last month and degree of 'outness'), sexual health (HIV/STI testing and diagnoses) and sexual behaviours in the previous 12 months. Sexual identity was assessed with a single measure ('What is your sexual orientation?' with the options of Gay, Bisexual, Straight and Other) and so is identity, rather than behaviourally derived. A measure of UAI with higher risk for HIV infection was created to include men who reported UAI with ≥ 2, casual and/or with unknown/discordant partners in the previous 12 months (compared with men reporting UAI with 0/1, regular and/or known/concordant partners only). Regularity of HIV testing was determined by combining responses to two questions which assessed current HIV status and frequency of HIV testing; to account for the absence of further testing once an HIV-positive diagnosis is received. Responses for this variable were 'Don't require testing', indicating a known HIV-positive status; and for those with a negative status or unknown status; 'testing at least yearly'; 'testing less often than yearly'; and 'never been tested'.

Data analyses

Data were analysed with IBM SPSS 21 by the first and last authors. Men with missing data on any of the regression variables were excluded from this analysis, leaving a sample size of $n = 1816$ participants across Scotland ($n = 896$, 49.3%), Wales ($n = 308$, 16.9%), NI ($n = 207$, 11.4%) and RoI ($n = 408$, 22.4%). Chi-square tests were used for bivariate comparisons. Variables significant at the bivariate level ($p < .05$) were entered into logistic regression models used to estimate odds ratios and 95% confidence intervals of NGI or GI for demographics, sexual risk behaviours, HIV/STI testing/results and gay community engagement.

Results

Bivariate analyses

A sizeable minority of the 1816 participants reported a NGI (18.3%; $n = 333$), the majority of whom (94.6%, $n = 315$) reported a bisexual identity, with the remaining 5.4% ($n = 18$) indicating a heterosexual identity. Table 1 reports the prevalence of each of the variables among the GI and NGI participants. Considering these analyses, relatively fewer NGI men were recruited in the Scottish sample than elsewhere (16% of those recruited from Scotland, 18.8% of those recruited from Wales, 23.2% of those recruited from NI and 20.6% of those recruited from the RoI). Although participant age profiles were broadly similar, there was a larger proportion of men aged ≥ 46 in the NGI group. NGI men were significantly more likely to report having a regular female partner than GI men. The majority of both GI and NGI men reported fewer than 10 male sex partners, but this prevalence was significantly higher among NGI men; this same pattern emerged with anal sex partners. Significantly fewer NGI men (5.7%) had ever been diagnosed with an STI than GI men (12.8%). NGI men were more likely to have never undergone an STI or HIV test, and were less likely to have a known HIV-positive status.

While the majority of GI men reported having used the gay scene in the last month, the majority of NGI men reported no such engagement and were significantly more likely to be further away from the nearest gay scene. GI men reported significantly higher feelings of being 'out' than NGI men.

Table 1. Characteristics of GI- and NGI-MSM.

	GI (%)	NGI (%)	χ^2
Country			
Scotland	50.7	42.9	8.075*
Wales	16.8	17.4	
NI	10.7	14.4	
RoI	21.8	25.2	
Age			
18–25	25.8	24.0	11.071**
26–35	25.9	20.4	
36–45	22.0	20.4	
46=<	26.2	35.1	
Relationship status			
Single	62.1	47.7	630.61***
Male Partner	36.9	9.3	
Female Partner	0.9	42.9	
Education			
Higher or less	34.2	39.0	2.814
Degree or more	65.8	61.0	
Employment			
Employed	70.5	71.5	2.222
Unemployed	7.3	8.1	
Inactive	6.3	4.0	
Student	15.9	16.2	
No partners			
<10	60.0	70.0	11.398**
10+	40.0	30.0	
No anal partners			
<10	78.6	89.8	21.825***
10+	21.4	10.2	
High risk UAI			
No	61.1	70.0	9.147**
Yes	38.9	30.0	
STI Diagnosis			
No	87.2	94.3	13.410***
Yes	12.8	5.7	
Recency of last STI test			
Never	27.3	44.7	42.430***
Within last year	47.2	31.3	
More than a year ago	25.5	23.7	
Regularity of HIV Test			
Test at least yearly	34.4	22.8	69.175***
Never	25.6	46.5	
Test less often than yearly	33.4	29.7	
Do not require testing	6.7	0.9	
Gay scene use			
No, never	36.1	58.9	58.749***
Yes	63.9	41.1	
Nearness to scene			
Near	57.1	45.9	13.761***
Far	42.9	54.1	
	$\bar{x}$ (s.d)	$\bar{x}$ (s.d)	
How 'out'	4.01 (1.19)	2.04 (1.25)	27.00***

Notes: GI, Gay identified men; NGI, non-gay identified men.
*$p < .05$.
**$p < .01$.
***$p < .001$.

Multivariate logistic regression analyses

A series of logistic regression models were estimated to separately investigate the relationship among NGI or GI with socio-demographics, sexual risk behaviours,

HIV/STI testing and gay community engagement, respectively (Table 2, Models 1–4). The first model indicated that men targeted in the NI and the RoI surveys had significantly higher odds of identifying as NGI, as did men aged 46 years and older. Model 2 indicated that greater numbers of anal sex partners (10 or more) was associated with lower odds of NGI. Model 3 indicated that men who had never been diagnosed with an STI had 1.8 times the odds of being NGI, but there were no significant associations with regularity of STI testing. Compared to those individuals who undertook HIV testing in line with BHIVA/BASH recommendations (i.e. yearly or more frequently; Clutterbuck et al., 2011), those who had never been tested had higher odds of reporting as NGI; additionally, men with a known HIV-positive status were less likely to report as NGI. In the fourth model, individuals who had not used the gay scene in the last month had significantly lower odds of reporting a NGI.

Finally, all indicator variables were included simultaneously in a fifth regression model to investigate their relative association with identity. In this model, significant associations emerged with country, age, number of anal sex partners, regularity of HIV testing and engagement with the gay scene. Men from NI and the RoI had higher odds of reporting NGI, as did men aged 46 years and older. Men with greater numbers of anal sex partners in the previous 12 months (10 or more) had lower odds of identifying as NGI, as did those men who reported engagement with the gay scene in the previous month. Men who had never had an HIV test had twice the odds of reporting a NGI, compared with those testing yearly; and men with a known HIV-positive diagnosis had lower odds of reporting as NGI.

Discussion

The findings reveal a small but notable proportion of MSM have non-gay identities, reporting either bisexual or heterosexual identity, with heterosexual identity the least frequently reported. In line with the previous research, (Myers et al., 1995; Pathela et al., 2006) the bivariate analyses indicated lower numbers of sexual partners and lower prevalence of risky sexual partnering practices among NGI men. Additionally, NGI men had lower rates of STI and HIV diagnoses, but also of testing, which confirms previous findings in this area (Lyons et al., 2012; Margolis et al., 2012; Pathela et al., 2006). NGI men were also less likely to be engaged in the gay scene, or to identify with the gay community, a consistent trend in the literature (Lyons et al., 2012; McLean, 2008). The final logistic regression model indicated that of all the variables considered, those most influential in distinguishing between NGI and GI men were country, age, number of anal sex partners in the previous 12 months, regularity of HIV testing and engagement with the gay scene in the previous month.

Older men, and those from NI and the RoI were more likely to be NGI which may reflect more traditional conceptualisations of the acceptability of homosexuality among these groups. For example, homosexuality has become increasingly acceptable in the last 50 years, with legalisation (1967), equal age of consent (2001), civil partnerships (2013) and now equal marriage (2014) reflecting increasing approval amongst wider British society (BSA, 2013). In contrast, NI is a highly religious, Christian society (Mitchell, 2006), and this is reflected in historically traditional and conservative attitudes towards sexual relations (Sneddon & Kremer, 1992), with a majority of respondents in the 1998 NI Life and Times Survey indicating that they viewed homosexual sex as morally wrong

Table 2. Logistic regression of NGI with demographics, community engagement, risk behaviours and testing behaviours, n = 1816.

	Model 1 Demographics	Model 2 Sexual behaviours	Model 3 HIV/STI testing	Model 4 Community engagement	Model 5 All variables
Country					
Scotland	–				–
Wales	1.158 (0.825–1.027)				1.082 (0.759–1.543)
NI	**1.705 (1.174–2.478)**				**1.644 (1.112–2.431)**
RoI	**1.404 (1.039–1.898)**				**1.412 (1.033–1.930)**
Age					
18–25	–				–
26–35	0.870 (0.610–1.240)				1.087 (0.749–1.579)
36–45	1.009 (0.706–1.442)				1.277 (0.873–1.867)
46=<	**1.532 (1.109–2.116)**				**1.762 (1.234–2.515)**
No partners					
<10		–			–
10+		0.936 (0.689–1.271)			1.072 (0.776–1.482)
No anal partners					
<10		–			–
10+		**0.478 (0.304–0.757)**			**0.584 (0.365–0.934)**
High risk UAI					
No		–			–
Yes		0.813 (0.621–1.064)			0.919 (0.692–1.221)
STI Diagnosis					
Yes		–	–		
No			**1.851 (1.109–3.087)**		1.564 (0.918–2.663)
Recency of last STI test					
Never			–		–
Within last year			0.936 (0.612–1.432)		1.064 (0.692–1.635)
More than a year ago			0.882 (0.601–1.293)		0.880 (0.595–1.300)
Regularity of HIV Test					
Test at least yearly			–		–
Never			**2.444 (1.567–3.812)**		**2.222 (1.409–3.505)**
Test less often than yearly			1.316 (0.903–1.917)		1.168 (0.793–1.721)
Do not require testing			**0.210 (0.065–0.677)**		**0.201 (0.062–0.657)**
Gay Scene Use					
No, never				–	–
Yes				**0.732 (0.546–0.962)**	**0.495 (0.383–0.640)**
Nearness to scene					
Far				–	–
Near				0.979 (0.733–1.308)	0.827 (0.641–1.068)

Note: Bold indicates significance; sexual orientation and 'How out' participant feels excluded due to high collinearity with other variables in model.

(Dowds, Robinson, Gray, & Heenan, 1999). Homosexual individuals in NI are particularly vulnerable to discrimination and homophobic violence both at an interpersonal and institutional levels, and at greater levels than in Great Britain (Jarman & Tennant, 2003). Furthermore, Berg, Ross, Weatherburn, and Schmidt (2013) reported that societal stigmatisation of homosexuality can increase internalisation of homo-negativity among MSM. Within this context, lower rates of GI in NI and the RoI may partially reflect heightened concerns about social censure and retaliation, or increased internalised homo-negativity in comparison with MSM from other areas.

Men with 10 or more anal sex partners were less likely to be NGI, suggesting lower sexual risk in terms of multi-partnering among NGI men. MSM who had a known HIV-positive status, were significantly less likely to report as NGI. This appears to imply that NGI men are less likely to be HIV positive than their GI counterparts, however, this must be interpreted carefully as NGI men were also much less likely to have ever been tested for HIV. Therefore, rather than reflecting a lower likelihood of a positive diagnosis, this may indicate potential for higher rates of undiagnosed infection amongst NGI men. Indeed, NGI men were also less likely to be engaged with the gay scene, this has been linked with greater HIV risk (Lelutiu-Weinberger et al., 2013). As safer sex and testing interventions are traditionally directed towards the gay scene (Lorenc et al., 2011), MSM who do not engage with these fora will be excluded from *in situ* interventions, and thus deprived of effective health promotion, intervention and treatment. Identity-driven HIV prevention, particularly where grab bag terms such as MSM are utilised, contribute to the creation and maintenance of blind spots and health inequalities, leaving some of the most excluded at highest risk, particularly in social media contexts where identities are emphasised and constructed in different ways. Berg et al. (2013) have also noted that MSM with higher internalised homo-negativity are less likely to participate in HIV testing; while the current research did not investigate self-stigmatisation among the MSM sample, further research may be useful in identifying if such internalising plays a role both in sexual identity and risky behaviours among NGI-MSM.

Limitations

A number of limitations of the current research must be noted. While the SMMASH survey included 2666 men, given the nature of online surveys and men's multiple profiles/use of multiple sites it is not possible to calculate a response rate; nor to appropriately gauge the representativeness of the current sample with the larger MSM population. However, given that historically research with MSM has been subject to sampling bias (Harry, 1986) in part due to recruitment primarily from those MSM engaged with the gay scene, it is suggested that the use of online/social media recruitment presents an opportunity to recruit and engage a more representative sample of MSM. Furthermore, a sizeable proportion of participants were excluded from the current analysis due to incomplete and missing data; however, there were no notable significant differences between the men included in the analysis and those excluded. The current research asked men to self-report their sexual orientation, but did not provide a mechanism to record multiple or fluid sexual identities, which may have restricted the responses made by participants, and may be subject to bias in responses. Both straight identifying and bisexual identifying MSM were included in this analysis in a single category of

NGI-MSM, while it would have been preferable to examine these two groups separately as the number of MSM reporting these identities was relatively low, and therefore to retain them within the sample, a strategic analytic decision was made to combine in a single category. Further research which seeks to explore this heterogeneity within the NGI-MSM category itself is warranted. Additionally, participants were not asked about the sex of their recent or historical sexual partners, therefore, the current study is unable to investigate how actual sexual partnering reflects self-reported sexual orientation. Further research which explores how both these components relate to sexual risk behaviours and sexual health is warranted. Finally, although the survey was targeted at men from four countries – Scotland, Wales, NI and the RoI, participants were not asked to indicate their normal/permanent country of residence, which may result in men from other countries having been included in the sample.

Conclusions

A sizeable proportion of homosexually active men in Celtic nations do not see themselves as gay and have weak or non-existent attachments to gay community networks and interventions which facilitate health promotion and the prevention of HIV and STIs. While their risk for HIV/STIs appears to be lower than GI men, they report lower levels of testing than GI men and still share a burden of preventable disease. The present study highlights considerable heterogeneity in the identities of MSM, and in the health behaviours and health risks faced by GI and NGI men. Current research, and interventions, which conform to narrow definitions and conceptualisations of MSM as 'gay' may, therefore, restrict our understanding of the health risks and needs of the MSM population, and result in interventions excluding men who do not identify within this narrow definition. Furthermore, evidence presented herein suggests a potential need for country specific health promotion for homosexually active men who are not gay identifying. This suggests a need to orient health promotion and clinical services in Celtic nations and outside of large metropolitan areas to the needs of homosexually active, heterosexual and bisexual men. Our research shows that hook-up apps, sites and social media such as Facebook are effective means for accessing populations who do not engage with gay scene based social networks within community settings, thus allowing access to a more representative sample of MSM to reflect the heterogeneity in identity within this population. Further research which investigates how these men use social media, as well as the interaction of age/generation and sexual identity would benefit our understanding of the online and offline lives and behaviours of this group, and assist in the development of interventions which meet the needs of those who currently are neglected.

Disclosure statement

No potential conflict of interest was reported by the authors.

ORCID

Kareena McAloney-Kocaman http://orcid.org/0000-0003-4561-9619

References

Berg, R. C., Ross, M. W., Weatherburn, P., & Schmidt, A. J. (2013). Structural and environmental factors are associated with internalised homonegativity in men who have sex with men: Findings from the European MSM internet survey (EMIS) in 38 countries. *Social Science and Medicine, 78*, 61–69. doi:10.1016/j.socscimed.2012.11.033

BSA-30. (2013). Personal relationships: Changing attitudes towards sex, marriage and parenthood. *British social attitudes 30 report*. Retrieved 12/2/15 from http://www.bsa-30.natcen.ac.uk/read-the-report/personal-relationships/homosexuality.aspx

Centers for Disease Control and Prevention. (2001). *HIV/AIDS surveillance report, 2001*. Atlanta, GA: U.S. Department of Health and Human Services, Centers for Disease Control and Prevention.

Clutterbuck, D. J., Flowers, P., Barber, T., Wilson, H., Nelson, M., Hedge, B., … Sullivan, A. K. (2011). *United Kingdom national guideline on safer sex advice in the GUM consultation*. London: Clinical Effectiveness Group, British Association of Sexual Health and HIV.

D'Augelli, A. R. (1994). Identity development and sexual orientation: Toward a model of lesbian, gay, and bisexual development. In E. Trickett, R. Watts, & D. Birman (Eds.), *Human diversity: Perspectives on people in context* (pp. 312–333). San Francisco, CA: Jossey-Bass.

Dowds, L., Robinson, G., Gray, A. M., & Heenan, D. (1999). *Men and women in Northern Ireland: Challenging the stereotypes*. Northern Ireland Life and Times Survey Research update no 1. Belfast: ARK.

Friedman, M. R., Wei, C., Klem, M. L., Silvestre, A. J., Markovic, N., & Stall, R. (2014). HIV infection and sexual risk among men who have sex with men and women (MSMW): A systematic review and meta-analysis. *Plos One, 9*(1), e87139. doi:10.1371/journal.pone.0087139

Goldbaum, G., Perdue, T., & Higgins, D. (1996). Non-gay identifying men who have sex with men: Formative research results from Seattle, Washington. *Public Health Reports, 111*(51), 36–40.

Goldbaum, G., Perdue, T., Wolitski, R., Rietmeijer, C., Hedrich, A., Wood, R., … Guenther-Grey, C. (1998). Differences in risk behavior and sources of AIDS information among gay, bisexual, and straight-identified men who have sex with men. *AIDS and Behavior, 2*(1), 13–21. doi:10.1023/A:1022399021926

Harry, J. (1986). Sampling gay men. *Journal of Sex Research, 22*(1), 21–34. doi:10.1080/00224498609551287

Jarman, N., & Tennant, A. (2003). *An acceptable prejudice? Homophobic violence and harassment in Northern Ireland*. Belfast: Institute for Conflict Research.

Kilmarx, P. H. (2009). Global epidemiology of HIV. *Current Opinion in HIV & AIDS, 4*(4), 240–246. doi:10.1097/COH.0b013e32832c06db

Lelutiu-Weinberger, C., Pachankis, J. E., Golub, S. A., Walker, J. J., Bamonte, A. J. & Parsons, J. T. (2013). Age cohort differences in the effects of gay-related stigma, anxiety and identification with the gay community on sexual risk and substance use. *AIDS Behavior, 17*, 340–349. doi:10.1007/s10461-011-0070-4

Lorenc, T., Marrero-Guillamón, I., Llewelly, A., Aggleton, P., Cooper, C., Lehmann, A., & Lyndsay, C. (2011). HIV testing among men who have sex with men (MSM): Systematic review of qualitative evidence. *Health Education Research, 26*(5), 834–846. doi: 10.1093/her/cyr064

Lyons, A. Pitts, M., Grierson, J., Smith, A., McNally, S., & Crouch, M. (2012). Sexual behaviour and HIV testing among bisexual men: A nationwide comparison of Australian bisexual-identifying and gay-identifying men. *AIDS Behavior, 16*, 1934–1943. doi:10.1007/s10461-012-0148-7

Margolis, A. D., Joseph, H., Belcher, L., Hirscfield, S., & Chiasson, M. A. (2012). 'Never testing for HIV' among men who have sex with men recruited from a sexual networking website, United States. *AIDS Behavior, 16*, 23–29. doi:10.1007/s10461-011-9883-4

McDaid, L., Li, J., Knussen, C., & Flowers, P. (2012). Sexually transmitted infection testing and self-reported diagnoses among a community sample of men who have sex with men in Scotland. *Sexually Transmitted Infections, 89*(3), 223–230. doi:10.1136/sextrans-2012-050605

McLean, K. (2008). Inside, outside, nowhere: Bisexual men and women in the gay and lesbian community. *Journal of Bisexuality, 8*(1–2), 63–80. doi:10.1080/15299710802143174

Mitchell, C. (2006). *Religion, identity and politics in Northern Ireland. Boundaries of belonging and belief*. Aldershot, England: Ashgate Publishing Ltd.

Myers, T., Allman, D., Jackson, E. A., & Orr, K. (1995). Variation in sexual orientations among men who have sex with men, and their current sexual practices. *Canadian Journal of Public Health, 86*, 384–388.

National Institute for Health and Clinical Excellence. (2011). *Increasing the uptake of HIV testing among men who have sex with men*. London: NICE.

Pathela, P., Hajat, A., Schillinger, J., Blank, S., Sell, R., & Mostashari, F. (2006). Discordance between sexual behavior and self-reported sexual identity: A population-based survey of New York City men. *Annals of Internal Medicine, 145*, 416–425. doi:10.7326/0003-4819-145-6-200609190-00005

Postmes, T., Spears, R., & Lea, M. (2002). Intergroup differentiation in computer-mediated communication: Effects of depersonalization. *Group Dynamics: Theory, Research, and Practice, 6* (1), 3–16. doi:10.1037/1089-2699.6.1.3

Public Health England. (2013). *Health protection report*: Sexually transmitted infections and chlamydia screening in England, *2012* (Rep. No. 7 (23)). Public Health England.

Reback, C. J., & Larkins, S. (2013). HIV risk behaviors among a sample of heterosexually identified men who occasionally have sex with another male and/or a transwoman. *Journal of Sex Research, 50*(2), 151–163. doi:10.1080/00224499.2011.632101

Sneddon, I., & Kremer, J. (1992). Sex behavior and attitudes of university students in Northern Ireland. *Archives of Sexual Behavior, 21*(3), 295–312. doi:10.1007/BF01542998

World Health Organization. (2011). *Guidelines: Prevention and treatment of HIV and other sexually transmitted infections among men who have sex with men and transgender people: Recommendations for a public health approach*. Geneva: World Health Organization, Department of HIV/AIDS.

'I am not a man': Trans-specific barriers and facilitators to PrEP acceptability among transgender women

Jae M. Sevelius, JoAnne Keatley, Nikki Calma and Emily Arnold

ABSTRACT
The frequent conflation of transgender ('trans') women with 'men who have sex with men (MSM)' in HIV prevention obscures trans women's unique gender identities, social and behavioural vulnerabilities, and their disproportionately high rates of HIV infection. Pre-exposure prophylaxis (PrEP) is an efficacious biomedical HIV prevention approach. However, trans women are underrepresented in PrEP research, and are often aggregated with MSM without consideration for their unique positions within sociocultural contexts. This study examined PrEP acceptability among trans women via three focus groups and nine individual interviews (total $N = 30$) in San Francisco. While knowledge of PrEP was low, interest was relatively high once participants were informed. Due to past negative healthcare experiences, ability to obtain PrEP from a trans-competent provider was cited as essential to PrEP uptake and adherence. Participants noted that PrEP could address situations in which trans women experience reduced power to negotiate safer sex, including sex work. Trans-specific barriers included lack of trans-inclusive marketing of PrEP, prioritisation of hormone use, and medical mistrust due to transphobia. Findings underscore the importance of disaggregating trans women from MSM in HIV prevention strategies to mitigate disparate risk among this highly vulnerable population.

Introduction

The behavioural category 'men who have sex with men (MSM)' has been in use in HIV-related public health literature since at least the early 1990s (Boellstorff, 2011). In an effort to acknowledge the fact that behaviours, not identities, put people at risk for HIV acquisition, epidemiologists advocated for a conceptual shift away from identity-based understandings of HIV risk. While it is true that sexual transmission of HIV depends on certain behaviours, use of the term 'MSM' as a behavioural risk category has been criticised for obscuring sociocultural heterogeneities within this population that are crucial to promoting sexual health and preventing HIV (Boellstorff, 2011; Young & Meyer, 2005). In an article critiquing the use of the behavioural categories 'MSM' and 'WSW' ('women who have sex with women') in HIV prevention literature, Young and Meyer (2005) discuss how these terms undermine the identities of sexual minorities, disregard social meanings of sexuality, and ultimately fail in their aim to describe sexual behaviour. While transgender women were not explicitly considered in their analysis, the implications of the erasure of sociocultural nuances within these terms are applicable to problematising the inclusion of transgender women within the behavioural category MSM.

While conceptualisations of gender and sexuality vary cross-culturally, the term 'transgender' has recently gained broader popularity in both the Global North and Global South. While the term originated and is currently more widely used in North America and Europe, the term is now being used to organise gender nonconforming people politically in other places such as South America (REDLACTRANS), South Africa (Gender DynamiX), Asia (TransgenderASIA), and the Middle East (MARSA). While culturally specific nuances of gender may not be fully captured by the term 'transgender', many activists all over the world find it a useful rubric under which to organise people who experience gender-based oppression (e.g. Global Action for Trans* Equality). Some organisers choose to shorten the term to 'trans' or 'trans*' to indicate inclusivity of other trans identities, such as transsexual.

In this paper, we will use the term 'trans women' to refer to people with a feminine and/or female gender identity who were assigned male sex at birth. We focus specifically on the implications of the aggregation of trans women within the behavioural risk group MSM in the sociocultural context of San Francisco, although our findings and discussion likely have wider applicability within the Global North, where resources for HIV prevention interventions may be more abundant than in other areas of the world.

Historically, trans women have been subsumed under the behavioural risk group 'MSM', obscuring their unique risks and prevention needs and hindering our understanding of accurate HIV prevalence and incidence rates globally. If considered at all, trans women are usually included in very small numbers or are referred to using the phrase 'MSM and transgender women', without disaggregation when presenting results or implications of research findings. While the advent of the MSM category aimed to avoid addressing the complexities of identities by describing behaviour, the imposition of the category on a heterogeneous group of people is certainly not devoid of cultural meaning. How we count and categorise people in public health research reveals a great deal about cultural attitudes and social constructions, and also shapes those attitudes and constructions (Young & Meyer, 2005). By subsuming trans women within the category MSM researchers convey several beliefs, including: (1) trans women are, in essence, men, (2) gender identity is not important in understanding sexual health and preventing HIV, and (3) trans women's sexual practices and experiences are essentially the same as those of men who are included in this category (Fiereck, 2013). None of these beliefs has been supported by the literature on trans women's sexual health, and overriding self-determined gender identity with public health notions of biology-driven sexual behaviour has likely exacerbated the HIV disparities experienced by trans women. In fact, gender affirmation (i.e. social and/or medical affirmation of one's gender identity) has been demonstrated to be a significant driver of both sexual risk taking as well as health care seeking behaviours among trans women (Colton Meier, Fitzgerald, Pardo, & Babcock, 2011; Nuttbrock, Rosenblum, & Blumenstein, 2002; Nuttbrock et al., 2009; Sevelius, 2013). Such psychosocial differences between trans women and MSM are important to fully characterise the disparities experienced by trans women, but cannot be elucidated in research that aggregates the two groups, privileging one sociocultural context over the other (Fiereck, 2013).

While trans people continue to be excluded from national data collection efforts, it is clear from meta-analyses of regional studies that trans women are disproportionately affected by HIV compared to all other groups. Internationally, trans women have 49 times higher odds of HIV infection compared to the general adult population (Baral et al., 2013) and in the USA they have the highest rates of new diagnoses by gender (2.1%, compared to 1.2% among men and 0.4% among women) (CDC, 2011). Because trans women's rates of HIV are higher than those of MSM, trans women may drive up the perceived prevalence among MSM in studies that aggregate trans women with MSM. Funding for HIV prevention efforts is then procured for MSM based on these HIV rates, but the programmes and prevention strategies that are subsequently developed are designed for men. Trans women's unique sociocultural issues and contexts of risk are not considered or addressed in prevention programming designed for men, and trans women often do not feel safe or welcome accessing these programmes. For example, although some MSM engage in sex work, due to pervasive economic marginalisation trans women have higher rates of lifetime engagement in sex work and it has been shown to be a prominent aspect of urban trans women's sociocultural context (Nadal, Davidoff, & Fujii-Doe, 2014). Furthermore, trans female sex workers have higher rates of HIV than non-trans male sex workers (Operario, Soma, & Underhill, 2008). Thus, sex work is a critical theme in HIV prevention programming for trans women, but is often minimally incorporated, if at all, into HIV prevention programming developed for MSM, even when that programming purports to be inclusive.

Recently, substantial attention has been paid to pre-exposure prophylaxis (PrEP), the newest and most promising biomedical HIV prevention intervention yet developed and tested. The first clinical trial of PrEP (the Chemoprophylaxis for HIV Prevention in Men study, also known as 'iPrEx') included high-risk MSM and trans women and found that PrEP reduced the risk of HIV acquisition by 44% (Grant et al., 2010). However, a subanalysis of the iPrEx data found no efficacy among the small subgroup of trans women in the study (Mascolini, 2011). Further analyses of the subgroup of trans women in iPrEx highlight unequal drug levels between MSM and trans women in the study. Lower levels of uptake and adherence among trans women likely contributed heavily to the differential rates of efficacy, but the interaction of PrEP with hormones cannot yet be fully ruled out due to the lack of pharmacokinetic studies (Deutsch et al., 2015). Of the seven clinical trials of PrEP for HIV prevention conducted to date, iPrEx is the only one with confirmed enrolment of trans women (Escudero et al., 2014).

Currently, there are no guidelines for PrEP demonstration projects that provide specific considerations for PrEP dissemination to trans women. While the World Health Organization guidance mentions trans women but does not consider their needs specifically, guidance from the Centers for Disease Control and Prevention fails to mention them at all (Centers for Disease Control and Prevention, 2011; World Health Organization, 2012). To date, PrEP demonstration projects have reported low or unclear levels of enrolment of trans women (Liu et al., 2014). Furthermore, a recently published study examined levels of knowledge, indications, and willingness to take PrEP among a population-based sample of 233 trans women in San Francisco (Wilson, Jin, Liu, & Raymond, 2015). Only 13.7% of their participants had heard of PrEP, despite the fact that San Francisco was a participating site in the three-city PrEP Demo Project and iPrEx results were widely disseminated locally. This is not surprising, due to the lack of trans-specific recruitment and retention strategies or data to guide trans-inclusive implementation. This finding underscores the fact that trans women are not reached by the same information networks as MSM and do not benefit from HIV prevention programming that is designed for MSM. The lack of attention to trans women's unique barriers to adherence in iPrEx and to the sociocultural context of trans women's lives that may affect PrEP uptake and adherence in demonstration projects exemplify how privileging the anatomy (or the assumed anatomy in the case of trans women who have had genital surgery) over sociocultural context of sexual risk results in HIV prevention strategies that perpetuate HIV-related disparities (Fiereck, 2013).

One published study of PrEP acceptability with adequate numbers of trans women was conducted in Chang Mai, Thailand (Yang et al., 2013). This study of 107 trans women and 131 MSM found that while overall PrEP acceptability was similar between the two groups, sexual behaviours, patterns of medication use, and correlates of PrEP acceptability significantly differed between the two groups. For example, trans women in the sample were more likely to exclusively engage in receptive anal sex, which may impact their HIV risk perception and thus their willingness to take PrEP (Yang et al., 2013).

The relative invisibility of trans women in studies of MSM has significant consequences for informing the structure of programming and access to PrEP. As the history of HIV prevention and treatment research has demonstrated, trans women have been left behind (Sevelius, Keatley, & Gutierrez-Mock, 2011), and they have higher rates of HIV than any group as well as higher rates of morbidity and mortality (Baral et al., 2013; Centers for Disease Control and Prevention, 2008; Herbst et al., 2008; San Francisco Department of Public Health, 2014). To date, PrEP research has repeated this pattern.

Purpose of the study

PrEP researchers have called for trans-specific research on PrEP knowledge and acceptability (Escudero et al., 2014; Golub, Gamarel, Rendina, Surace, & Lelutiu-Weinberger, 2013). To date, no published qualitative studies of facilitators and barriers to PrEP uptake have disaggregated trans women from MSM to examine the unique interests and concerns expressed by trans women. Our main objective for this study was to address this gap in the literature by exploring trans-specific facilitators and barriers to PrEP acceptability among a sample of urban trans women at risk for HIV acquisition.

Methods

From January to June 2014, the study team recruited adult participants from community-based organisations and service sites in the San Francisco Bay Area and via snowball sampling. We conducted three focus groups and nine individual qualitative interviews with trans women (total $N = 30$ unique participants) focused on their knowledge of, interest in, perceptions of, and concerns about PrEP as an HIV prevention strategy. Each focus group had seven participants, for a total of 21 focus group participants. Nine participants completed individual interviews. While focus groups are useful to explore community norms, individual interviews allowed participants to express personal preferences. Because we wished to document both, we used both methodologies. Interviews lasted approximately 60 minutes; focus groups ranged from 60 to 90 minutes. In-depth interviews were conducted by trained peer staff at a community-based organisation and focus groups were conducted by a trained peer facilitator. Many of the focus group members knew each other prior to participation due to tightly knit social networks among trans women in the San Francisco Bay Area. Topics included current knowledge about PrEP, appropriateness of PrEP as an HIV prevention strategy for trans women, thoughts about accessing and remaining adherent to PrEP, concerns about PrEP, efficacy of PrEP, stigma related to taking PrEP, willingness to regularly see a healthcare provider and test for HIV, and experiences and interactions with medical and pharmacy-based providers. Participants provided verbal consent and received a $30 stipend to help defray transportation costs and time. All study procedures were reviewed and approved by the University of California San Francisco Committee on Human Research.

The in-depth interviews and focus groups were recorded and transcribed verbatim by a professional transcriptionist. Project staff also took extensive notes during focus group discussions, to capture the tone of the group, body language of the participants, and flow of the discussion and topics. All transcripts and notes were analysed using concept analysis (Walker & Avant, 2005). Concept analysis is a useful approach to analysing qualitative data collected to answer questions that are guided by a central concept and are relatively structured. For our study, we were particularly interested in learning about trans women's unique perspectives on PrEP acceptability, which was the organising principle guiding the endeavour. Codes or major themes in the data were derived from interview and focus group guides, with flexibility for in vivo codes to emerge during the analytic process. Example codes included 'interest in/willingness to take PrEP', 'problems with MSM focus', and 'HIV stigma'. The first and senior authors read a subset of two interview transcripts and notes to create potential codes. We then met to discuss the codes and their use in three different interview transcripts. Based on these discussions, we found some variability in our coding and identified additional emergent themes in the data, which we took into account in our next iteration of the codebook. Using the revised codebook to code one additional transcript, we then finalised the codebook. With the establishment of the codebook, each individual interview and focus group transcript was coded using Atlas.ti by the first author and senior author. The team compared coding strategies within two transcripts, identified segments where coding was discrepant, and used subsequent meetings to clarify use of the codes and create more consistency in their application across the dataset. Once the data were coded, we generated reports of segments associated with a code of interest. These reports were synthesised to facilitate discussion of the findings then elaborated upon in analytic memos. Analytic memos were written for focus group transcripts to illuminate community norms and for individual interview transcripts to compare experiences of trans women across the sample. For example, analytic memos included notes about issues such as community-level beliefs about HIV stigma as it intersects with transphobia, and comparisons of differing individual experiences with medication management. We have chosen quotes from participants that are reflective of the variety of perspectives that trans women expressed, to provide a sense of the range of perspectives.

Eligibility criteria included being at least 18 years of age, sexually active within the past 3 months, assigned male sex at birth and reporting gender identity as female, transgender female, or another trans identity indicating that they did not identify as male. Participants ranged in age from 21 to 51, with a mean age of 36. The majority ($n = 22$, 74%) self-identified as a person of colour (see Table 1).

Results

Knowledge of and interest in PrEP

Across both the focus groups and individual interviews, participants reported very little knowledge of PrEP (only one participant had extensive knowledge of PrEP because she worked in HIV prevention); many confused PrEP with post-exposure prophylaxis. None of the participants reported having ever taken PrEP, none reported knowing of any trans woman who had taken or was taking PrEP, and none of the trans women had a medical provider ever mention or offer PrEP to them. During an interview, one participant became angry when she learned of PrEP because her doctor had not mentioned it to her, despite knowing she was engaging in risky sexual activities and was also an HIV doctor.

> You can't just – Oh, we're going to give you drugs after you get HIV. That's not okay. That's really cruel, in fact. Like, if a doctor is going to be keeping himself in the dark about something – like, it's one thing to not know about it, it's another thing to know about it and not learn about it or tell your patients about it. That's just awful. [Participant 1]

While knowledge of PrEP was low, once participants were informed about PrEP, interest in PrEP use as an HIV prevention strategy was relatively high. Many participants stated that they would be willing to get tested for HIV every three months and see their doctor monthly in order to be on PrEP.

> When I first initially heard of the concept, my first thoughts I guess would be under the stigma umbrella. 'Oh, so it's an HIV med', is the first thing I thought. Yes, that was my

Table 1. Demographics.

	N (%)
Race/ethnicity	
African-American	5 (17)
Latina	6 (20)
White	8 (26)
Multiracial	11 (36)
Mean age	36 (range 21–51)
Education	
Less than high school	8 (27)
High school/GED	8 (27)
Some college	11 (37)
College or tech degree	3 (10)
Post-graduate	0 (0)
Housing status	
Stably housed	12 (40)
Unstably housed/Marginally housed	18 (60)

first impression. Then after that, I was like – when I got a little more informed about the situation, I said, 'oh wow, this would be a really great alternative for somebody.' [Participant 7]

Barriers and facilitators to PrEP acceptability

Some of the barriers and facilitators to PrEP uptake and acceptability identified by the participants are common to many populations affected by HIV, such as concerns about cost, potential side effects, and wanting additional education about the risk of drug resistance if one were to become positive. Because the aim of this study is to address the gap in knowledge about trans-specific barriers and facilitators to PrEP uptake and acceptability, our findings focus on issues that were raised that are unique or especially relevant to the sociocultural context of trans women's lives.

Facilitators to PrEP acceptability

Access to a trans-competent PrEP provider. Being able to obtain PrEP from a trans-competent provider was the most often cited facilitator to PrEP acceptability, and was noted by several participants as a prerequisite to consideration of PrEP use. Furthermore, the possibility of obtaining PrEP from one's current provider with whom one already has a positive relationship was noted as an ideal scenario to limit the number of medical appointments she would need to manage. Because hormone use requires regular clinic visits, the majority of participants stated that being able to incorporate PrEP-related monitoring into these regular visits would greatly facilitate their willingness to take PrEP. Focus group participants explained that trans women often avoid clinics that are not known to be trans-informed, so being able to access PrEP at a clinic that already has a trans-specific programme in place, including hormone provision, would facilitate uptake among those who are not currently connected to care.

> Sometimes just to find a doctor that's trans-friendly and make sure that we're on our right hormones is hard enough. I think there would be trans women who would be scared [to take PrEP] because its all about finding that right doctor. Having a good relationship with your doctor, I think, is a very good help – a very good healthy thing. [Focus group 2]

Those who had access to culturally competent care for transgender individuals saw few barriers in asking their providers about PrEP. Because they already had an established relationship with their provider, and in many cases saw their provider regularly (as often as once a month), they were more open to the idea of asking for PrEP. One stated,

> I would be totally okay. Plus, we're in a closed room, so it's not like we're in some crowded tunnel with just curtains. It's a private, intimate doctor/patient setting. So I would be totally willing to ask him, because it's his job. [Participant 6]

Being able to get PrEP from the trans-competent primary care doctors they are already seeing, in a private setting, was a strong facilitator to PrEP acceptability.

Risk perception. Engagement in sex work, either in the past or currently, was frequently mentioned by our participants and protection during sex work was a primary perceived benefit of PrEP use. Focus group participants discussed how PrEP could empower sex workers to take charge of protecting themselves from HIV, without having to rely on their ability to convince a 'date' to wear a condom. In those cases where a date was willing to pay more for sex without a condom and the woman needed the money, participants felt that by taking PrEP they could have a level of protection that was not available to them before.

> Some of us, you know, we do sex work on the side, and some us, you know, we're like, part of that kind of like, marginalized community and we don't really have that much opportunity to employment. So we end up trying to make a quick buck with sex work and that's a lot of exposure, and that's a risk. And I think that's one of the reasons why I would go for it. [Participant 6]

Low power to negotiate safer sex. Even outside of sex work encounters, participants described feeling that they have less power to negotiate safer sex due to transphobia and social isolation. Several participants described feeling like trans women do not have as much say over their selection of partners and thus have riskier sex with riskier partners.

> When you tell people you're trans and what this and that means ... they don't want you – they don't want any thing to do with us. Let alone when we find someone who wants something to do with us, we're there. It doesn't matter if it's right or wrong, it's just – we're more willing to go with the wrong person because it's harder to find someone who will accept us. And that's why I think [PrEP] would be a good thing to do. [Focus group 2]

This participant reflected on the general sense that, due to transphobia, trans women have limited options in terms of partner selection, later alluding to the fact that gay men are more likely to serosort, but trans women often feel they do not have that option. Another participant later responded that even asking a partner about his HIV status can feel precarious because he may get offended and not want to have sex with her. Furthermore, because trans women are at disproportionate risk for sexual and intimate partner violence, some described not always having control over the sexual encounter due to fear of or actual retaliatory violence.

Other facilitators. Another particularly powerful perspective came from a participant who reflected on wanting to stay healthy so she will be alive when her family comes around to accepting her.

> If it's a way to maintain or take care of myself, then if I'm sexually active, then taking PrEP is just – its taking care of my body, and it's knowing that I'm going to live longer, and I'm going to be around for when my family loves me and cares about me and accepts me, and they want to be there for me, and they want to know me for me. They are trying to be open-minded to more. And God forbid, when the day comes, I don't want to be dead. I want to be known that I'm here. I love you guys, and I'm here. [Focus group 2]

For her, PrEP represents hope for the future in terms of a longer, healthier life so that she can be there to express her love when her family is finally open to getting to know her.

For some participants, the fact that they already took daily medications, namely their hormones, adding PrEP to their routine was described as relatively straightforward as long as PrEP did not interfere with the effect of hormones. 'I take hormones, so I could probably just take it with that if they're not going to react in a bad way with the hormones' [Participant 5].

Barriers to PrEP acceptability

Participants also described a number of barriers that would prevent them from taking PrEP as it is currently being provided, particularly in the San Francisco Bay Area.

Marketing of PrEP is not trans-inclusive. One of the most prominent barriers was the general perception that PrEP was for gay men, and in particular, white, high socioeconomic status, gay men. In San Francisco, outreach efforts and community education efforts regarding PrEP have been primarily targeted to gay men, which was reflected in our data.

> To me, this PrEP thing is a white gay man's thing, Okay? And it's for like, the Castro community … It's for people that have stability and maybe have money. … And you know, some of us [who are trans], we don't know where we're going to be tomorrow, or what we're going to be doing … some of us may not even have a stable place to live, let alone take PrEP. [Focus group 1]

The participant points to the fact that PrEP is seen as a prevention option for those who are stable and have money and a secure future. Many of our participants did not have that sense of security and stability. The lack of trans-specific services, including providing PrEP within a programme that acknowledges their resource-constrained lives, is apparent.

Another participant explained that she has not heard trans women discuss PrEP, and that the potential it has to reduce the risk of contracting HIV make it an essential conversation. In contrast to the silence she observes around PrEP in trans communities, she speculates that PrEP is widely discussed and promoted among gay men. Additionally, the fact that so few of our participants had heard of PrEP despite extensive outreach campaigns in San Francisco supports the notion that trans women are not reached by MSM information sources and social networks.

> I would love to see stats on trans involvement [with PrEP] and I would like to see it talked about a little more because trans women, just being trans women, are at risk for HIV, AIDS and STDS. So anything that can detour that risk, definitely needs to be had in broader conversations … and brought to the same plateau as it has been [discussed] in the gay community. Because, I'm pretty sure it's being talked about like it's the holy grail over in the gayborhood. But it's not being talked about over here in Transtasia. [Participant 7]

Another participant worried that the lack of discussion and promotion of PrEP in the trans community was due to a dynamic of gay men wanting to maintain control of HIV-related resources for prevention and treatment. She describes an experience where in the context of a clinic that purports to provide PrEP and other sexual health services to both gay men and trans women, staff still tend to treat her as 'just another guy.' She explains how this dynamic leaves her feeling marginalised, disrespected, and disregarded.

> I feel like it's a sort of, 'we want to keep this for ourselves' kind of thing. Sometimes there is cattiness between gay men and trans women … specifically because most see us as gay men and most don't understand that we're women and most don't treat us as such … So, I have gone to [clinic in San Francisco that provides PrEP] before for testing and I felt completely uncomfortable because I am the only woman sitting there, the only trans woman sitting there, and yet they see me as just another guy. It's like, it's not fair … So, I feel like there's a certain sense of 'oh, we want this for ourselves' or 'we need it more.' Maybe on some level they do, but they shouldn't have a monopoly on HIV meds or HIV prevention because no one deserves to go through this … .Everyone has the right to the same healthcare. [Participant 1]

Concerns about interactions with hormones and prioritisation of hormone therapy. Perhaps the single most compelling issue that trans women expressed regarding potential uptake of PrEP was the felt need to prioritise their hormone therapy at all costs. Many wondered whether Truvada would interfere with hormone therapy, and many participants stated that if PrEP undermined the effectiveness of their hormone regimens they would immediately stop PrEP. Upon learning more specifics about PrEP, it was common for women to immediately ask, 'How is it going to interact with HRT? Is it going to harm that in any way? Is it going to disrupt the process?' [Focus group 5] Another interview participant put it bluntly:

> If it stopped my hormone progress, I would be irate because I like to look pretty and pretty is a soft face. And if hormones do not give me that soft face while taking a pill that's supposed to stop something that condoms do pretty fine just by themselves, then I would probably try to sue … That would definitely make me stop instantaneously. I'd be like [snaps fingers], I am off the pill. [Participant 3]

Managing multiple appointments and medications. Many participants noted that because they have so many other medical appointments fitting 'one more in' would be burdensome. One participant explained that she was tired of being 'poked and prodded' at doctor's offices, due to a great deal of medical monitoring. For these participants, PrEP was less appealing due to the need to submit to yet more medical monitoring.

> Because I'm on so much regimens now I think that squeezing in one more doctor's appointment to take care of my health, would be one more issue that I don't think I could handle … I'm constantly getting poked and prodded for hormones … I'm beginning to feel like a damn horse at the vet's office. Look at my teeth, let me count how many years I have, put me out to pasture, and leave me alone! [Focus group 3]

Although many recognised the convenience of adding PrEP to their 'cocktail' of pills in the morning, some participants were concerned about the long-term effects of taking and managing multiple pills. This, in conjunction with the need to see the doctor regularly and be monitored for side effects, gave some participants pause.

> It sounds like a good idea but the only thing I have is that right now with my hormones and my other meds, I'm taking 13 pills in the morning and 7 at night. And what is that doing to my liver and my other organs? With – I take 22 pills a day. And then, on top of that, it seems like it would be more work … .it seems like it would be more of a hassle. [Participant 4]

Medical mistrust due to transphobia. Focus group participants noted that many trans women generally avoid medical settings, due to prior experiences of transphobia during interactions with providers, clinic staff, and other patients in waiting rooms. Many reported that personnel in medical settings had been disrespectful and they had experienced transphobic or incompetent treatment, such as being misgendered or being called by one's legal name instead of their preferred name. Importantly for providers of PrEP, many of our participants had explicit concerns about discussing sexual risk behaviours with doctors.

> My poor provider doesn't know how to handle me, honey. I mean, my poor doctor, I think I break his brain every time I see that man … so any conversations surrounding [sex] ends up

with a bit of discomfort on his part. So, I try to figure out, one, how does a man who specializes in helping transwomen not know what these things are, and two when I actually talk about my self advocacy or my self education on these types of things, why doesn't he really know how to [explore these topics with me]? So, how can you help me with getting beyond this point? It's a major challenge. [Focus group 5]

Another participant agreed, and suggested that trans women take a more active role in educating themselves about their sexual health and well-being.

> I don't like going to a professional place and then I tell you – you're my professional doctor and you work with trans people – and then I tell you, well, because I got a dick yeah, I fuck too, when you look at me like I'm crazy ... It seems like we have to educate ourselves and each other because half of these doctors, to me, it doesn't seem like they know what they're talking about. [Focus group 1]

Even if they do have a trans-friendly care provider, many trans women avoid medical settings because of the transphobia they may encounter from other patients in the waiting room. 'A lot of trans women do not even have a primary care physician, for whatever reason: stigma, prejudice, the waiting in the waiting room dealing with people staring, all of it' [Focus group 2].

HIV-related stigma, and its intersection with transphobia. Some participants were concerned that if someone found out they were taking HIV medications, they would be perceived as being HIV-positive. Many participants felt that HIV stigma is strong within trans communities, especially among those engaged in sex work, and that HIV status is sometimes used against those in the highly competitive and close-knit social environment of sex work.

> Within the trans community, I don't think I would take it upon myself to dish my T that, hey, I'm taking PrEP as a precaution because it may come out to them as, she's covering up for the fact that she's finally contracted HIV, and now we get to read her [insult her] and terrorize her. [If] I was taking PrEP, and I, kind of, just wanted to tell somebody, it wouldn't be anybody in the trans community. That's for damn sure. And it wouldn't be anybody in California either. [Focus group 2]

Some participants felt that the combination of transphobia and HIV stigma often results in trans women being perceived as 'vectors' [Participant 7] and that having PrEP specifically marketed to them was a way of saying 'you all have to take these meds so you all don't keep passing out HIV' [Participant 7]. Many participants felt that the risk of being perceived as having HIV or engaging in risky sexual behaviour was especially daunting for many trans women, who are often already socially marginalised and isolated. They feared that their friends or family might find out they were taking HIV medications, or that their doctor or even the pharmacist would judge them.

> You don't want to come out every time you get a prescription. And sometimes, being transgender in and of itself is difficult when I am constantly having to identify. Here it's safe ... but out there, I just want to be stealth. Not that I'm ashamed of it, but I don't want people to know. Because when I say that, they're like, 'Oh, I know what's in your pants'. That's what it comes down to. So, I think, being trans and having access to that medication kind of go together because we already have a bad rep[utation] when it comes to sex. And it's like, I don't want to be seen as a ho ... I wouldn't want to be seen as a whore because I'm

picking this up. Not that people who do sex work are bad, but I am talking about the stigmatized version of a whore [and] I don't want to be seen as that. [Participant 1]

As this participant explains, trans women do not want to have to 'come out' every time they go to a pharmacy to pick up medications such as PrEP because of the stigmatised narratives that they feel circulate around trans women and sex work.

Life instability and substance use. Some women reflected on times in their lives, or in the lives of other trans women they knew, when they did not think they had the stability or the resources to manage the complexity of PrEP use. In terms of housing, only 40% ($n = 12$) of our participants reported being currently stably housed (see Table 1). When basic life needs such as housing and food were not secure, participants speculated that something like PrEP would not likely be treated as a priority.

> Food's more important right now than something that might take years for it to do something to me. Unfortunately, that's the reality of the situation for some people ... If you're not HIV positive ... there's really not a lot of resources for you ... For me, I have to work my ass off to get on as many housing lists as possible to make my GA [General Assistance] last and to eat, or on top of that to clothe myself or pay a phone bill. [Participant 7]

Due to economic marginalisation and competing priorities, some women did not feel that self-protection would be an adequate incentive to use PrEP because of the cost in terms of money, time, and energy. Some participants felt that PrEP use by trans women should therefore be incentivised.

> I also think that transgender women probably would not use it, unless, like she said, there's an incentive. I mean, how many girls in this room know someone working the street who is not taking care of herself? [Focus group 3]

Participants felt that the women who are engaged in sex work would likely weigh the cost of their time and energy against what they could make on the street.

Participants also explained that keeping regular medical appointments could be difficult for those living in uncertain circumstances. Many women had unstable housing and were concerned about making ends meet, which took precedence over keeping medical appointments.

> They don't have time to go to the doctor ... because it's taking away from time that they could be using trying to catch a date ... You know, they don't have time for the doctor because they're worried about paying for their, you know, their hotel room for the night. So, the doctor is not an option. [Focus group 2]

For others, there were concerns about substance use and how addiction might interfere with their ability to take PrEP daily and maintain the regimen that would make it effective.

Our participants were quite thoughtful regarding integrating PrEP into their complex lives and offered many insights and suggestions for overcoming some of the barriers that they and other women like them might experience in accessing this innovative HIV prevention modality.

Discussion

This study demonstrates the importance of the unique sociocultural context of trans women's lives when considering how PrEP might best be marketed to them as a tool for HIV prevention. Even in San Francisco, where the largest PrEP clinic in the world is located, where HIV prevention services are abundant, and where one of the first PrEP demonstration clinics was located, very few of the trans women we interviewed had ever heard of PrEP. This finding clearly demonstrates how disseminating information through MSM sources and networks does not reach trans women. Our findings support the notion that the behavioural risk group 'MSM' implies a homogeneity that does not exist among this group. Thinking solely in behavioural terms causes us to ignore social networks and communities that are important sources of information, norms, and values, and that provide resources for health promotion strategies.

Our participants cited multiple trans-specific barriers and facilitators to PrEP acceptability, including uptake and adherence, which have not previously been elucidated in observational studies that have aggregated them with MSM. For example, trans women who are engaged in sex work may view PrEP as an empowering tool to increase their control over HIV prevention in their lives. Because sex work is more prevalent in the lives of trans women due to social and economic marginalisation, efforts to roll out PrEP to trans women may benefit from incorporating messaging about HIV prevention during sex work. Overall, our participants felt it is vitally important that PrEP messaging and information be delivered via trans-specific networks with trans women's unique concerns and life contexts in mind. Community-based strategies such as community mobilisation to increase knowledge and trust of information about PrEP among trans women should be explored.

Furthermore, trans women do not benefit from programming and services that are designed for MSM or offered through clinics that primarily serve MSM. Our participants, like most trans women, did not feel comfortable accessing programmes and services designed for men (Bauer et al., 2009). Accessing services for men, being treated as a man, and not having one's own unique issues addressed during health care, can feel extremely alienating and even humiliating for trans women (Sevelius, Patouhas, Keatley, & Johnson, 2014; Sevelius, Carrico, & Johnson, 2010). Trans women, their advocates, and public health researchers have issued a strong call for the disaggregation of trans women from MSM (Baral et al., 2013; Poteat et al., 2014; Santos et al., 2014), as the importance of incorporating gender-affirming practices in addressing HIV among transgender women is becoming increasingly recognised (Sevelius, 2013; Sevelius, Patouhas, et al., 2014).

Our participants identified the difficulty in and importance of finding trans-competent providers as a powerful facilitator to increasing the acceptability of PrEP. In the rollout of PrEP to trans women, it is essential that we identify and/or train health care providers who are comfortable and competent in providing health care to trans women, including hormone provision. While there is no evidence to suggest that PrEP interacts with commonly used feminising hormone regimens, and evidence from studies of antiretroviral interactions with hormonal contraceptives have been reassuring (Whiteman et al., 2015), no direct study of these interactions has been conducted to date with trans women. Providers and clinics that serve MSM are not necessarily equipped to recruit, retain, and provide care to trans women. Guidelines developed for the implementation of PrEP need to consider trans women's unique barriers and facilitators to uptake, especially the prioritisation of hormone use and engagement in sex work. Multi-modal interventions are recommended for uptake and adherence support, but should consider culturally unique barriers to adherence to maximise effectiveness with trans women (Marcus et al., 2014; Sevelius, Saberi, & Johnson, 2014). There are opportunities to leverage unique facilitators for uptake among trans women that to date have not previously been recognised or utilised to augment HIV prevention efforts among this highly vulnerable group. Furthermore, many of the guidelines cited in these documents are not applicable to trans women's lives. Risk assessment tools, adherence support, and retention strategies are being developed without consideration of trans women's unique issues and are not validated for use with trans women (Marcus et al., 2014).

In addition to the development of trans-specific services, the possibility of offering PrEP and other HIV prevention services to trans women through non-transgender women's clinics and providers needs to be explored. Trans women are women first and foremost, and share more in common with non-transgender women than they do with men in terms of contextually situated psychosocial drivers of HIV risk. These drivers include experiences of trauma, domestic and sexual violence, misogyny, survival sex work, sexual objectification, and unequal power in relationships to negotiate safer sex (Coe et al., 2012; Grant et al., 2011; Machtinger, Haberer, Wilson, & Weiss, 2012; Sevelius, Patouhas, et al., 2014). The effect of these drivers on uptake and adherence to PrEP must be explored in the context of PrEP demonstration projects that are truly inclusive of and/or marketed specifically to trans women. Many women-focused HIV prevention services have sought to be more trans-inclusive, but there are currently no data or guidance available. While trans-specific services are important to continue to develop, it is also critical to develop effective programming for trans women within existing programmes. Many regions of the world do not have the resources nor the number of trans women to justify funding and developing separate trans-specific programming, but need to know how to effectively serve trans women as risk for acquiring HIV in their communities. Similarly, there is anecdotal evidence that some trans men who have sex with men ('TMSM') are interested in PrEP for HIV prevention, but the gaps in knowledge about HIV risk and prevention needs for TMSM are arguably even greater than those for trans women.

This study represents a convenience sample of trans women in San Francisco at risk for HIV acquisition and the results may only be generalisable to similar urban contexts within the USA. However, these findings clearly indicate that public health efforts cannot adequately address the HIV epidemic among trans women as long as they remain aggregated, and thus invisible, under the MSM behavioural risk category in HIV prevention research and programming.

Disclosure statement

No potential conflict of interest was reported by the authors.

Funding

This work was supported by California HIV/AIDS Research Program Community Collaborative Award [CR10-SF-421].

References

Baral, S. D., Poteat, T., Stromdahl, S., Wirtz, A. L., Guadamuz, T. E., & Beyrer, C. (2013). Worldwide burden of HIV in transgender women: A systematic review and meta-analysis. *Lancet Infectious Diseases*, *13*(3), 214–222. doi:10.1016/S1473-3099(12)70315-8 S1473-3099(12)70315-8 [pii]

Bauer, G., Hammond, R., Travers, R., Kaay, M., Hohenadel, K., & Boyce, M. (2009). "I don't think this is theoretical; this is our lives": How erasure impacts health care for transgender people. *Journal of the Association of Nurses in AIDS Care, 20*(5), 348–361. doi:10.1016/j.jana.2009.07.004

Boellstorff, T. (2011). But do not identify as gay: A proleptic genealogy of the MSM category. *Cultural Anthropology, 26,* 287–312. doi:10.1111/j.1548-1360.2011.01100.x

Centers for Disease Control and Prevention. (2008). *HIV incidence. Morbidity and mortality weekly report.* Retrieved from http://www.cdc.gov/hiv/topics/surveillance/incidence.htm

Centers for Disease Control and Prevention. (2011). Interim guidance: Pre-exposure prophylaxis for the prevention of HIV infection in men who have sex with men. *Morbidity and Mortality Weekly Report, 60*(3), 65–68.

Coe, A. B., Moczygemba, L. R., Gatewood, S. B. S., Osborn, R. D., Matzke, G. R., & Goode, J.-V. R. (2012). Medication adherence challenges among patients experiencing homelessness in a behavioral health clinic. *Research in Social and Administrative Pharmacy.* Retrieved from http://dx.doi.org/10.1016/j.sapharm.2012.11.004

Colton Meier, S. L., Fitzgerald, K. M., Pardo, S. T., & Babcock, J. (2011). The effects of hormonal gender affirmation treatment on mental health in female-to-male transsexuals. *Journal of Gay & Lesbian Mental Health, 15*(3), 281–299. doi:10.1080/19359705.2011.581195

Deutsch, M., Glidden, D., Sevelius, J., Keatley, J., McMahan, V., Guanira, J., ... Grant, R. M. (2015). Preexposure chemoprophylaxis for HIV prevention in transgender women: A subgroup analysis of the iPrEx trial. *The Lancet HIV, 2*(12), e512–e519. doi:10.1016/S2352-3018(15)00206-4

Escudero, D. J., Kerr, T., Operario, D., Socías, M. E., Sued, O., & Marshall, B. D. L. (2014). Inclusion of trans women in pre-exposure prophylaxis trials: A review. *AIDS Care, 27*(5), 637–641. doi:10.1080/09540121.2014.986051

Fiereck, K. (2013). Cultural conundrums: The ethics of epidemiology and the problems of population in implementing pre-exposure prophylaxis. *Developing World Bioethics* (1471–8847. (Electronic)). doi:10.1111/dewb.12034

Golub, S. A., Gamarel, K. E., Rendina, H. J., Surace, A., & Lelutiu-Weinberger, C. L. (2013). From efficacy to effectiveness: Facilitators and barriers to PrEP acceptability and motivations for adherence among MSM and transgender women in New York City. *AIDS Patient Care STDS, 27*(4), 248–254. doi:10.1089/apc.2012.0419

Grant, J., Mottet, L., Tanis, J., Harrison, J., Herman, J., & Keisling, M. (2011). *Injustice at every turn: A report of the national transgender discrimination survey.* Washington. Retrieved from http://www.thetaskforce.org/static_html/downloads/reports/reports/ntds_full.pdf

Grant, R., Lama, J. R., Anderson, P. L., McMahan, V., Liu, A. Y., Vargas, L., ... Glidden, D. V. (2010). Preexposure chemoprophylaxis for HIV prevention in men who have sex with men. *New England Journal of Medicine, 363*(27), 2587–2599. doi:10.1056/NEJMoa1011205

Herbst, J., Jacobs, E., Finlayson, T., McKleroy, V., Neumann, M., & Crepaz, N. (2008). Estimating HIV prevalence and risk behaviors of transgender persons in the United States: A systematic review. *AIDS and Behavior, 12*(1), 1–17. doi:10.1007/s10461-007-9299-3

Liu, A., Cohen, S., Follansbee, S., Cohan, D., Weber, S., Sachdev, D., & Buchbinder, S. (2014). Early experiences implementing pre-exposure rrophylaxis (PrEP) for HIV prevention in San Francisco. *PLoS Medicine, 11*(3), e1001613. doi:10.1371/journal.pmed.1001613

Machtinger, E., Haberer, J., Wilson, T., & Weiss, D. (2012). Recent trauma is associated with antiretroviral failure and HIV transmission risk behavior among HIV-positive women and female-identified transgenders. *AIDS and Behavior, 16*(8), 2160–2170. doi:10.1007/s10461-012-0158-5

Marcus, J. L., Buisker, T., Horvath, T., Amico, K. R., Fuchs, J. D., Buchbinder, S. P., ... Liu, A. Y. (2014). Helping our patients take HIV pre-exposure prophylaxis (PrEP): A systematic review of adherence interventions. *HIV Medicine, 15*(7), 385–395. doi:10.1111/hiv.12132

Mascolini, M. (2011). *TDF/FTC PrEP durable in MSM, but MSM and transgender responses differ.* Paper presented at the 6th IAS conference on HIV pathogenesis, treatment and prevention, Rome, Italy.

Nadal, K., Davidoff, K., & Fujii-Doe, W. (2014). Transgender women and the sex work industry: Roots in systemic, institutional, and interpersonal discrimination. *Journal of Trauma & Dissociation, 15*(2), 169–183. doi:10.1080/15299732.2014.867572

Nuttbrock, L., Bockting, W., Hwahng, S., Rosenblum, A., Mason, M., Macri, M., & Becker, J. (2009). Gender identity affirmation among male-to-female transgender persons: A life course analysis across types of relationships and cultural/lifestyle factors. *Sexual and Relationship Therapy*, 24 (2), 108–125. doi:110.1080/14681990902926764

Nuttbrock, L., Rosenblum, A., & Blumenstein, R. (2002). Transgender identity affirmation and mental health. *International Journal of Transgenderism*, 6(4).Retrieved from http://www.iiav.nl/ezines/web/ijt/97-03/numbers/symposion/ijtvo06no04_03.htm

Operario, D., Soma, T., & Underhill, K. (2008). Sex work and HIV status among transgender women: Systematic review and meta-analysis. *Journal of Acquired Immune Deficiency Syndromes*, 48(1), 97–103. doi:10.1097/QAI.0b013e31816e3971

Poteat, T., Wirtz, A. L., Radix, A., Borquez, A., Silva-Santisteban, A., Deutsch, M. B., ... Operario, D. (2014). HIV risk and preventive interventions in transgender women sex workers. *Lancet*. doi:10.1016/S0140-6736(14)60833-3

San Francisco Department of Public Health. (2014). *HIV/AIDS annual epidemiology report*. San Francisco. Retrieved from https://www.sfdph.org/dph/files/reports/RptsHIVAIDS/HIV-EpidemiologyAnnualReport-2014.pdf

Santos, G.-M., Wilson, E. C., Rapues, J., Macias, O., Packer, T., & Raymond, H. F. (2014). HIV treatment cascade among transgender women in a San Francisco respondent driven sampling study. *Sexually Transmitted Infections*. doi:10.1136/sextrans-2013-051342

Sevelius, J. (2013). Gender affirmation: A framework for conceptualizing risk behavior among transgender women of color. *Sex Roles*, 68(11–12), 675–689. doi:10.1007/s11199-012-0216-5

Sevelius, J., Carrico, A., & Johnson, M. (2010). Antiretroviral therapy adherence among transgender women living with HIV. *Journal of the Association of Nurses in AIDS Care*, 21(3), 256–264. doi:10.1016/j.jana.2010.01.005

Sevelius, J., Keatley, J., & Gutierrez-Mock, L. (2011). HIV/AIDS programming in the United States: Considerations affecting transgender women and girls. *Women's Health Issues*, 21(6, Suppl), S278–S282. doi:10.1016/j.whi.2011.08.001

Sevelius, J., Patouhas, E., Keatley, J., & Johnson, M. (2014). Barriers and facilitators to engagement and retention in care among transgender women living with human immunodeficiency virus. *Annals of Behavioral Medicine*, 47(1), 5–16. doi:10.1007/s12160-013-9565-8

Sevelius, J., Saberi, P., & Johnson, M. (2014). Correlates of antiretroviral adherence and viral load among transgender women living with HIV. *AIDS Care*, 1–7. doi:10.1080/09540121.2014.896451

Walker, L. O., & Avant, K. C. (2005). *Strategies for theory construction in nursing* (4th ed.). Upper Saddle River, NJ: Pearson/Prentice Hall.

Whiteman, M. K., Jeng, G., Samarina, A., Akatova, N., Martirosyan, M., Kissin, D. M., ... Jamieson, D. J. (2015). Associations of hormonal contraceptive use with measures of HIV disease progression and antiretroviral therapy effectiveness. *Contraception*. http://dx.doi.org/10.1016/j.contraception.2015.07.003

Wilson, E. C., Jin, H., Liu, A., & Raymond, H. F. (2015). Knowledge, indications and willingness to take pre-exposure prophylaxis among transwomen in San Francisco, 2013. *PLoS ONE*, 10(6), e0128971. doi:10.1371/journal.pone.0128971

World Health Organization. (2012). *Guidance on Pre-Exposure Oral Prophylaxis (PrEP) for serodiscordant couples, men and transgender women who have sex with men at high risk of HIV: Recommendations for use in the context of demonstration projects*. Retrieved from http://www.who.int/hiv/pub/guidance_prep/en/

Yang, D., Chariyalertsak, C., Wongthanee, A., Kawichai, S., Yotruean, K., Saokhieo, P., ... Chariyalertsak, S. (2013). Acceptability of pre-exposure prophylaxis among men who have sex with men and transgender women in Northern Thailand. *PLoS ONE*, 8(10). doi:10.1371/journal.pone.0076650

Young, R. M., & Meyer, I. H. (2005). The trouble With "MSM" and "WSW": Erasure of the sexual-minority person in public health discourse. *American Journal of Public Health*, 95(7), 1144–1149. doi:10.2105/AJPH.2004.046714

'Proyecto Orgullo', an HIV prevention, empowerment and community mobilisation intervention for gay men and transgender women in Callao/Lima, Peru

Andres Maiorana, Susan Kegeles, Ximena Salazar, Kelika Konda, Alfonso Silva-Santisteban and Carlos Cáceres

ABSTRACT
We used qualitative, quantitative, and observational methods to assess the feasibility, acceptability, and potential efficacy of *Proyecto Orgullo* (PO), a pilot community mobilisation intervention to decrease sexual risk, promote health-seeking behaviours, and facilitate personal and community empowerment among gay men (GM) and transgender women (TW) in Peru. PO was adapted from Mpowerment and *Hermanos de Luna y Sol*, two US interventions. PO included six interrelated core elements: (1) Self-reflection Small Group sessions; (2) Supporting peers in HIV prevention; (3) Mobilisation Activities addressing HIV, GM/TW issues, and community empowerment; (4) A Core Group (staff + GM/TW volunteers) designing/implementing those activities; (5) A Project Space; (6) Publicity. PO included specific components for TW, but promoted that GM/TW, who historically have not worked well together, collaborate for a common goal. We found that PO was embraced by GM/TW. PO positively influenced GM/TW's HIV prevention beliefs, self-efficacy, and behaviours; provided social support and created community; facilitated individual and community empowerment; achieved that GM/TW collaborate; and established a functional Community Centre for socialising/ conducting mobilisation activities. Community mobilisation strategies, lacking from HIV prevention efforts in Peru but considered key to HIV prevention, can help improve health-seeking behaviours and consolidate social norms supporting preventive behaviours among GM/TW.

Background

HIV among men who have sex with men and transgender women in Peru

Peru has a concentrated HIV epidemic, in which 12% of men who have sex with men (MSM) and 30% of transgender women (TW) are estimated to be living with HIV; and HIV incidence remains high at 5% (León et al, 2013). Most HIV/AIDS cases in Peru (78%) have been reported in Lima, the capital city (population 8 million). Fifty-five per cent of new HIV infections occur among MSM/TW (PanAmerican Health Organization, 2009). Prevalence of other sexually transmitted infections (STIs) is also high (León et al, 2013; Silva-Santisteban et al., 2012). Approximately 48% of MSM/TW report unprotected anal intercourse (UAI), with many of those MSM/TW residing in low-income areas (Clark et al., 2014; PanAmerican Health Organization, 2009). Socially marginalised and low-income MSM/TW have been identified for being at high risk for HIV (Clark et al., 2007; Snowden et al., 2010). Knowledge of HIV status among MSM/TW is not associated with UAI, and over 52% of sex acts with partners of unknown serostatus are unprotected (Clark et al., 2014). Fewer than 40% of MSM/TW were tested in the past year (Lee et al., 2013), and only 65% report ever having tested for HIV (Clark et al., 2014), even though testing and antiretroviral treatment are free through the Ministry of Health. A recent analysis (Cáceres, Konda, et al., 2014) found low testing rates, with only an estimated 27% of HIV+ MSM/TW aware of their status, and an estimated 18% of HIV+ MSM/TW virally suppressed. The low testing frequency explains late HIV diagnoses and entry into care (Crabtree-Ramirez et al., 2011), which implies increased infectivity.

HIV prevention for Peruvian MSM/TW: the need for a new approach

HIV prevention efforts for MSM/TW in Peru have varied little in 15 years and neglect broadly accepted approaches, such as seeking to change social norms and the combination of biomedical, behavioural, and social/community interventions (Auerbach, Parkhurst, & Cáceres, 2011; Schwartlander et al., 2011). Peru's national strategy lacks attention to the conceptualisation of HIV prevention and care as a continuum (Berg, 2009; Hardon, 2005). The Global Fund to Fight HIV/AIDS, Tuberculosis, and Malaria (GF) provided funding for nine years for prevention programmes targeting MSM/TW, including outreach through a small number of peer promoters for referrals to STI clinics for condom provision, syndromic management of STIs, and HIV testing. Unfortunately, there is little evidence that GF projects in Peru influenced HIV incidence (Cáceres, Borquez, Silva-Santisteban, Guanira, & Hallett, 2014). Messages from promoters have changed little over time and fail to empower MSM/TW to make informed decisions and develop negotiating skills related to real-life issues influencing their HIV vulnerability, for example, lack of HIV status disclosure because of stigma (Salazar et al., 2013). Neither promoters nor healthcare providers counsel HIV+ MSM/TW on Positive Prevention (Myers et al., 2010; Nagaraj et al., 2013). Prevention efforts for MSM/TW in Peru do not facilitate personal and community empowerment and have lacked a strategy to influence social norms, increase social support, and foster community mobilisation (Cáceres & Mendoza, 2009). Clearly, a new approach to HIV prevention for MSM/TW is needed.

We developed Proyecto Orgullo (PO) (Project Pride), a community mobilisation intervention to decrease sexual risk behaviour and increase HIV testing among Peruvian gay men (GM) and TW. Community mobilisation strategies are designed to engage community members to take action towards a mutual goal, are increasingly seen as core components of combination HIV prevention programmes (Auerbach et al., 2011), and may create social contexts that help optimise health and well-being, including sexual risk reduction (Campbell & Cornish, 2010; Coetzee et al., 2004). Community mobilisation interventions for HIV prevention have demonstrated promise in increasing safer sex (Berg, 2009; Schwartlander et al., 2011), improving services, and increasing HIV testing

(Jana, Basu, Rotheram-Borus, & Newman, 2004). To our knowledge, PO was the first intervention conducted in Peru that utilised community mobilisation methods to change social norms, increase social support, and facilitate GM/TW's empowerment around safer sex, HIV testing, and health (Coates, Richter, & Cáceres, 2008). The aims of this paper are to assess the feasibility and acceptability of PO and to examine the process of implementation and potential efficacy of the intervention on HIV risk among GM/TW.

Development of PO

To develop PO, we conducted extensive formative research, including reviewing previous research we and others had conducted on Peruvian MSM/TW; working with a Community Advisory Board (CAB) of Peruvian activists with expertise working with GM and TW; and drawing upon the guiding principles and core elements underlying the Mpowerment Project (MP) and methods from *Hermanos de Luna y Sol* (HLS) to determine how best to address HIV risk for GM and TW in Peru. Through interviews and focus groups with GM/TW and CAB input during our formative research, we found considerable interest in an MP and HLS approach to HIV prevention, particularly regarding opportunities to discuss issues that affect GM/TW's vulnerability to HIV and lack of HIV testing, such as homophobia/transphobia, societal stigma, and poor treatment by healthcare providers. MP is a well-established multi-level intervention for young gay and bisexual men who support each other regarding sexual risk reduction and HIV testing, community mobilisation, and individual and community empowerment. MP's efficacy in decreasing unprotected sex and increasing HIV testing has been tested through two randomised, controlled trials (Hays, Rebchook, & Kegeles, 2003; Kegeles, Hays, & Coates, 1996; Kegeles, Rebchook, Hays, & Pollack, 2002). HLS is a small group (SG) HIV prevention intervention for Spanish mono-lingual Latino gay male immigrants to the US (Díaz, 2007) that focuses on individual empowerment and self-critical analysis. HLS' aims are to: provide experiences of social support and enhanced self-esteem; promote critical awareness of the social and cultural forces that impact men's lives; increase sexual self-knowledge and recognition of the sexual contexts and personal vulnerabilities that limit men's ability to practice safer sex; and facilitate community involvement to support a sense of increased personal agency (Díaz, Ayala, Bein, Henne, & Marin, 2001; Díaz, Ayala, & Bein, 2004). The development of PO remained consistent with the theoretical premises of MP and HLS, many of which are the same.

The research team included Peruvian researchers from Universidad Peruana Cayetano Heredia (UPCH) and US researchers from the University of California, San Francisco (UCSF), and the University of California, Los Angeles (UCLA) with substantial expertise in HIV prevention research with MSM/TW from low socioeconomic strata in Peru. This team has been collaborating effectively for the last 12 years on other studies. The specific implementation activities part of the intervention were conducted by the team at UPCH and UCLA established in Lima, while UCSF researchers also participated in the design, implementation, monitoring, and evaluation of the intervention during regular trips to Peru and communication via phone and email. Dr Kegeles, who developed MP, was intrinsically involved in the development of PO, while Dr Díaz, who developed HLS, has retired from research but provided consultations at the beginning of the project.

Table 1. PO guiding principles.

(1) Multilevel approach to HIV prevention: addressing issues at the individual/social/community/structural levels
(2) Social focus: relating HIV risk reduction to the development of self-esteem, life skills, and supportive social interactions
(3) Community-building: creating healthy social support networks and health-promoting settings (Kretzmann & McKnight, 1993; Minkler, 1990)
(4) Peer-based: peers as change agents (Cialdini, 1993; Rosen & Solomon, 1985)
(5) Empowerment philosophy: building a sense of agency and the community's ability to address their own issues (Freire, 1974; Freire & Faundez, 1989; Rappaport, 1981)
(6) Diffusion of messages: informal communication and modeling by peers promote community change and social norms encouraging HIV prevention (Rogers, 2003)
(7) Positive focus on sexuality and self-acceptance: building pride in sexual and gender expression

Table 2. PO core elements.

(1) Small Groups (SG): four group sessions of peer-led, 2–3 hour meetings with 8–10 GM or TW focused on empowerment, self-reflection, sexual/gender identity, societal/internalised homophobia/transphobia, social support, HIV risk, HIV testing and treatment, sexual communication skills. Participants first recruited through community-based organisations in Callao, and later by participants inviting friends
(2) Informal Outreach: in the SG, participants learned skills to talk to peers about HIV prevention. Training included role-plays, asking participants to talk to peers and problem-solving those conversations at the following session; reinforced in the mobilisation activities and via posters in the PO Centre, texting, and Facebook
(3) Formal Outreach: mobilisation activities helped build a community in which GM/TW support each other and analyse issues that render them vulnerable to HIV. All activities addressed HIV prevention
(4) *Grupo Impulsor* (GI) (Leadership Group): comprised GM/TW participants and Coordinators (paid staff) and empowered to make decisions, analysed issues facing GM/TW, designed and implemented project activities, and helped diffuse HIV prevention messages in the community
(5) Community Centre: a locale to conduct project activities, promote healthy sexual behaviours and build community; had drop-in hours, TV, DVD, and computers. Information, referrals, safer sex materials, and condoms were available
(6) Publicity: conducted through word of mouth, distribution of materials, and social media

The seven principles guiding PO and MP, based on underlying theories, are described in Table 1, and are reflected in the six PO core elements, which are designed to function synergistically and are described in Table 2.

In this article, we refer to the homosexual men in the intervention as GM, and not MSM, since in order to feel comfortable participating in the project, they needed to self-identify, to a degree, as gay. We use the term TW to refer to the biological men in the intervention who self-identified as women. We believe this was the first intervention in Peru that had specific components for TW separate from the needs of GM, while actively promoting that GM and TW collaborate for a common goal.

The formative research revealed the need to create separate but parallel curricula for the four-session SG intervention component with GM and TW. The sessions for TW included issues such as internalised transphobia, the risks of using silicones and hormones for body modifications, and risk reduction in the context of sex with heterosexually identified men. The team and the CAB considered that GM and TW would feel more comfortable attending separate groups aimed at self-reflection. TW in Peru have less skills, education, and financial resources, and are more disenfranchised than GM. In addition, historically GM and TW in Peru have not worked well together, reflecting the stigma and judgment toward TW by some GM who consider TW's behaviour 'vulgar', and the social exclusion and internalised transphobia among TW that makes them feel intimidated by GM, whom they often consider as to have more education and social privilege. The specific components for TW we developed for the intervention were informed by the Guidelines for Multisectorial Work for and with Transgender Populations in Peru (Salazar & Villayzán,

2010), the Theory of gender and power (Connell, 1987), and the 'Gender affirmation: A framework for conceptualising risk behavior among transgender women' (Sevelius, 2013). We believe that this is the first intervention in Peru that had specific components for TW separate from the needs of GM, while actively promoting cooperation among GM and TW to attain the common goal of HIV prevention.

Implementation of PO

We conducted a full pilot of PO with GM/TW age 18–45 for 9 months. With the CAB's input, we selected Callao, part of metropolitan Lima and the main port of Peru, to conduct the pilot. Callao (900,000 inhabitants) is predominantly a lower income area with its own identity. The CAB included members of gay and transgender small community organisations in Callao (which neither had a physical project space, nor conducted any activities), whose buy-in was key to recruitment and PO implementation.

We hired four part-time Coordinators (a TW, two GM, and a heterosexual man) with previous experience working with the GM/TW communities and HIV/STI issues to facilitate the SG, staff the Community Centre, and work with the *Grupo Impulsor* (GI), the group that serves as the decision-making body of the project. We trained the Coordinators on all aspects of the intervention, and supervised them through weekly meetings in order to monitor implementation and to ensure that the intervention core elements were implemented with fidelity.

We started conducting the pilot in June 2012, beginning with an SG to attract participants to PO. The GI started functioning in July 2012 with participants who had finished the first wave of SG (the four sessions of the SG curricula). Participants who attended consecutive waves of the SG were invited to participate in the community mobilisation activities and, if interested, in the GI. All core elements were implemented concomitantly between July 2012 and March 2013. Most activities were implemented at the Community Centre. Due to the distances within Callao, we provided a small transportation reimbursement to attend the SG and the GI. Participants were not provided a financial incentive other than transportation and refreshments.

Methods

We used a combination of qualitative, observational, and quantitative methods to evaluate the intervention. The study was approved by the IRBs at UPCH, UCSF, and UCLA.

Data collection and analysis

We collected qualitative data using a semi-structured interview guide to examine the experiences of the Coordinators implementing, and of GM/TW participating in the intervention. During the last two months of the pilot, we conducted 25 semi-structured interviews with a purposive sample of GM/TW participants in the SG, the GI, and mobilisation activities, and a debriefing group with eight GI members. Interview and debriefing group participants provided informed consent and received the equivalent of $3.50 for their participation. We asked about their perceptions and experiences with intervention components they had participated in, and if participation influenced them to be more reflective about their sexual risk and to support their peers in reducing sexual risk. We also interviewed the four Coordinators at the end of the intervention to assess their perceptions of the intervention and implementation challenges. All interviews were audio-recorded and transcribed verbatim into Spanish. We also made phone calls to 22 participants to find out why they had stopped attending the SG. We collected demographic data and neighbourhood of residence within Callao of participants in the intervention. We observed 50% of the SG, 80% of the GI meetings, and 50% of the mobilisation activities using an observation checklist to assess the completion of objectives of the intervention activities. Observations were unobtrusive to the participants in the intervention. Notes from the observations and 30 supervisory meetings with the Coordinators helped to inform the development of the interview guides above and complemented data from the interviews.

Our analysis of the qualitative data was iterative and was informed by the Framework Method (data immersion, identifying a thematic framework to classify data, assigning text segments to established codes, and defining concepts to interpret excerpted data) applied in health research (Ritchie & Spencer, 1993). Interview transcripts were entered into Atlas ti™, a qualitative analysis software to organise and code the data. First, three analysts, including Andres Maiorana (AM), this paper's first author, individually read a subset of interviews and assigned preliminary codes to those interviews. Analysts then compared their initial codes and together finalised a codebook that they applied to all the interviews. Coding discrepancies were resolved through discussion. Then analysts summarised the coded data and met periodically to discuss the findings. For data verification, AM read all the interview transcripts and reviewed all data summaries. Data from all sources were triangulated to identify domains for interpretation. Those domains were based on a priori issues (such as those included in the interview guides) and salient themes emerging from the data. Demographic data were entered into Excel spreadsheets and used to assess recruitment, intervention reach, and retention. Demographic data helped to inform the rest of our data.

Findings

We have organised our findings into two sections. The first section examines the feasibility and acceptability of PO with respect to the six core elements. The second section examines evidence of how the intervention may have influenced health-seeking behaviours and HIV risk among GM/TW in Callao. Both sections also highlight how the pilot propelled the processes of self-reflection and personal and community empowerment important for change and inherent to a community mobilisation intervention. We use fictitious names for the participants quoted in this section.

Feasibility and acceptability of PO

A variety of evidence indicates that the intervention was feasible, acceptable and embraced by GM/TW, including the number of participants and their engagement in the SG; the number of GI members and the issues they discussed in the meetings; and the number, content, and diversity of mobilisation activities. The intended processes of individual and community empowerment and mobilisation appear to have occurred. While it takes time to start up a multicomponent intervention, in nine months PO established its presence and attracted GM/TW to participate. The pilot was successful in achieving the goal of having GM and TW collaborate together.

(a) Self-reflection and individual empowerment through the SG

In total, 68 GM and 47 TW ($N = 115$), average age 33, from 5 out of the 6 Callao neighbourhoods (except the farthest and wealthiest), attended the different waves of the SG. Eighty-seven per cent reported having completed high school (95% GM, 73% TW). Self-reports on occupation were more vague. Only a few reported being students. Most reported some form of employment (full, part-time, or sporadic.) Some TW supported themselves through sex work. Based on our observations, most participants were low income. Participants who identified as TW encompassed a diversity and fluidity of self-presentations, including using makeup, different gender enhancements and bodily modifications, and dressing and identifying as women either part- or full-time.

We observed that the sessions were very effective in facilitating introspection to explore issues many of the participants reported having never considered or talked about before, such as identity, stigma, relationships, and HIV. Maricarmen, a TW we interviewed, related that the sharing of experiences and the way the Coordinators motivated and encouraged participants created a trusting atmosphere conducive to learning and self-growth. Mixing participants of different ages worked because they socialise together and consider themselves part of the same community. Younger participants learned from older participants' resilience and how they coped with negative experiences, while older participants learned from younger ones who may be more open about their sexuality and/or gender identification.

For GM, watching segments of the television programme 'Queer as folk' (2000–2005) (http://www.sho.com/sho/queer-as-folk/home) enabled them to discuss the impact of HIV on their lives. For TW, watching the video *Silicone industrial* (2011) (https://www.youtube.com/watch?v=scvSX9CanqA) provided the framework to discuss using silicones and/or hormones. Afterwards, some of them reported that they had decided to wait injecting silicones for bodily modifications. Alfredo, a GM, recalled how the SG helped him act upon stigma. He told a co-worker who always made homophobic remarks that the stereotypes of weakness and irresponsibility he attributed to GM rather applied to him because of how he mistreated his wife and did not take responsibility for his children. Also because of participating in the SG, Pepe, another GM, recounted how he came out to his future brother-in-law by telling him that the 'friend' his mother was introducing to the brother-in-law was in fact the participant's partner.

In general, participants were very engaged in the SG's discussions and exercises. Most GM (80.9%) attended all four sessions. However, only 57% of TW attended the four sessions, even if we scheduled them at different times and days. When we called those TW to ask why they had stopped attending most of them referred to work obligations, either as hairdressers or doing sex work. However, the Coordinators' impression was that some TW stopped attending because they felt intimidated by what they perceived as long sessions or abstract concepts. Because of the high attrition, after five waves we stopped conducting SG with TW and instead implemented 'Martes Femeninos' (MF) (Feminine Tuesdays) which consisted of weekly workshops led by the TW Coordinator. MF provided an opportunity to cover much of the same content of the SG, but in the context of learning specific information about human rights and body feminisation or a new skill (knitting, manicure, pedicure, and makeup), TW potentially could use to produce an income. Attendance at MF was consistent and averaged 10 TW.

(b) Talking to friends through Informal Outreach

Diffusion of the intervention and its messages in the community occurred. Consistent with the core element of Informal Outreach, participants spoke to friends about prevention and the project, setting in motion a diffusion process of communicating with and encouraging each other about risk-reduction. The following quotes illustrate participants' responses when asked about their conversations related to HIV prevention with friends:

> I was talking to someone [and she said] 'I didn't use a condom.' I tell her: Look, you already did it, you enjoyed it, now you have to go to be tested three months from now. I told her that the world will not end, that there are people who survive with the illness for a long time, follow their treatment and do well. Because if we lost our head in that moment now it is time to be aware, because if you do not take care, value, love yourself, no one will do it for you. So, I am saying this because I appreciate you and you are my friend. (Mariana, TW)

> They were surprised about what I was telling them, and how diseases are transmitted, they didn't know that there were health care places where they can go. (Juan, GM)/ In the last conversation I had with six trans, I explained ... about the project, for our rights, and the benefits we could have for our own future. (Shakira, TW)/ I have told them what we talked about in the sessions, about self-care and the correct way of using a condom. (José, GM)/ I give them condoms because they don't have any. And I tell the truth, that if I don't have a condom I don't feel safe having sex. I tell them that one can get any type of disease [referring to STIs], and not just HIV. (Miguel, GM)

Based on referrals and attendance, we know that participants talked to their friends about PO, invited them to the SG, mobilisation activities, and the Community Centre. In one case, for example, we observed that the male partner of a TW first used to just drop her off, while later he participated himself and helped with small tasks at the centre, reflecting more openness and comfort. In addition, a couple of TW reported that they brought their dates to Movie Night in order to, 'be sure they also get a prevention message ... .'

(c) Community mobilisation: GM and TW working together through the Grupo Impulsor

The GI met weekly for a total of 32 meetings. Attendance was scarce at first, but gradually increased, including among TW, whose participation at the beginning was tentative. A few elements helped coalesce and facilitated the functioning of the GI, and the Coordinators' role was key. The Coordinators, themselves part of the GI, facilitated or co-facilitated the GI meetings. While the presence and previous experience of a few members of the existing gay and transgender organisations in Callao in the GI was welcome, the Coordinators, especially at the beginning, worked to remind all members about the goals of PO and that at the GI meetings everyone was equal, regardless of their external affiliation. The Coordinators regularly emphasised the project's ground rules, that included mutual respect and listening to each other. Referring to the growth and participation in the GI, Daniel, a GM we interviewed stated: 'In the GI everyone gives their opinion, and every day there are more and more participants in the meetings. They start loosening up and start giving their opinions and exchanging ideas.' The Coordinators trained GI members to plan and organise mobilisation events, and helped them discover they could do things for themselves, such as developing a script for a speech and speaking in public in front of a group of peers or community authorities, something most of them had never done before, and being able to say, 'Hello we are here from Proyecto Orgullo.' Progressively, members took more responsibility and became more committed as they saw the results of their efforts reflected in activities they organised, and as they transformed the rented space into a Community Centre they claimed their own. Referring to her work with the GI and the innovation of the project, Camila, a TW, said, 'I like this group because it makes us meet and participate in many things that have never been done in Callao before.'

The Coordinators applied and built on a few concepts, implicit in PO's guiding principles: (1) the need for GM and TW to work together and support each other to build a stronger community; (2) the GI members as the decision-makers of the project (instead of the Coordinators telling them what to do); and (3) that since the project's resources were limited they had to rely on themselves. Referring to GM/TW collaborating, a Coordinator stated that PO achieved what previously had not been accomplished in Lima. He recalled that at the beginning of the project there was little interest in working together since TW and GM did not see much commonality among themselves, other than living in the same district. This was reflected in aggressive comments and captious jokes exchanged between GM and TW during the first few GI meetings. While jokes continued being part of the meetings, their tone changed, and the barbs previously exchanged stopped or greatly diminished. The process of working together was slow and one of building trust and interacting. It made a difference that they shared a space to socialise and realise that the issues affecting the two communities were similar, and that perhaps it did not matter that GM may be a little more educated or that TW may have less skills. Consistent with their role, the Coordinators modelled behaviours demonstrating how to work together, and that GM and TW were of equal importance within the project. Arturo stated that at first he was a little annoyed because TW can be 'escandalosas' (scandalous or outrageous), but that later he got used to working with them. Tito said: 'Now they [TW] are my friends. Without even realizing it I have become friends with the ones who participate [in the GI].' Some TW also emphasised the respect and unity. Dina stated: 'At least in the context of the GI meetings, I have seen a lot of communication. I have never seen funny faces, but I have seen praise instead. We have treated each other affectionately.'

The Coordinators worked for the GI not to depend on the project's resources. A Coordinator recalled that at first, GI participants asked, '*Y la Cayetano que va a dar?* [And Cayetano, the university, what is it going to give?]'. While the concept and practice of cooperativism is widespread in Peru, she explained that GM/TW are used to receiving large incentives from the GF and non-governmental organisations to participate in HIV prevention studies or activities. The Coordinators, instead, tried to instil the concept that the GI needed to self-manage, in order for them to continue working by themselves when the project ended. In addition, the Coordinators made it explicit and transparent what financial resources the project could provide, besides renting and furnishing the community centre. The GI members adapted to that and functioned with the available resources. As a reflection of self-management and community empowerment, they found resources themselves for the mobilisation activities and the Community Centre.

For example, GI members brought desserts to sell at 'Karaoke Night' in order to buy Christmas ornaments for the Centre. For the 'Chocolatada' before Christmas, they obtained donations of milk, chocolate, sugar, and pannetones. At 'MF', they paid for some of the materials for the beauty workshops and, through community contacts, asked for assistance from the 'First Lady' (the sister of the mayor) of Callao, who provided an instructor for those workshops through the municipality. There were some challenges with the GI, such as that some members who also worked with organisations were used to a more vertical and hierarchical way of functioning. Punctuality to attend the GI meetings, perhaps reflecting cultural norms, remained an issue throughout.

(d) Community mobilisation activities
A process of community mobilisation took place through different activities designed and run by the participants. The total number of activities conducted during the pilot intervention was 53. The fewest number of participants in the activities was four, and the largest number was 35. The GI organised weekly small-size activities such as GM/TW-themed 'Movie Night', regular medium-sized activities such as 'Bingo and Karaoke Night', and large size events to coincide with particular dates such as Christmas. Medium and large size activities were always jointly held for TW and GM in order to build community and concentrate on issues that both communities face. A typical weekly calendar included activities Saturday afternoons and every evening but Sundays. All activities included some aspect of HIV prevention. For example, films at Movie Night were followed by a discussion about the film facilitated first by a Coordinator and later in the project by GI members. The idea for Friday discussion groups came from the GI as a need to talk about topics that could not be elaborated upon during the SG or large mobilisation activities. Bingo and Karaoke Nights functioned as social opportunities to share food, sing, and dance, integrating HIV prevention messages and encouraging participants to do informal outreach. 'Sábados Gigantes' included organising PO activities. One of the Coordinators recalled that *Sábados* slowly became like an open house where the two communities could interact, use the computer, learn to use Facebook, design flyers for activities, and during lunch talk about different topics, including HIV. While more complicated to organise, outings had the highest attendance. HIV prevention messages and community building exercises were incorporated into outings. For these events, the project rented a bus and provided a small breakfast, but attendees brought their own lunch. For some GM/TW, these outings provided the rare opportunity to visit non-urban areas, to which they otherwise would not have access because of lack of financial resources to get there, or because the fear of stigma or violence may cause some TW not to travel relatively long distances by themselves using public transportation.

(e) Community centre
For participants the space was their home. Consistent with one of the principles of PO of creating health-promoting settings, the Centre became a point of reference, was essential to support a sense of ownership in PO and the process of community empowerment, and contributed to community building and the visibility of the project. The PO Centre provided GM/TW with a sense of belonging to a community with its own space. Participants became invested in improving and decorating the space, thus transforming it into their own social space. Willy referred to feeling freer at the community centre:

> Sure, you become friends and open up, you know this is your space and you feel freer, more comfortable, and you can talk about your things .... This is my space and I can talk more freely. I know that the person next to me is my peer and he won't criticize me, won't disclose what I saying, because it is understood that what we talk about here is confidential and stays with us.

Elisa commented on the centre providing a healthy space, an alternative to getting drunk:

> I like it. It is not large but at least you have a place where to enjoy yourself in a good way. You are not with those bad ideas, you are not thinking only in the fun, in drinking, getting drunk, the bad company. You don't see that here, the space is comfortable.

Contrary to previous experiences in Peru to establish similar centres for GM, the consensus among the Coordinators was that the PO Community Centre was feasible and functional because of that sense of belonging and investment in it developed by the participants. We observed one instance, for example, when Tatiana arrived at the space while two other TW walked by and asked her what she was doing there. She responded, 'here is my home', referring to PO, and added, 'how come you don't know *Proyecto Orgullo*'? That conversation resulted in that one of those two TW passers-by started going to PO activities.

Participants took home condoms and lubricants, but we found that the project's supply of condoms at the PO Centre was unable to meet the demand. We also found that there was no need to open the centre on Sundays since GM and TW go out on Saturday night and use Sunday to rest. Through PO, members of existing organisations learned the importance of a community space and how to organise it, opening the way for them to seek funding and consider having their own space and activities.

(f) Publicity

Ongoing publicity was essential to promote the project. Word of mouth, another indication of diffusion of the intervention within the community, worked very well to attract participants to PO. The GI members and the Coordinators designed flyers and cards to promote the project and specific activities. Those were distributed at venues attracting GM/TW such as hair salons and volleyball fields. One of the Coordinators managed the project page on Facebook, which is very popular in Peru. While GM/TW may not own a computer, they access the web at Internet booths. Because most GM/TW own a cell phone, calling or texting them to remind them of activities worked well. A challenge, however, is that because they use pre-paid cell phones, their numbers may change, or they may lose or have their phones stolen. There are no GM/TW bars or discos in Callao for venue-based outreach.

Health-seeking behaviours, HIV risk, and HIV testing

While the period of implementation was too short to quantify change, our findings suggest that PO positively influenced participants' beliefs, self-efficacy, intentions, and behaviours related to health and HIV. A couple of GM we interviewed summarised how the project achieved its aims by emphasising personal empowerment and community mobilisation, and compared it to HIV prevention efforts by promoters, which they perceived as more directive or even authoritative. Federico noted: 'The project helps sensitize and provides information, not directly like they come and give you condoms, but through information, discussions, games, which is a basic way of helping.' Enrique explained:

> The job of the promoters is to help persons get an HIV test, go for medical check-ups, and have condoms. But PO is different, it is more sociable, for communication, assertiveness, participation. For example, 'Who knows how to make a brochure?' 'Me, me'. 'Then, when can you come?' They arrive and do the work. It is participation, not an obligation, [instead of], 'Tomorrow you have to go to take an HIV test.'

An important goal of the SG was to clarify information about HIV, examine reasons for getting tested for HIV, create skills for correct condom use, and think more creatively about safer sex and testing. We observed that many participants still had misconceptions about HIV transmission and prevention. Participants welcomed the chance to practice the proper way of using a condom by putting a condom on a dildo. Surprisingly, we observed that many of them did not know how to do so. Role plays allowed participants to practise how to talk to their partners about safer sex and condom negotiation. During those role plays, participants actively discussed different sexual risk scenarios we presented. In one case, they responded to a TW who always used condoms for sex work but was reluctant to ask her partner to use condoms because she trusted him, telling her she needed to always use condoms to take care of herself. Reflecting trust and a newly gained confidence, we observed that several participants, while at first reluctant, disclosed their HIV+ status during group activities.

We also found indications that PO positively affected HIV testing and sexual risk. For example, a GI member reported that she started using condoms because of being part of PO, and a GM showed a Coordinator that he carried condoms with him, stated that he was grateful for the SG for talking about condoms, and that he now was trying to use them. Four GM approached different GI members to inquire about HIV testing. The GI members provided them with referrals and messages about the importance of seeking medical care if HIV+. One GI member accompanied one of those men to get tested. Another GI member accompanied a second man to get tested and, upon learning he was HIV+, to his first appointment for medical care. Thus, PO promoted HIV testing and GI members also served, informally, to link newly tested HIV+ individuals to care.

Discussion and conclusion

Corresponding to one of the goals of this special issue of Global Public Health, this paper presents empirical research aimed at re-conceptualising HIV prevention and health promotion for disenfranchised sexual and gender minorities. With PO, we tested a multi-level HIV community mobilisation intervention relevant to the needs, values, and social reality of low-income GM/TW in Peru that focused on the multiple dynamics and societal factors that make TW and GM vulnerable to HIV, including gender, sexuality, stigma, homophobia, and transphobia. The pilot of PO was significant because we found the intervention to be feasible, accepted, and well received by GM/TW, and because it stimulated the processes important for change and inherent to community mobilisation strategies. We found that the PO core elements are well suited for delivering HIV prevention and health-promoting content and that those core elements worked synergistically to produce the intended processes of individual and community empowerment and mobilisation. Because of the short duration of the pilot and the time it takes for community-level interventions to have an effect, a pre- and post-quantitative outcome evaluation was not appropriate. Consistent with qualitative methods, our findings cannot be generalised, but we believe that the findings related to the implementation and feasibility of PO and the lessons learned below can inform similar interventions not just in Peru but internationally.

Lessons learned

We learned a number of things from this pilot: (a) PO demonstrated that a successful community intervention must not be implemented top-down, but bottom-up by the community, and that disenfranchised, low-income GM/TW at high risk for HIV can be engaged and motivated to participating without financial incentives in an intervention that responded to their needs; (b) In some cases, TW's social and economic marginalisation proved challenging to their participation, but tailoring the format and content of the activities specific for TW to their needs helped to increase their engagement. Future interventions with TW who engage in sex work may consider the framework for factors increasing HIV vulnerability proposed by Poteat et al (2015). While our resources and timeline to do so were limited, future interventions need not only to contribute to the development of TW's skills to find employment, but also attempt to create employment opportunities at large where TW will not be further discriminated against or marginalised; (c) PO focused on transgender and gay-related issues separately, as well as together as sexual minorities who face similar societal stigma and internalised oppression. At the start of the pilot, GM and TW held some cross-group ambivalence about each other. The intervention ultimately altered that dynamic and helped to engage GM/TW to work together for a common goal; (d) The role of the Coordinators was crucial not only in facilitating the process of GM and TW working together, but for maintaining fidelity to the guiding principles, implementing the core elements synergistically, and the overall success of the intervention; (e) Community mobilisation interventions such as PO may be particularly relevant in areas or countries where transgender or gay communities are not well-developed and other opportunities to discuss and reflect about health issues, their social vulnerability, and the diversity of their non-normative sexual and gender expressions may not exist.

Implications for future research

Our findings do not provide conclusive evidence, but they do point to the potential feasibility and acceptability of the intervention. They indicate the need for further research using a combination of biomedical, behavioural, social/community, and structural strategies, and engaging the health system to address some of the barriers that exist at that level. Structural obstacles to health-seeking behaviours and HIV prevention and care remain in Peru, including: a lack of sensitive health services for GM/TW, the separation and lack of linkage between HIV testing services and HIV care, and facilities' lack of capacity to retain or re-engage patients in HIV care (Scherr-Williams et al., 2013).

While we were implementing PO, international consensus was growing about the need to address the Continuum of Care and Prevention (Berg, 2009; Hardon, 2005) and the role of treatment and viral suppression in prevention (Hall et al., 2013). In Peru, where the majority of people living with HIV are not virally suppressed, focusing on sexual risk reduction among both HIV+ and HIV− individuals, increased HIV testing, and engagement in care will contribute to a decrease in HIV incidence, besides reducing morbidity and mortality. Considering that in most of Latin America HIV prevalence is generally over 10% (Bastos, Cáceres, Galvao, Veras, & Castilho, 2008; Miller, Buckingham, Sanchez-Dominguez, Morales-Miranda, Paz-Bailey, 2013), that the HIV epidemic is concentrated among GM/TW, and that those GM/TW are affected by the same vulnerabilities, health disparities, and social and structural issues as in Peru, this future research will provide evidence of broader international relevance and may influence the development of meaningful policies and programmes. PO could be applied to such research because it targets multilevel issues and its design is inherently flexible, allowing adaptations and fluidity while still adhering to its core elements.

Interventions that facilitate personal and community empowerment by helping GM/TW critically analyse their needs and challenges can create opportunities for them to define issues and develop action plans to carry out solutions. Such interventions could operate synergistically with individual-level or clinically oriented programmes to help maximise prevention and healthcare engagement outcomes. Our findings suggest that community mobilisation strategies that respond to the lived realities of GM/TW in Peru are feasible and may help GM/TW build community, contribute to enhance sexual health and health in general, decrease vulnerability and risk of HIV transmission, affirm sexual and gender identities, and develop a sense of agency in their lives.

Acknowledgements

We are extremely grateful to the participants in this study, the members of the Community Advisory Board, Clara Sandoval and Elizabeth Lugo at Universidad Peruana Cayetano Heredia, and the four Coordinators for their efforts implementing the study.

Disclosure statement

No potential conflict of interest was reported by the authors.

Funding

This work was supported by the National Institutes of Mental Health [grant number R34 MH086330].

References

Auerbach, J. D., Parkhurst, J. O., & Cáceres, C. F. (2011). Addressing social drivers of HIV/AIDS for the long-term response: Conceptual and methodological considerations. [Review]. *Global Public Health*, 6(Suppl. 3), S293–S309. doi:10.1080/17441692.2011.594451

Bastos, F. I., Cáceres, C., Galvao, J., Veras, M. A., & Castilho, E. A. (2008). AIDS in Latin America: Assessing the current status of the epidemic and the ongoing response. *International Journal of Epidemiology*, 37(4), 729–737. doi:10.1093/ije/dyn127

Berg, R. (2009). The effectiveness of behavioural and psychosocial HIV/STI prevention interventions for MSM in Europe: A systematic review. *European Surveillance, 14*(48). Retrieved from http://www.eurosurveillance.org/images/dynamic/EE/V14N48/art19430.pdf

Cáceres, C. F., Borquez, A., Silva-Santisteban, A., Guanira, J., & Hallett, T. (2014, July 20–25). *Introducing mathematical modeling to assess HIV programmatic impact on an epidemic concentrated on MSM/transwomen in a middle-income country.* Poster at 20th International AIDS Conference, Melbourne, Australia.

Cáceres, C. F., Konda, K., Silva-Santisteban, A., Salazar, X., Romero, L., León, S., & Klausner, J. D. (2014). The continuum of HIV care in Peru – Where are we now? Key lessons from an estimation in the context of very limited data. *AIDS Research and Human Retroviruses, 30*(Suppl. 1), A109. doi:10.1089/aid.2014.5206.abstract

Cáceres, C. F., & Mendoza, W. (2009). The national response to the HIV/AIDS epidemic in Peru: Accomplishments and gaps – a review. [Review]. *Journal of Acquired Immune Deficiency Syndrome, 51*(Suppl. 1), S60–S66. doi:10.1097/QAI.0b013e3181a66208

Campbell, C., & Cornish, F. (2010). Towards a "fourth generation" of approaches to HIV/AIDS management: Creating contexts for effective community mobilisation. *AIDS Care, 22*(Suppl. 2), 1569–1579. doi:10.1080/09540121.2010.525812

Cialdini, R. B. (1993). *Influence: Science and practice* (3rd ed.). New York, NY: Harpercollins College.

Clark, J. L., Cáceres, C. F., Lescano, A. G., Konda, K. A., Leon, S. R., Jones, F. R., ... Coates, T. J., NIMH STD/HIV Collaborative Prevention Trial. (2007). Prevalence of same-sex sexual behavior and associated characteristics among low-income urban males in Peru. *PLoS One, 2*(8), e778. doi:10.1371/journal.pone.0000778

Clark, J. L., Konda, K. A., Silva-Santisteban, A., Peinado, J., Lama, J. R., Kusunoki, L., ... Sanchez, J. (2014). Sampling methodologies for epidemiologic surveillance of men who have sex with men and transgender women in Latin America: An empiric comparison of convenience sampling, time space sampling, and respondent driven sampling. *AIDS & Behavior, 18*(12), 2338–2348. doi:10.1007/s10461-013-0680-0

Coates, T. J., Richter, L., & Cáceres, C. (2008). Behavioural strategies to reduce HIV transmission: How to make them work better. *Lancet, 372*(9639), 669–684. doi:10.1016/S0140-6736(08)60886-7

Coetzee, D., Boulle, A., Hildebrand, K., Asselman, V., Van Cutsem, G., & Goemaere, E. (2004). Promoting adherence to antiretroviral therapy: The experience from a primary care setting in Khayelitsha, South Africa. *Aids, 18*(Suppl. 3), S27–S31. Retrieved from http://www.ncbi.nlm.nih.gov/pubmed/15322481

Connell, R. W. (1987). *Gender and power: Society, the person and sexual politics.* Stanford, CA: Stanford University Press.

Crabtree-Ramirez, B., Caro-Vega, Y., Shepherd, B. E., Wehbe, F., Cesar, C., Cortés, C., ... Sierra Madero, J. (2011). Cross-sectional analysis of late HAART initiation in Latin America and the Caribbean: Late testers and late presenters. *PLoS One, 6*(5), e20272. doi:10.1371/journal.pone.0020272

Díaz, R. M. (2007). *Hermanos de Luna y Sol, Program evaluation report.* Submitted to San Francisco Department of Health. San Francisco, CA: Mission Neighborhood Health Centre (MNHC).

Díaz, R. M., Ayala, G., & Bein, E. (2004). Sexual risk as an outcome of social oppression: Data from a probability sample of Latino gay men in three US cities. *Cultural Diversity & Ethnic Minority Psychology, 10*(3), 255267. doi:10.1037/1099-9809.10.3.255

Díaz, R. M., Ayala, G., Bein, E., Henne, J., & Marin, B. V. (2001). The impact of homophobia, poverty, and racism on the mental health of gay and bisexual Latino men: Findings from 3 US cities. *American Journal of Public Health, 91*(6) 927–932. Retrieved from http://www.ncbi.nlm.nih.gov/pmc/articles/PMC1446470/

Freire, P. (1974). *Pedagogy of the oppressed.* New York, NY: The Seabury Press.

Freire, P., & Faundez, A. (1989). *Learning to question: A pedagogy of liberation.* New York, NY: Continuum.

Hall, H. I., Frazier, E. L., Rhodes, P., Holtgrave, D. R., Furlow-Parmley, C., Tang, T., ... Skarbinski, J. (2013). Differences in human immunodeficiency virus care and treatment among subpopulations in the United States. *JAMA Internal Medicine, 173*(14), 1337–1344. doi:10.1001/jamainternmed.2013.6841

Hardon, A. (2005). Confronting the HIV/AIDS epidemic in sub-Saharan Africa: Policy versus practice. *International Social Science Journal, 57*, 601–608. doi:10.1111/j.1468-2451.2005.00577

Hays, R. B., Rebchook, G. M., & Kegeles, S. M. (2003). The Mpowerment Project: Community-building with young gay and bisexual men to prevent HIV. *American Journal of Community Psychology, 31*, 301–312.

Jana, S., Basu, I., Rotheram-Borus, M. J., & Newman, P. A. (2004). The Sonagachi Project: A sustainable community intervention program. *AIDS Education & Prevention, 16*(5), 405–414.

Kegeles, S. M., Hays, R. B., & Coates, T. J. (1996). The Mpowerment Project: A community-level HIV prevention intervention for young gay men. *American Journal of Public Health, 86*(8), 1129–1136.

Kegeles, S. M., Rebchook, G. M., Hays, R. B., & Pollack, L. M. (2002). *Staving off increases in young gay/bisexual men's risk behavior in the HAART era*. Presentation at the The XIV International AIDS Conference, July, Barcelona, Spain.

Kretzmann, J. P., & McKnight, J. L. (1993). *Building communities from the inside out: A path toward finding and mobilizing a community's assets*. Chicago, IL: ACTA.

Lee, S., Deiss, R., Segura, E., Clark, J., Lake, J., Konda, K., & Coates, T. (2013). *Low HIV testing frequency and high-risk behavior among MSM/TW in Lima, Peru*. Paper presented at the APHA, Boston, MA.

León, S. R., Klausner, J. D., Konda, K. A., Flores, J. A., Silva-Santisteban, A., Galea, J. T., ... Cáceres, C. F. (2013). High rates of chlamydia and gonorrhea infection in anal and pharyngeal sites in men who have sex with men (MSM) and transgender women (TW) in Lima Peru. *Sexually Transmitted Infections, 89*, A184. doi:10.1136/sextrans-2013-051184.0577

Miller, W. M., Buckingham, L., Sanchez-Dominguez, M. S., Morales-Miranda, S., & Paz-Bailey, G. (2013). Systematic review of HIV prevalence studies among key populations in Latin America and the Caribbean. *Salud pública de Mexico, 55*(Suppl 1), S65–S78. Retrieved from http://www.scielosp.org/pdf/spm/v55s1/a10v55s1.pdf

Minkler, M. (1990). Improving health through community organisation. In K. Glanz, F. M. Lewis, & B. K. Rimer (Eds.), *Health behavior and health education: Theory, research, and practice* (pp. 287–301). San Francisco, CA: Jossey-Bass.

Myers, J. J., Shade, S. B., Rose, C. D., Koester, K., Maiorana, A., Malitz, F. E., ... Morin, S. F. (2010). Interventions delivered in clinical settings are effective in reducing risk of HIV transmission among people living with HIV: Results from the health resources and services administration (HRSA)'s special projects of national significance initiative. *AIDS & Behavior, 14*(3), 483–492. doi:10.1007/s10461-010-9679-y

Nagaraj, S., Segura, E. R., Peinado, J., Konda, KA., Segura, P., Casapia, M., ... Peruvian HIV Sentinel Surveillance Working Group. (2013). A cross-sectional study of knowledge of sex partner serostatus among high-risk Peruvian men who have sex with men and transgender women: Implications for HIV prevention. *BMC Public Health, 13*, 181. doi:10.1186/1471-2458-13-181

PanAmerican Health Organization. (2009). *Modos de Transmisión del VIH en América Latina: Resultados de la aplicación del modelo* [Modes of HIV transmission in Latin America: Results from applying a model].

Poteat, T., Wirtz, A. L., Radix, A., Borquez, A., Silva-Santisteban, A., Deutsch, M. B., ... Operario, D. (2015). HIV risk and preventive interventions in transgender women sex workers. *Lancet, 385* (9964), 274–286. doi:10.1016/S0140-6736(14)60833-3

Queer as folk [Television series]. (2000–2005). Retrieved from http://www.sho.com/sho/queer-as-folk/home

Rappaport, J. (1981). In praise of paradox: A social policy of empowerment over prevention. *American Journal of Community Psychology, 9*(1), 1–25.

Ritchie, J., & Spencer, L. (1993). Qualitative data analysis for applied policy research. In A. Bryman & R. G. Burgess (Eds.), *Analyzing qualitative data* (pp. 173–194). London: Routledge.

Rogers, E. M. (2003). *Diffusion of innovations* (5th ed.). New York, NY: Free Press.
Rosen, J. C., & Solomon, L. J. (Eds.). (1985). *Prevention in health psychology.* Hanover, NH: University Press of New England.
Salazar, X., & Villayzán, J. (2010). *Outlines for multisectorial work with transgender populations, human rights, sex work and HIV/AIDS.* Lima: Instituto de Estudios en Salud, Sexualidad y Desarrollo Humano, REDLACTRANS, United Nations Population Fund.
Salazar, X., Villayzán, J., Anamaría, P., Sandoval, C., Ceccarelli, M. A., Prada, P. P., ... Cáceres, C. F. (2013). *" ... Y me di cuenta de que el SIDA no es sinónimo de muerte" – Diagnóstico del Acceso a Servicios de Prevención de Salud Sexual y Reproductiva por parte de Personas Viviendo con VIH* [" ... And I realized that AIDS is not a death sentence" – diagnostic of access to sexual and reproductive health prevention services by persons living with HIV]. Instituto de Estudios en Salud, Sexualidad y Desarrollo Humano, UNAIDS, REDTRANS, Peruanos Positivos.
Scherr-Williams, A., Konda, K., Fuchs, J., Clark, J., Segura, P., Gonzalez, P., & Duerr, A. (2013, October). *Overcoming barriers to HIV testing among men who have sex with men and transgender women in Lima, Peru: A qualitative analysis.* Poster session presented at the annual meeting of the HIV Vaccine Trials Network, Barcelona.
Schwartlander, B., Stover, J., Hallett, T., Atun, R., Avila, C., Gouws, E., ... Investment Framework Study. (2011). Towards an improved investment approach for an effective response to HIV/AIDS. *Lancet, 377*(9782), 2031–2041. doi:10.1016/S0140-6736(11)60702-2
Sevelius, J. M. (2013). Gender affirmation: A framework for conceptualizing risk behavior among transgender women of color. *Sex Roles, 68*(11–12), 675–689. Retrieved from http://www.ncbi.nlm.nih.gov/pmc/articles/PMC3667985/
Silicone Industrial (part 1–4) (2011). Jornal SBT Brasilia, Primera Edição [TV series]. Retrieved from https://www.youtube.com/watch?v=scvSX9CanqA
Silva-Santisteban, A., Raymond, H. F., Salazar, X., Villayzan, J., Leon, S., McFarland, W., & Cáceres, C. F. (2012). Understanding the HIV/AIDS epidemic in transgender women of Lima, Peru: Results from a sero-epidemiologic study using respondent driven sampling. *AIDS & Behavior, 16*(4), 872–881. doi:10.1007/s10461-011-0053-5
Snowden, J. M., Konda, K. A., León, S. R., Girón, J. M., Escobar, G., Coates, T. J., ... NIMH STD/HIV Collaborative Prevention Trial. (2010). Recent syphilis infection prevalence and risk factors among male low-income populations in coastal Peruvian cities. *Sexually Transmitted Diseases, 37*(2), 75–80. doi:10.1097/OLQ.0b013e3181c03434

Index

Note: **Boldface** page numbers refer to tables & italic page numbers refer to figures. Page numbers followed by "n" refer to endnotes.

Abidjan, Côte d'Ivoire: language and politics of 'MSM health' in 181–3; sexual and gender minority organising in 179–81
aceite de avion 168
Adams, Vincanne 179
After-Nine sexual partners: gay men relationships with 140–1, 143; in Mpumalanga 144
AIDS 84, 121, 131; GPA in prevention 87, 91–2; policies 92, 93; programmes 92–6
AIDS and Men who have Sex with Men 92
American Foundation for AIDS Research (amfAR) 96–9, 101n9
American Psychiatric Association (APA) 50
amfAR *see* American Foundation for AIDS Research
anal intercourse 7
APA *see* American Psychiatric Association
Apartheid 135, 136
Arc-en-Ciel 180, 183, 185

Bangladesh, 2012 Country Progress Report 96
Barbara 182
behavioural category, men who have sex with men 242
'behaviourally bisexual men' 89
behaviours, risk reduction 200–1
Berg, R. C. 238
biological essentialism 33
biologically male 9
biological sex designation 195
bisexual identity 109, 110
bisexual men 7
Black gay community 220
Black masculinity 120
Black men, Mississippi: HIV for 120; same-gender-loving 120, 121, **123–4**, 129–31
Black men who have sex with men (BMSM) 18, 25, 119–21, 208, 209, 225–7, 245; data analysis 211–12; data collection method **212**; fund 243; incidence rates 208; multiple dimensions of identity 213, **214–17**, 217; procedures 211; selection of participants 210–11; sex back into HIV prevention 224–5; social and sexual subjectivities 222–4; social reality 223
Black trans women 26
BMSM *see* Black men who have sex with men
Boellstorff, T. 6, 8, 185
buchas, trans men and 149–52, 154, 155, 158–9
Bull, S. S. 75

Carrillo, Héctor 3
CBPR *see* community-based participatory research
CDA *see* critical discourse analysis
Centers for Disease Control and Prevention 244
cervical cancer screening 50
cisgender 159n1; non-cisgender 157, 158
Claver 178, 180, 183, 184, 186, 187
Community Advisory Board (CAB) 260
community-based participatory research (CBPR) 65
community-based programmes, HIV prevention 225–7
community centre **261**, 267–8
community mobilisation: activities 267; *grupo impulsor* 265–7; interventions for HIV prevention 259; strategies 259
condomless receptive anal intercourse 14
condoms 219; use of 21, 23, 25; water-based lubricants with 201
conventional masculinity, constraints of 113–14
Craigslist.org 107
Crawley, S. 150
critical discourse analysis (CDA) 72
cultural context, of Puerto Rican trans men and buchas 149–50

Declaration of Commitment on HIV/AIDS 93–4, 99
DerSimonian-Laird random effects model 36
Devor, A. H. 157

INDEX

digital revolution 232
discrimination: multiple levels of 198; societal 193; violence and 171; work-related 171
down low (DL) 105, 107, 115; Black men on 120; duality of 128; paradox of 127–8; stigmatisation of 130
Dowsett, G. W. 77
drug use 21–2

enacted stigma 23, 26
'End of AIDS' 1
'epistemic violence' 71
epistemology 80n2
exchange 141–42

female-to-male (FTM) transgender 48–9; anatomical changes 63; cervical cancer screening 50; community engagement 65; gaps and opportunities 60–1; gay identity 64; gender affirmation 63; health surveillance systems 61–2; heterogeneity of sexual partners 50; human rights 64–5; literature review of 50–1, 60; non-binary gender identities 62–3; in North America 50; psychosocial dynamics 64; sex and gender pathways 62; sexual behaviours 49, 50, **52–9**, 62, 63–4; sexual health risks 64; sexual practices 50, 64; sexual risk indicators **52–9**; transgenderism 49
femininity 3; *travesti* 169–70
Finnemore, Martha 85
Fish, J. 145
Forces Républicaines de Côte d'Ivoire (FRCI) 184
formal outreach, Proyecto Orgullo **261**
Foucault, Michel 72
Friedman, M. R. 232
frontal sex 63

gay communities: in Mpumalanga 143; sexual and gender diversity within 138–40
gay-identified men 64; after-nine sexual partners, relationships with 140–1, 143; in Mpumalanga 145; narratives 138; relationships 136
gay identified MSM (GI-MSM) 231–3, **235**
gender 62, 141–42; affirmation 22, 49, 63; behaviours 62; beliefs 62; diversity within gay communities 138–40; dysphoria 49; expression 13; fluidity 221; inequalities 9, 219; performance 155–6, 213, **214–17**, 217–21; relations, heteronormative models for 158; role trigger 60; and sexuality 176; sexual scripts 126–7; transition 49
gender-based violence 9
gender identity 11, 13, 49, 62–3; Malaysia's *mak nyah* community 195–9, 202; and sexual orientation **153**
genetically male 8
GI-MSM *see* gay identified MSM
Global AIDS Strategy 1992 90

Global Fund 86, 98, 100n7
Global Programme on AIDS (GPA) 85, 86, 99, 100n3; decision-making structure of 87, 89–90; emphasis on divided epidemic 87; international funding for 91–2; NGO development 88; prevention of AIDS 87; Social and Behavioural Research Unit 88, 91; stakeholder meetings 89, 90
Goldbaum, G. 233
GPA *see* Global Programme on AIDS
grupo impulsor (GI), Proyecto Orgullo **261**, 262; community mobilisation 265–7

Halberstam, J. 150
Hale, C. 150
healthcare access, and utilisation 199–200, 202
health discourse, MSM label in public 136
health-seeking behaviour 268–9
health surveillance systems 61–2
Henrickson, M. 77
Hermanos de Luna y Sol (HLS) 260
heteroflexibility, notion of 106–7, 109, 115
heterogeneity: of MSM 233; South Africa 136
heteronormativity 75, 109
heterosexuality 106, 109, 116; conventional masculinity 113–14; meanings of sex with men 112–13; pleasing women 114; romantic attraction toward women and men 110–12
'hijra' 40
HIV 119, 121, 125, 130, 131, 193, 201; acquisition 244; among men who have sex with men 258–9; risk behaviours 120, 202, 268–9; testing 268–9; vulnerability to 23, **24**, 177
'HIV-positive MSM' 74
HIV-related stigma 252–3
HLS *see Hermanos de Luna y Sol*
Hoffman, Amanda 3
homosexuality 7, 71, 74, 135, 238
hormone replacement therapy (HRT) 194
hormone therapy 12, 251
Horvath, K. 71
HRT *see* hormone replacement therapy
hybridity, concept of 78
hyperfemininity 12
hypermasculinity 12, 126–7
hysterectomy 63

IDIs *see* indepth interviews
indepth interviews (IDIs) 19–20, 23; enacted stigma and violence 23, 26; HIV vulnerabilities 23, **24**; relationship challenges **24**; sexuality 23, **24**
informal outreach, Proyecto Orgullo **261**; talking to friends through 265
Institute of Medicine, LGBT Health Report 34
International AIDS Conferences 87, 88
International Lesbian and Gay Association 87–8
international organisations 85

INDEX

'Internet-Using MSM' 73
Intersectionality and Syndemic Theory 18, 24
intersectionality theory 120, 122, 131, 145
intimacy, unrequited desire for 142

Jocelyn 185
Joint United Nations Programme on HIV/AIDS (UNAIDS) 85, 86, 92–4, 99

'*kathoey*' 2, 40
key populations, in HIV epidemiology 32, 34, 40–2
Khan, O. A. 7
Khan, S. 7
Ko, N.-Y. 74

Lebanon: Euro-Atlantic context 10, 12; trans feminine individuals 10–12
Lelutiu-Weinberger, C. 233
Lesbian, Gay, Bisexual, and Transgender (LGBT) 121, 131
life instability and substance use 253
Lima, Peru: *travesti* identity in 164, 167–8; *travesti*'s femininity 169; *see also* transgender female identity (Lima, Peru)
Lorway, R. 145

Malawi: AIDS programming in 90–1; HIV prevalence among MSM 96–7; 2015 Progress Report 97
Malaysia's *mak nyah* community 192–4; background on Malaysia 194; data collection 195; gender identity 195–9, 202; healthcare access and utilisation 199–200, 202; health concerns *203*; limitations 204–5; participant references with demographics *196*; risk reduction behaviours 200–1; sex workers 198, 200, 202, 204
male body 7
male–male sexuality 7
male sex workers 32
male-to-female (MTF) transgender 48, 193
Mann, Jonathan 87
MARI *see* Minority HIV/AIDS Research Initiative
masculinity, Black 120
McCune, J. Q 130
medical gender affirmation 63
Medicare 26
'Men4Men (casual encounters)' 107–8
'Men4Men (relationships)' 107–8
men who have sex with both men and women (MSMW) 232
men who have sex with men (MSM) 85, 105, 114–16, 119, 120, 122, 129; anal intercourse 7; behavioural category 106, 242; bisexual men 7; bivariate analyses 234; categories 6–7; data analyses 234; deployment of 176, 177; design and participants 233; discontents 96–7; donor programmes and policies 97–9; euphemism for gay 106; Euro-Atlantic contexts 7; gender expression among 143; heterogeneity of 233; heterosexual and bisexual identifying 233; homosexuality 7; identities and labels associated with *124*; label in public health discourse 136; language and politics of 181–3; limitations 238–9; making of 185–7; male body 7; male–male sexuality 7; measurement 233–4; multivariate logistic regression analyses 235–6; in national aids programmes 94–6; non-Euro-Atlantic contexts 7; non-gay-identified 107; penile–vaginal penetration 9; population 232; as programming priority 86; racial stereotypes 115; sexual behaviour 7; sexual identities diversity within 121–31; sexual orientation/identity 7; sexual practices 7; straight *see* straight MSM; straight-identified 105–6; transition probability matrix for **95**
men who use the Internet to seek sex with men (MISM) 80n1; category of 71, 72, 76–8; cause-and-effect analyses 73; databases 72; as discursive formations 72; epistemological analysis 71, 72; HIV prevention, intervention for 74; multiple prevention strategies for 74; operationalisation of 71; predominant notion of 71; public health researchers 79; reflexivity 80; sexuality discourses on 75; sexual networking for 74; as a stable 73–4; STI prevention, intervention for 74; subjectivities of 75
meta-analysis 32, 38; and sensitivity analysis 36, **37**
Meyer, I. H. 7, 8, 77, 143, 243
Middle East and North Africa (MENA) 10–12
migrant trans feminine people 10
Minority HIV/AIDS Research Initiative (MARI) 121
Mississippi, Black men in *see* Black men, Mississippi
Mocombe, P. C. 130
Money, John 7
Mpumalanga: After-Nine sexual partners in 144; gay men in 145
MSM *see* men who have sex with men
MSM Initiative 97–8, 100n6
MSMW *see* men who have sex with both men and women
Muslim TGW risk imprisonment 194

narratives, resistance 128–9
national AIDS programmes 93, 94–6
National HIV Behavioral Surveillance (NHBS) 18–20; demographic information of participants 20, **21**; drug use 21–2; HIV status 22; implications for data collection 26–7; MSM and trans women in 24–5; sexuality 20–1

INDEX

Naz Foundation International 96
NGI-MSM *see* non-gay (bisexual/heterosexual) identified MSM
NHBS *see* National HIV Behavioral Surveillance
non-binary gender identities 62–3
non-cisgender 157, 158
non-exclusively straight men 106, 107, 109, 111–12, 114
non-gay identified (NGI) 236, 238; After-Nine men 145; logistic regression of **237**; men 234
non-gay (bisexual/heterosexual) identified MSM (NGI-MSM) 231–2, **235**
non-governmental organisations (NGOs) 177; as sites of social ordering 183–5
North America, transgenderism 49

online interviews 108
oophorectomy 63
opposite sex 49
orchiectomy 9

Parker, R. 71, 78
penile–anal sex 14
penile–vaginal penetration 9
PEPFAR programmes 98–9
Peruvian MSM/TW: HIV prevention for 259–60; transgender women in 258–9
Petchesky, R. P. 120
power, gay men 141–2
PR *see* Puerto Rico
pre-exposure prophylaxis (PrEP) 4, 210, 218–22, 225, 253–5; barriers to 250–3; clinical trial of 244; demographics **247**; facilitators to 248–9; for HIV prevention 244; knowledge of and interest in 247–8; purpose of the study 245; study methods 245–7
PrEP *see* pre-exposure prophylaxis
Proyecto Orgullo (PO) 259; core elements **261**; data collection and analysis 262–3; development 260–2; feasibility and acceptability 263–8; guiding principles **261**; implementation 262
public health discourse, MSM label in 136
publicity 268
Puerto Rico (PR) 148; *see also* trans men and buchas

queer heterosexualities 109
queer-identified communities 64

race and ethnicity 3
racial community, sense of 220
receptive anal intercourse 14
reflexive epidemiology 32–3; context–policy intersections 39–40; co-occurring epidemics 40; critical engagement model 43; gender identity and sexual orientation 33–5; global North context 40–1; limitations 41–2;
measurement and reporting problems 38; meta-analysis 32, 36, **37**, 38; politics of exportation 40–1; sensitivity analysis 36, **37**; systematic review 35; transactional sex, HIV prevalence by 36, **37**
Reid, Graeme 183
resistance narratives 128–9
risk behaviours, in HIV 200–2
Rosser, B. R. S. 71
Ross, M. W. 238

safer sex 249
same-gender-loving (SGL) 120, 213; Black men 120–2, **123–4**, 129–31
San Francisco, trans feminine individuals 12–14
Schmidt, A. J. 238
secular laws 194
self-reflection 265–5
sense of racial community 220
sensitivity analysis 36, **37**
sex 62, 141–42; binary model 8; epistemological changes 8; Euro-Atlantic conceptualisations 8; and gender pathways 62; social construction 8
sex-gender-sexuality, Jordan-Young's metaphor 34
sexual activity 71
sexual and gender diversity, study method 176–8; interviews 178–9; MSM category in public health 179; participant observation 179; research participants 178
sexual behaviour 7, 49, 122
sexual desire 219
sexual diversity, within gay communities 138–40
sexual encounters 142
sexual experiences 71
sexual fluidity 221
sexual health risks 50, 64
sexual hierarchy 122
sexual identities diversity 64, 122–31, 143–6, 213, **214–17**, 217–21; analysis 137–8; analytic approach and data analysis 122; participants and procedures 121, 136–7
sexual intercourse 135
sexuality 71; behavioural aspects of 73; discourses, deployment of 75; essentialising replacement for 73–4; and gender identities 3, 4, 33–5; and HIV 22; indepth interviews 23, **24**; National HIV Surveillance analysis 20–1; social and cultural aspects of 73; in transnational context 74–5; transnational dynamics of 71
sexually transmitted infections (STIs) 48, 121, 193, 201, 232, 259
sexual minority populations 72, 120
sexual objectification 13
Sexual Orientation and Gender Identity (SOGI) 98
sexual orientation/identity 7, 49; gender identity and **153**

INDEX

sexual performance 217–21
sexual position 213, 217
sexual practices 7, 50, 64
sexual relationships 169–70
sexual risk behaviors 13, 62, 63–4, 73
sexual roles **214–17**
sexual scripts, gendered 126–7
sexual subjectivities 222–4
sex work 23, 25, 34; in Spain 39
SGL *see* same-gender-loving
small groups (SG), Proyecto Orgullo **261**; self-reflection and individual empowerment through 264–5
social desirability hierarchy 122
social exclusion 75
social interactions 213
Social Media, MSM and Sexual Health (SMMASH) study 233, 238
social reality, of HIV prevention methods 223
social subjectivities 222–4
societal discrimination 193
SOGI *see* Sexual Orientation and Gender Identity
South Africa: heterogeneity 136; sexual identities diversity, study method 136–8, 143–6
Spain, sex work in 39
Special Programme on AIDS 87
Stata© software 20
STI *see* sexually transmitted infections
stigmatisation 210; of down-low 130; HIV-related 252–3
STIs *see* sexually transmitted infections
Stoller, Robert 7
straight MSM 109–10
street-based sex work 23

Taiwanese men, online behavioural survey 74
testosterone therapy 63
TGW *see* transgender women
TMSM *see* trans men who have sex with men
transactional sex practices 35; HIV prevalence by 36, **37**
trans-competent PrEP provider 248
trans feminine individuals 8; in Beirut, Lebanon 10–12; gender binary 10, 12, 13; gender expression 13; gender identity 11, 13; HIV infection 10; hormones 12; hyperfemininity 12; hypermasculinity 12; in Middle East and North Africa (MENA) 10–12; penile–anal sex 14; penile–vaginal penetration 9; receptive anal intercourse 14; recruitment 10–11; sexual risk behaviour 13; transition related health care 12, 13; in United States 12–14
transgender 2, 3, 149, 150, 243; affirmation 49; dysphoria 49; gay-identified men 64; gender identity 49, 62–3; identity and sexuality 49–50; identity in health surveillance systems 61–2; medical treatment 49; non-binary gender identities 62–3; opposite sex 49; queer-identified communities 64; sexual identities 64; sexual orientation 49; trans masculine 49
transgender female identity (Lima, Peru) 164–5; analysis 165–6; becoming travesti 167–8; body transformation 168–9; implications for HIV prevention 172–3; limitations 173–4; participant characteristics **166**; sexual relationships 169–70; terminology 166–7; violence and discrimination 171
transgenderism 49; North America 49; Western Europe 49
transgender persons 192; male-to-female 193
Transgender Supplement Questionnaire (TSQ) 19, 20; demographic information **21**, 22; gender affirmation 22; implications for data collection 26–7; MSM and trans women in 24–5; sexuality and HIV 22
transgender women (TGW) 9, 172, 193; community 194; Muslim, risk imprisonment 194; in Peru 258–9
transition 49
trans masculine 49
trans men and buchas (Puerto Rico) 149–50; bodily representation and gender performance 155–6; community, health-related issues 150–1; data analysis 153; ethnographic field note excerpt 154–5; ethnographic procedures 151–2; female biological processes 157–8; intersections and distinctions between 150; socio-demographic characteristics **152**; study methods 151–3; vulnerabilities of 150
trans men who have sex with men (TMSM) 51, 60, 255
transphobia 193, 251–3
transsexuality 33–4
trans women 148, 149, 243
travesti 40; femininity 169; identity 164, 167–8
true transsexuals 49
TSQ *see* Transgender Supplement Questionnaire
2001 Global Strategy Framework on HIV/AIDS 92

UAI *see* unprotected anal intercourse
UNAIDS *see* Joint United Nations Programme on HIV/AIDS
UN Country Progress Reports 85, 96
UNDP 92
UNGASS Country Progress Reports 86, 93
UN General Assembly 87
UNICEF 92
United Nations General Assembly Special Session on HIV/AIDS 93
United States: HIV prevalence in 17; secondary data analysis 18; trans feminine individuals 12–14
unprotected anal intercourse (UAI) 232, 234, 259
unprotected receptive anal intercourse 14
unprotected sexual relations 76

279

INDEX

US Food and Drug Administration 18
US President's Emergency Plan For AIDS Relief (PEPFAR) 86, 98–9, 101n8

vaginal sex 63
Valentine, D. 144
violence: and discrimination 171; enacted stigma and 23, 26

water-based lubricants with condoms 201
Watney, Simon 225
Weatherburn, P. 238
Weber, L. 121
Wei, C. 74
West, C. 155
Western Europe, transgenderism 49

WHO *see* World Health Organization
women: attracted to 110–12; pleasing 114
work-related discrimination 171
World Bank 92
World Health Assembly 87
World Health Organization (WHO) 85, 87; consolidated guidelines for key populations 18; HIV guidelines for key populations 34; Homosexual Response Studies 88

Ybarra, M. L. 75
Young, R. M. 7, 8, 77, 143, 243

Zimmerman, D. H. 155
Zou, H. 74